D1824953

INDICTED!

Best Wishes
Always
Nancy Henderson

EXPOSING A NATIONAL SCANDAL

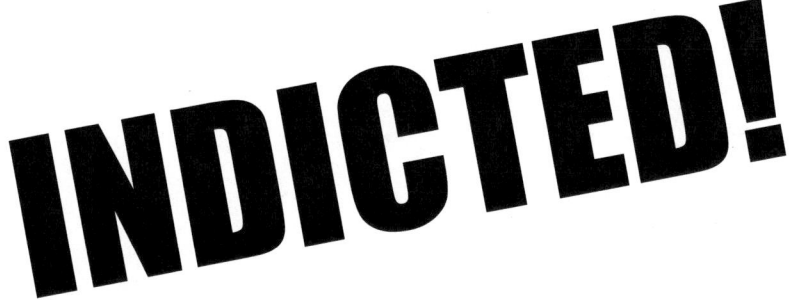

INDICTED!

THE PEOPLE
VS
THE MEDICAL
& DRUG CARTEL

by ATTORNEY JAMES HENDERSON

MANAGING THE SYMPTOMS OF DISEASE
IS BIG BUSINESS

Tate Publishing & Enterprises

Published by Tate Publishing & Enterprises, LLC
127 E. Trade Center Terrace | Mustang, Oklahoma 73064 USA
1.888.361.9473 | www.tatepublishing.com

Tate Publishing is committed to excellence in the publishing industry. The company reflects the philosophy established by the founders, based on Psalm 68:11,
"The Lord gave the word and great was the company of those who published it."

Book design copyright © 2008 by Tate Publishing, LLC. All rights reserved.

Published in the United States of America

ISBN: 978-1-60604-325-7
1. Medical: Ethics   2. Medical: Nutrition
09.02.27

CONTENTS

Dedication

To the Creator,
Our Great Lawgiver, Physician, and Custodian
of the Health, Healing, and Happiness
of those who Serve Him in Love
and Obey His Laws of Life
Divinely Imprinted into the Fabric of Nature.
To the valiant pioneers in
Nutritional medicine in this modern age,
who, standing firm in the tradition of the great Hippocrates
and risking their careers and reputations, are courageously
attempting to hold back the tide of a New Dark Age in Medicine.

PREFACE

Today pharmaceutical medical science is primarily devoted to a search for ways to avoid the consequences of our intemperate lifestyles and eating habits. It perpetuates the delusion that we can continue to violate the laws of life and not suffer the inevitable consequences. It is not primarily concerned with *teaching* the patient to live in harmony with natural law—although this is the *root* meaning of the Greek word for doctor, *to teach*. Modern medicine pays lip service to the fact that for over twenty-five hundred years, Hippocrates (460–377 BC) has been recognized as the Father of Medicine. He raised medicine to heights unsurpassed and not yet recovered since the obscurantism of the Dark Ages.

What modern medicine fails to tell you is that Hippocrates was the Father of *nutritional* medicine and that this greatest of geniuses in the history of medicine *shunned* the use of poisonous drugs in the healing of the sick, even *prohibiting them,* in his *Oath of Medical Ethics.* [1] Modern medicine would have you believe that Hippocrates was the Father of *pharmaceutical* medicine, but this is 180 degrees away from the truth. Furthermore, in the healing of the sick and diseased, Hippocrates taught that *food* was the *best medicine,* to be administered along with fresh air, exercise, cleanliness, and adequate rest. Moreover, Hippocrates *defined* medicine as the art of discovering the best foods for maintaining and restoring health. Referring to the art of preparing and using *health-restoring foods,* he stated, "To such a discovery and investigation what more suitable name could one give than that of Medicine?" [2]

In 400 BC Hippocrates wrote this appeal to physicians:

Wherefore it appears to me necessary to every physician to be skilled in nature, and strive to know, if he would wish to perform his duties, what man is in relation to the articles of food and drink, and to his other occupations, and what are the effects of each of them to everyone. [3]

Whoever pays no attention to these things [the preparation of wholesome food to maintain and restore health], or, paying attention, does not comprehend them, how can he understand the diseases which befall a man? For, by every one of these things, a man is affected and changed this way or that, and the whole of his life is subjected to them, whether in health, convalescence, or disease. *Nothing else, then, can be more important or more necessary to know than these things.* [4] [Emphasis added.]

In emphasizing nutrition as the basis of good health and good medicine, Hippocrates was in express agreement with Moses, the chronicler of the early history of man, whom Western civilization recognizes as the *great lawgiver.* He is so depicted in the artistic relief above the benches of the Supreme Court of the United States. Moses wrote that the Creator designed man's diet.

> And God said, "See, I have given you every herb that yields seed which is on the face of the earth, and every tree whose fruit yields seed; to you it shall be for food."
>
> Genesis 1: 29

God created the laws of man's being; designing that he should live in harmony with these laws of life. These laws include the consumption for pleasure and nutrition of wholesome foods designed to strengthen the human body. Today our profit-driven food industry has refined, adulterated, and denatured the natural foods God provided. Dr. Nancy Appleton stated that because of consuming these refined and denatured foods, such as refined sugar, we are experiencing all of the chronic degenerative diseases known to man. God recognized at the Fall of Man that the ravishes of sin and lawlessness would bring diseases upon men. So he added to man's original diet the herbs of the field: *greens and vegetables.* "And you shall eat the herb of the field."(Genesis 3: 18). In adding green herbs and vegetables to the diet of sinful men, God acted the part of the first *nutritional* physician. Moreover, God made it clear to humankind through Moses that if they were to obey his laws of life, they would be free of the common diseases that befall men.

> If you diligently heed the voice of the Lord your God and do what is right in His sight, give ear to His commandments and keep all His statutes, *I will put none of the diseases on you, which I have brought on the Egyptians.* For I am the Lord who heals you. [Emphasis added.]
>
> Exodus 15: 26

It is not that God brings diseases upon men; this statement is but simply a recognition of the fact that God is the author of the laws of man's being, and that he has so designed man and the universe that everything has a consequence. Cause follows effect with unvarying certainty. If you obey the laws of life, you would be substantially free of diseases in this sinful earth. Obedience and disobedience have their own built-in consequences. If you violate the laws of life, you would reap the harvest of your actions in the form of disease, suffering, and death. Modern medicine has substantially turned its back upon the Hippocratic and Mosaic concept that cooperating with the natural laws of life is the *best approach* to both the prevention of disease and the restoration of health.

Today the medical establishment has *redefined* medicine in terms of drugs and surgery. They advocate that only drugs can cure or prevent diseases. [5] But man does not suffer diseases from the lack of a drug in his system. Modern medicine and its cartel companions in the petro-chemical industry and state and federal governments are feverishly working behind the scenes to *discredit* and *outlaw* the practice of *nutritional* medicine; thus creating a *monopoly* for the use of pharmaceutical drugs in medicine. After decades of an undeclared war upon nutritional medicine by the medical Cartel, the consequences are being seen. By the suppression of the truth about the relationship between food and disease and of the many natural ways of restoring health through nutrition, America is reaping a harvest of chronic degenerative diseases. They are now pandemic. The apostle Paul warned of the consequences to those "who suppress the truth in unrighteousness" (Romans 1: 18).

Having turned its back on the science of true medicine, America has lost its wisdom in responding to this pandemic. The whole structure of our medical establishment is geared toward treating the *symptoms* of disease while failing to eradicate the root causes of the diseases. Our system is geared toward managing *disease* not *health*. We do not have a healthcare system. We have a disease management system—one based on the maximization of profits. It is an irrational system based on faulty science.

Suppressing the symptom of a disease while refusing to treat the underlying cause makes as much sense as removing the red light on the dashboard of a vehicle that indicates an engine dysfunction and continuing to run the engine. Eventually the engine will quit on you. The red light was only the *symptom* of a deeper underlying problem. Cutting out the symptom does not fix the engine. Yet we act as though it does in the treatment of chronic degenerative diseases! The symptomatic treatment of disease is addicting. It provides a false sense of well-being and increased energy, but underneath the disease still lurks. For example, cancer is *not* the mass or lump. The lump is only the *symptom* of a deeper metabolic dysfunction; removing it will not cure the cancerous condition of the body. Likewise, high blood sugar is only a *symptom* of a metabolic dysfunction, which disables the efficacy of insulin. Artificially lowering the blood-sugar level will not cure diabetes or impede the corrosive effect of saturated fat, which is one of the underlying causes of diabetes.

In no other area is modern medicine further from Hippocratic medicine than in its understanding of the causes of disease and its cure. Modern medicine holds that disease is *caused* by an *external agent,* such as a germ or a condition. Drug-based medicine's response is to identify the germ and devise pharmaceutical *silver bullets* to destroy the germ or administer a drug to reverse the condition, while doing next to nothing to restore the healthy functioning of the organism. But Hippocrates taught that disease was a dysfunction of the *entire* organism; and that health can be best restored by treating the *whole* organism; that by providing it with proper nutrition, the body would heal itself without the intervention of harmful drugs. [6] Modern medicine has no faith in the ability of God's natural laws imprinted in the fabric of nature to heal the organism. In restoring our health, *we the people* must decide whether we believe "In the Pill we trust" or "In God we trust."

The erroneous concepts that diseases are caused by external agents and that the body is unable to heal itself are at the core of the differences between nutritional medicine and pharmaceutical medicine. Nutritional medicine, following in the footsteps of Hippocrates, holds that disease and the pathogen are the *results* of a metabolic dysfunction and the consequent impairment of the immune system of the *whole* organism. It holds that if we restore the health of the organism by nutrition and appropriate lifestyle changes, the body will heal itself. The future of America's health is dependent upon returning to the medical science and teachings of Hippocrates.

The conflict between pharmaceutical medicine and dissenting nutritional physicians is rapidly intensifying. The first has the power of government and industrial wealth behind it; the latter have only truth and fidelity to the facts of nature to fall back on. There is a not-so-quiet civil war occurring between these two conceptions of medicine. This trial will answer the question whether pharmaceutical medicine is a false, irrational science masquerading under the sanction of a powerful industrial and medical cartel in league with conniving governmental agencies. Medical experts—from Paracelsus and Sir Francis Bacon in the sixteenth and seventeenth centuries to Max Gerson, the twentieth century's foremost medical genius—will present the case for restoring the empirical science and nutritional medicine advocated by Hippocrates.

This author, an attorney and not a physician, offers no medical opinions of his own. The testimony presented will not constitute the practice of medicine. The presentation of evidence will constitute merely a contest, a battle between the experts. The goal is to *reform* medicine by *indicting* its most egregious errors. In this trial, you the people, who have the most to lose, convened into a vast national jury, will be the final arbiters of the truth. What is that truth?

Pharmaceutical medicine as applied to the treatment of chronic degenerative diseases, a practice shunned by the great Hippocrates, is bad medicine generated by a false concept of science.

Nutritional medicine, based upon true empirical science, strives to uphold the legacy of Hippocrates in the treatment of chronic degenerative diseases.

A powerful medical and industrial cartel in league with big government has written the rules, establishing a medical monopoly in pharmaceutical medicine while seeking to disparage and outlaw nutritional medicine.

The rules of the game permit drug companies to manufacture and physicians to administer in non-emergency situations, powerful and pernicious drugs to manage, but not cure, the symptoms of chronic degenerative diseases—drugs whose side effects are often worse than the disease, thus often inflicting irreparable damage to their unsuspecting patients.

THE INDICTMENT

Count 1:

PROFITEERING WITH OUR HEALTH

Ladies and gentlemen of the jury, today you are installed as a panel of impartial jurors to preside over a case that concerns your vital interests. Drastic times call for drastic measures. William Penn contended that a jury has the right and perhaps the duty to disregard any law that is in violation of our dearly held rights and privileges. Today you are being asked to return a verdict of indictment upon a vast network of interconnected political and commercial institutions that are preying on our health and our pocket books. In the docket is a cartel of institutions: the pharmaceutical industry, the medical industry, the processed food manufacturers, and governmental institutions that have robbed us of our medical freedom and our health. The evidence will show that the conduct of this Cartel threatens to bankrupt our nation.

My discourse will not constitute the practice of medicine—it is an *indictment* of certain aspects of modern medicine, in particular the use of pharmaceutical medicine to manage the symptoms of chronic degenerative diseases, without seriously attempting to cure these diseases. I will marshal the evidence so as to demonstrate that modern medicine has been diverted from its original purpose—to restore, to heal, to eliminate the causes of degenerative diseases, and to instruct the patient how to live in harmony with the laws of life. Today medicine has struck a Faustian bargain with the pharmaceutical and chemical industries and with big government. The *management* of the *symptoms* of disease has become *big business*—to the long-term detriment of the patient. Drug treatment of the symptoms of chronic degenerative diseases leaves the *causes* of the disease intact while seeking to *avoid* the consequences of violating the laws of health and life.

Throughout the presentation of the evidence against the defendants, I will deftly lead you, the jury, into an in-depth study of the causes of six chronic degenerative diseases. You will find that they are all primarily lifestyle diseases. The villains undermining our health are well known to you. They are excessive saturated animal fat, excessive animal protein, refined foods (such as white sugar and white bread) in our diets, inactivity, alcohol, and nicotine. We will then compare and contrast the management (hence their perpetuation) of these diseases by conventional medicine with the nutritional cure of these diseases by natural remedies, which seek to reverse their causes.

Ladies and gentlemen of the jury, drugs never cure chronic degenerative diseases. [1], [2] They cannot by their very nature. They are not designed to. They target only the symptoms of the disease, not its causes. A drug is a poison. Physicians seek to manage chronic degenerative diseases by a slow and measured release of a variety of poisons into our bodies, hoping to suppress one or two symptoms of the disease before doing the patient irreparable harm. Unfortunately, many of these poisons wreck havoc with our immune systems, the body's frontline mechanism for fighting disease. Drugs only mask the *symptoms* of the disease, while the destructive course of the disease silently rages on—until you, the patient, finally expire. [3] In America today, we do not have a *healthcare* system. We have a *disease man-agement* system. The evidence will show that virtually all of these chronic generative diseases can be prevented, and in most cases reversed, by living in harmony with the natural laws of life and nutrition. And all of this can be accomplished at a fraction of the cost of the pharmaceutical or surgical treatment of disease.

Ladies and gentlemen of the jury, the evidence will also show that, influenced by the drug companies, the physicians of today dare not cure the chronic degenerative diseases rampant in our society by eliminating their causes. [4] The physician's livelihood and the perpetuation of the enor-mous disease-management industry depend on keeping the patient *depen-dent*—essentially sick. We have become skilled at managing diseases—at a price. At a price tag of over two trillion dollars and climbing, we manage the lifestyle diseases of our civilization—diseases such as arthritis, cancer, heart disease, diabetes, high blood pressure, and osteoporosis.

The evidence will further show that over the last 150 years, a vast body of scientific information has been accumulated by skilled and devoted physicians and researchers, demonstrating that chronic generative diseases are primarily caused by a diet of rich foods—essentially refined, enervated, and debased foods—and an abundance of animal-based products. These unwholesome foods result in multiple systems and organs breaking down in the human body; and chronic degenerative diseases like cancer, heart diseases, arthritis, osteoporosis, and high blood pressure is the natural sequelae. [5] That body of scientific evidence also demonstrates that a plant-based diet of whole foods not only prevents but also can arrest, and in many cases reverse, these same chronic degenerative diseases. [6]

Yet in the face of this body of scientific evidence, the medical establishment, in cohorts with the chemical, industrial, and refined-foods cartel, does not endorse a dietary approach to the cure of chronic degenerative diseases. The reason is obvious as it is tragic: the nutritional treatment of disease competes with the standard menu of pills, concoctions, and expensive surgical procedures. Ladies and gentlemen of the jury, this is nothing short of criminal and morally reprehensible. [7] The renowned nutritional researcher, Dr. T. Colin Campbell and co-author Thomas Campbell, commented on the suppression of nutritional modalities by the medical establishment in their seminal work, *The China Study:*

As far as I am concerned, this is nothing short of criminal. We, the public, turn to doctors and hospitals in times of great need. For them to provide care that is *knowingly less than optimal, that doesn't protect our health, doesn't heal our diseases and costs us tens of thousands of dollars is morally inexcusable.* [8] [Emphasis added.]

One high-ranking member of the medical establishment admitted "if word gets out" that members of certain medical establishments often turn to a plant-based diet to arrest and reverse their chronic degenerative diseases, yet do not permit their institutions to "treat the common herd" with these same natural methods, "we would be open for a lawsuit." [9] Ladies and gentlemen, that time has come. It is your sacred duty to study the evidence as it is presented in this case and courageously indict this medical and industrial cartel for criminal conduct and profiteering with your health and the health of our nation.

After you have reviewed the evidence and have spent time deliberated among yourselves, I will ask you to bring back a verdict of *indictment* against a government-sponsored profiteering Cartel consisting of the medical, refined foods, and pharmaceutical industries. The profits of death threaten to bankrupt our country and ruin our health. We must and we will regain our medical freedom and our health—our lives depend upon it. This is your task today. You must not shrink from it. You must not be intimidated by the power or wealth of the defendants nor be swayed by their specious rationalizations.

Ladies and gentlemen, we have today the choice to regain our medical freedom. The path we must follow is simple. By conforming our lives to the natural and moral laws God designed us to live by, we can become, and remain, substantially disease-free as the great Hippocrates, the Father of medicine taught. Thus, ultimately our destiny lies within our power. If we disregard the laws of life and health, we become vulnerable to disease and, once stricken, would be tempted to place ourselves under the care of the drug dispensers. William Penn is reputed to have said:

Those people who are not governed by God will be ruled by tyrants.

When we live within the laws of life designed by our Creator, we are governed by God. The choice is ours: to be guided by the Life-Giver or hoodwinked by the dispensers of false hope.

Ladies and gentlemen of the jury, this indictment is not against all aspects of modern medicine. America has the finest emergency care system, as well as the most advanced trauma and surgical care in the world. Let us keep it so. The indictment is against the conventional methods of treating chronic degenerative diseases. Nor is this indictment against individual doctors. Often they are well-meaning, hard-working individuals. But they are the victims of a corrupt system that denies them the essential knowledge about the relationship between food and disease. Dr. Campbell observed that the nutritional training of doctors is not merely inadequate; it is practically nonexistent. [10] He stated that in 1985, the National Research Council reported that physicians receive on average only two credits of nutrition training during their four years of medical school. [11]. A survey of the literature by nutritionist Jeffrey Novick in 2001 revealed that seven years after this landmark 1985 study by the National Academy of Sciences (which concluded that nutrition education in US medical schools was inadequate and that only 25% of medical schools had such courses), there was a "downward trend in the number of medical schools offering a required course in nutrition and a decline in the number of medical schools teaching nutrition (Young, 1992)." [12]

If doctors are ignorant of the relationship between food and disease, how can they cure these chronic diseases? How can they adequately and intelligently instruct their patients?

Count 2:

REAPING AN EPIDEMIC OF CHRONIC DEGENERATIVE DISEASES

The evidence will show that drug-based conventional medicine has retreated from its ancient and sacred oath. I refer to the injunction of Hippocrates, the Father of medicine, to all physicians: *first do no harm.* [1] The well-respected historian of medicine, Harris Coulter, after reviewing the history of medicine from the days of Hippocrates to the present, concluded that the epidemic of chronic degenerative diseases we are experiencing today is largely iatrogenic—that is to say, *physician induced.* [2] Physicians, he stated, are contributing to this epidemic of chronic diseases by their disdain for nutritional medicine, while relying on pharmaceutical drugs that treat only symptoms, leaving intact, and in some cases even aggravating, the underlying degenerative disease. Harris Coulter stated in his fourth volume of *Divided Legacy:*

> The major drug diseases, as will be shown below, are coextensive with the principal chronic diseases afflicting the populations of the twentieth-century industrialized societies: allergic hypertension, hypertension, ulcers, deafness, asthma, heart disease, mental illness, cancer, diabetes, congenital defects, neurologic disorders, and arteriosclerosis. To what extent, therefore, does drug use contribute to chronic disease? Or, in other words, how much chronic disease is really drug disease? [3]

Coulter then proceeded to marshal the facts to answer his own question. He stated that in the immediate post-World War II period of the 1950s, chronic degenerative disease affected only 30% of the population. [4] But by 1978, 80% of all illnesses in America were chronic degenerative diseases. [5] Did poor nutrition and unhealthy lifestyles cause this gigantic rise in chronic diseases in twenty-eight short years? Only in part, Coulter contended. He stated that drugs compound these diseases while resulting in *new* chronic diseases.

> While chronic diseases can be generated by congenital weaknesses, exposure to morbific influences, poor nutrition, fatigue, emotional stress and shock, overwork, and the like, the therapeutic drugs used to treat acute conditions are no less important as causal factors. Treatment suppresses and transforms diseases and symptoms, whereupon the new entities are "treated" with other therapeutic drugs, generating new chronic disease entities, some known to medical science, others nameless.

> There is no alternative explanation for the late twentieth-century epidemic of chronic disease in the old and its rapid increase in the young. [6]

Ladies and gentlemen of the jury, Harris Coulter was correct when he asserted that that modern drug-oriented medicine undermines our health because it is based upon a false system of therapeutics—that chronic degenerative diseases can be treated by drugs. Ladies and gentlemen, this is our Maginot line—the line separating pharmaceutical medicine from nutritional medicine. The gulf between these two forms of medical therapeutics is broad and deep. They are virtually polar opposites. One system is based on a false rationalistic concept of science and the other on the empirical science of Hippocrates and Sir Francis Bacon.

The erroneous drug-based medical approach attempts to treat chronic degenerative diseases by use of poisonous substances, which manifest symptoms *contrary* to the symptoms exhibited by the disease. The purpose of these drugs is to *suppress* the symptoms of the disease, not to *cure* the disease. But the real effect of these drugs is to aggravate and worsen the original disease because the underlying causes go untreated. Suppression of the symptoms of a disease provides only a temporary illusion of health. The drugs not only aggravate the disease but also weaken the immune system, the patient's natural and God-given first-line-of-defense against disease. The result is that the patient is abused, the healthcare system is fleeced, and society reaps a harvest of chronic degenerative diseases.

In the late twentieth century, when the Rationalistic [allopathic] medicine has been granted a quasi-monopoly on what is called "healthcare", absorbing an ever-expanding proportion of the national wealth and, abetted by a drug industry flourishing as never before in human history, this guiding concept of pharmacology has become a theoretical shambles, while the practice is in many respects a menace to health. The contrary medicine is an assault on the patient's organism, especially the immune system. The ensuing epidemic of drug diseases and drug-induced chronic diseases apparently represents the price civilization must pay for an active and flourishing allopathic profession and pharmaceutical industry. [7]

The evidence will show that the harvest of rationalistic Allopathic medicine is truly frightening. Coulter will testify that in 1988 one-third of all hospital deaths (620,000) were caused in whole or part by drug side effects and iatrogenic, that is, doctor-induced diseases. [8] This represents more deaths annually than were caused by our great Civil War of 1861–1865; the total for that carnage was, approixmately 618,000. Consider also this comparison. We lost approximately 58,000 troops in Vietnam over a ten-year period. But in one year, 1988, we lost as many patients to doctor-induced deaths as would have been caused by over 10 Vietnams! This frightful carnage is either ignored or accepted with calm resignation. America seems to have lost its collective ability to reason from cause to effect. Despite ample evidence that drug-based modern medicine is not very effective, especially in the treatment of chronic degenerative diseases, the public at large, like unthinking sheep, continue to bow to the dictates and prescriptions of a Medical Deity, which is foisted on us by government agencies— the institutions that should be protecting our lives and liberty

Under the reign of the lancet and pill, America is dying. Dr. Julian Whitaker observed that despite having the most brilliant emergency healthcare system in the world, and spending over two trillion dollars annually on health care, America is the sickest Western nation on earth in terms of chronic degenerative diseases. [9] The evidence will show that an epidemic of chronic degenerative diseases is sweeping America. Consider these sobering facts:

* Over 69 million Americans suffer from some form of cardiovascular disease. [10]

* Every year, over 1.5 million Americans have heart attacks and 80 million Americans have cholesterol levels that require some degree of medical treatment. [11]

* 60 million Americans have high blood pressure and it is the most common reason people go to the doctor. [12]

* An estimated 10 million Americans are diabetic, and another 20 million have impaired glucose tolerance that may lead to full blown diabetes. [13], [14]

* Approximately 40% of Americans are overweight; 25% of these are clinically obese, requiring some degree of medical management. [15]

* About 50 million Americans have osteoarthritis and another Two and a half million suffer from rheumatoid arthritis. [16]

* More than 20 million people in America suffer from osteoporosis or *porous bones.* [17]

Through their seminal work, *The China Study*, Drs. T. Colin Campbell and Thomas M. Campbell will testify that the leading causes of death in the year 2000, including death by medical care (totaled and itemized), were as follows [18]:

Heart diseases . . . . (710,760 deaths)
Cancer . . . . (553,091)
Medical care errors . . . . (225,400)

Strokes . . . . (167,661)
Chronic lower-respiratory diseases . . . . (122,009)
Adverse drug effects . . . . (106,000)
Accidents . . . . (97,900)
Hospital-borne infections . . . . (80,000)
Diabetes mellitus . . . . (69,301)
Influenza and pneumonia . . . . (65,313)
Alzheimer's disease . . . . (49,558)
Other preventable hospital errors . . . . (20,000)
Unnecessary surgery . . . . (12,000)
Medication errors . . . . (7,400)

Notice that the primary causes of death are all lifestyle related. We are killing ourselves with our knives and forks, literally. Ladies and gentlemen of the jury, to combat this epidemic of disease and death, this frightening plague of apocalyptic proportions sweeping our land, modern conventional medicine has constructed an elaborate and costly system for *managing* without curing or reversing, these chronic degenerative diseases. But the evidence shows that with 450,000 preventable deaths in the year 2000, this gigantic medical establishment has become the *third leading* cause of preventable death itself! [19]

Ladies and gentlemen, if it is indeed true that many of today's chronic degenerative diseases are pandemic because of the actions of physicians, then there is something very wrong with modern pharmaceutical medicine. This is the dark side of modern medicine, which no one in the medical establishment wishes to acknowledge or alter. Indeed the medical establishment has the weight of the law on their side. The evidence will show that never before in the history of medicine has governmental power intervened on the side of a medical system that preys upon and wrecks havoc upon its citizens.

Ladies and gentlemen of the jury, the evidence will show that modern medicine has fallen a long way from its guiding star, the great Hippocrates, whom we have many times stated enjoined physicians to, "first, do no harm." [20] The questions we must ask ourselves are sobering:

* If America has the finest healthcare system in the world, why are epidemics of disease sweeping America?

* Why is the treatment of diseases itself the third leading cause of death in America? Is medical science failing us?

* How did we get to this abysmal condition in an era that boasts great scientific advances?

* Could there be something wrong with our very conception of what science is?

* What is the true role of medicine—to manage disease or to get people well?

* Is pharmaceutical medicine part of the problem—in leading people to expect a quick fix for their indulgences rather than to make lifestyle changes?

* Is not the chief goal of medicine to prevent people from getting sick and diseased in the first place?

If a primary function of medical science, as Hippocrates taught, is to teach people how to avoid sickness and disease, then conventional medicine is failing society. Before we can hope to reverse the epidemic of diseases in this country, we must discover the true causes of chronic diseases. This discovery will help us understand why modern conventional medicine is hopelessly failing to stem the tide of these modern plagues.

Ladies and gentlemen of the jury, it was to cast *the light of commonsense* on these important issues that this trial has convened. I would remind you that you have been installed as judges of the facts to preside over matters that concern your vital interests. At the beginning of this trial you will hear the charges and the indictment being brought against that vast network of interconnected political and commercial institutions that are preying on our health and our pocket-books, and have robbed us of our medical freedom. The head of this profiteering Cartel is the pharmaceutical and chemical industries conjoined with big government bureaucracies. To our hurt they have set up a medical monopoly whose modus operandi is to *manage* the *symptoms* of disease instead of *curing* or *reversing* chronic degenerative diseases. Contrary to popular belief, physicians have long lost control of the medical profession. In many respects they are little more than sale representatives of the drug industry.

Ladies and gentlemen, mark this well—you have the power and ability to pass judgment on the efficacy of the theories and practices of conventional medicine. Let no one deceive you. The true scientific criterion for validating all theories and medical practices is to judge them by the objective facts of experience and the natural laws of nature that are open for all to discover. By this standard you must judge the efficacy of the practice of drug therapy to mask, but not cure, the symptoms of chronic degenerative diseases. You have it in your power to alter the course of the law of the land.

As you review the evidence, ask yourself these questions about conventional drug therapy:

* Does it do harm?

* Does experience demonstrate that often the "treatment" is worse than the disease?

* Does it suppress symptoms while *aggravating* the underlying chronic degenerative disease?

* Does it suppress and often destroy the body's immune system and hence the ability of the body to heal itself?

* Is this form of medicine geared to generating profits and not to restoring health?

* Are there safer, non-lethal ways of restoring the health of America?

Count 3:

A NEW DARK AGE: A FALSELY RATIONALISTIC SCIENCE DOMINATES MODERN MEDICINE

Ladies and gentlemen you will hear testimony on the nature of science and how to distinguish between true science and a false science masquerading under garments that deceive and lie. Critizing medical science's desire to *manage*, at a *handsome profit*, chronic degenerative disease, rather than *cure* the disease, Dr. Caldwell Esselstyn (past champion of radical mastectomy, until he learned the role of diet in the causation of cancer), may have hit on the cause for the failure of modern scientific medicine to treat chronic degenerative diseases when he wrote, " It's just so grippingly unbelievable to think that we are being led around by people who *refuse to believe the obvious!*" [1]

The key phrase is "refuse to believe the obvious." The evidence is there. It is being ignored, and, in many ways, suppressed. To refuse to believe the obvious takes us to the very heart of the dispute—one of true science against false science.

Ladies and gentlemen of the jury, to understand the failure of modern medicine in the treatment of chronic degenerative diseases, one must understand the failure of modern science. It is that simple. This may come as a shock to you, but not all that *passes* for science is science. Much of what we call science today was once derided and ridiculed by Sir Francis Bacon and other early modern empirical scientists as scholastic obscurantism and metaphysical superstition. This false science was the basis of the political correctness of the Dark Ages. Historians and scientists have labeled it *rationalistic science* because it seeks to rationalize away common-sense and the stubborn facts of sense perception. Today, in the great age of technology, this false conception of science is again passing itself off as true science. Technology is not exactly the same thing as science in the empirical sense. Sure, we have learned to discover, but we are spending the scientific capital built up by past centuries, for we have largely forsaken the path of pure empirical science. It follows that if we have strayed from the path of pure science, then we have abandoned the road to true medical science.

A definition of terms is in order. Throughout this discourse the term *empirical* will be use to refer to a method of inquiry which looks to the facts of nature to validate man's theories about the operations of nature. It will be expanded to describe a process of inquiry that acknowledges that man is able to look at nature and discover what God was thinking when he created the universe and imprinted his laws upon the fabric of created things. Thus, *empiricism* is compatible with and is a vital part of a biblical worldview, which holds that God created the Universe and man to exist under the same set of laws; consequently, man is able, under the tutelage of his Creator, to discover the operations of nature by objective inquiry. To recognize that God is the source of all knowledge, understanding, and wisdom is the first step in understanding the operations of nature

Likewise, the term *rationalistic* will be broadened to refer to a human-centered, as opposed to a God-centered, process of reasoning. Francis Schaefer defined *rationalism* in his insightful book, *Escape From Reason*, as the intellectual process by which man, rejecting any input from God, begins absolutely and totally from himself, gathers information concerning the particulars of nature, and formulates his own universals and theories about reality. [2] The central idea is that in formulating his theories about reality, rationalistic man looks only to himself and his intellect for answers. Intellectually man thinks and acts autonomously—without any reference to God. This is the dominant worldview today, and it was the legacy of both the Renaissance and French Enlightenment of the eighteenth century.

Ladies and gentlemen of the jury, the testimony will show that rationalism in science and medicine leads to false theories about the nature of man and the universe because it puts *rationalistic theories* above the *facts* of nature in arriving at knowledge. Typically *rationalistic science* selectively uses *some* of the facts of nature in formulating its answers. Thus there are elements of truth and self-deception in rationalism. This is the secret of its power over the gullible imagination: it *seems* to work—but only on the surface. Rejecting the evidence of God's existence in nature, this system of thought emphatically rejects the laws of nature and the laws of God as normative because they conflict with man's own ideas.

This, in sum, is the reason why rationalistic science and its counterpart, pharmaceutical medicine, refuse to acknowledge the healing power inherent in the organism. The laws of God imprinted into nature are the source of the healing power of nature. However, rationalistic science and medicine is in rebellion from God and his laws. Their solutions to the problem of sickness are to devise man-made solutions. Perceiving man as a purely materialistic being, rationalistic physicians look to chemistry as the laboratory out of which they fashion their tools to fight disease and sickness. They are not disposed to follow the natural paths to healing that God ordained in nature. The products of this type of thinking are variously termed rationalistic science, rationalistic medicine, and rationalistic philosophy; each of these disciplines produce a *false* theory of reality which is in conflict with the facts of nature.

Ladies and gentlemen, Harris Coulter, the medical historian earlier introduced to you, will testify that modern rationalist medicine gained the support of government by equating itself with scientific medicine. However, he argues that the only medical therapeutic doctrines that are truly curative and hence can be regarded as genuinely scientific medicine, are those based on *empirical* traditions. This embraces much of modern medicine such as our superior emergency and trauma-care medicine, orthopedic medicine, and infectious-disease medicine. It also embraces such disciplines as nutritional medicine, homoeopathy, osteopathy, naturopathy, and chiropractic medicine. The latter forms of medicine have been derisively labeled by conventional medicine as alternative medicine and have been more or less suppressed or discouraged during the twentieth century.

As copiously illustrated in earlier pages, the medicines generated by Rationalist doctrine are, on the whole not therapeutically efficacious and often actively harmful. The rising burden of side effects, adverse reactions, chronic disease, and immune-system destruction is the result of a pathologically hypertrophied Rationalism being given free rein in late twentieth-century industrial societies, bolstered by seemingly impregnable institutional support and fed by seemingly unlimited public funds. [3]

Medicine in its very nature should be a pursuit of the truth of what conditions generate health and life and what conditions and activities result in disease and death to man. Many scientific historians have recognized that medicine is the oldest scientific activity of man. If our *science* is false, our *medicine* will be false, because it is based on a false science. Modern rationalistic medicine is not scientific because it does not follow the methodology of science for the discovery of truth. It is based on false science and false ideologies that have no basis in fact. While not all modern medicine has followed the rationalistic path, pharmaceutical medicine, in its vain quest to treat or rather manage chronic degenerative disease with chemical poisons is based on this false science. To clear up confusion in our thinking, we must note the inversion of terminology that has occurred. The false *rationalistic* and *unscientific* medicine is regarded today as *scientific* medicine while the really *true* empirically based scientific medicine of Hippocrates and Paracelsus has been labeled as *false* and *unscientific* or, with some degree of facetiousness, it is referred to as *alternative* medicine.

Mark this well, ladies and gentlemen of the jury, the modern empirical science of Sir Francis Bacon and Isaac Newton, is, to a substantial degree, not being practiced today by either the scientific community or the medical establishment. The reason is very simple to understand, yet profoundly significant. One's concept of science (which is defined as the orderly and systematic pursuit of knowledge) is shaped by one's *worldview*. All man's beliefs—his science, his medicine, his knowledge, his laws, and his institutions—are shaped by his worldview. When science is shaped by a creationist worldview, it is empirical and genuine; and consequently medicine is empirical and genuine, striving to discover and come into compliance with divine laws implanted in man and nature. When so-called science is shaped by an atheistic or materialistic worldview, it degenerates into rationalistic and false science. Consequently, when medicine is rationalistic, it is sometimes destructive to the patient, for it tends to disregard the divine laws implanted in nature and in the fabric of man's being. Because much of *modern science* has been diverted from its true course, *modern medicine*, its stepchild, has been similarly derailed.

Ladies and gentlemen of the jury, for you to fully comprehend the failure of much of modern science and modern medicine, you must appreciate the crisis we are facing today in our *theory of knowledge*. Now please follow me here. By theory of knowledge, I mean how we come to *know* things and how we *verify* our knowledge. In slow and gradual steps our generation has slipped back into the Dark Ages in our thinking and in our science. We have lost the ability to verify knowledge, to discern truth from error, the false from the true; and this has profoundly altered our conception of what true science is. During the Dark Ages, knowledge was *verified* by the *authority of the Church* and by the *authority of rationalistic scholars* acting under the aegis of the Church. In those dark days, *opinion* was passed off as truth.

Count 4:

TURNING THE WHEEL OF KNOWLEDGE BACKWARDS: WORLDVIEWS DO MATTER

Ladies and gentlemen, let us delve a little deeper into the conflicting worldviews behind true and false science and how they relate to one's theory of knowledge. The time invested into this enquiry will pay great dividends, for it will help us unmask the false rationalistic science that is driving modern pharmaceutical medicine. It may be politically correct science, but it is nonetheless destructive. The evidence will show that it was the Sixteenth-century Reformation that taught men first to question, and then to challenge, this type of *politically correct* knowledge which destroys everything in its path, including science and medicine. A century before Sir Francis Bacon, the Reformation ushered in a revolution in the theory of knowledge when it abandoned a pagan worldview for a biblical one. The Great Sixteenth-century Reformation is usually only associated with the reform of religion and theology in the Christian Church. However, to confine it so narrowly is a great mistake. The same principles and concepts that transformed religion also transformed medicine, science, law, and the art and theory of government. Historians generally acknowledge that the modern world was born when the pagan worldview of Plato and Aristotle, which had been championed by an authoritarian Church and its Scholastic system, was overthrown and replaced by a biblical worldview.

When the Reformers said that the *facts* of Scripture (the plain reading of the Word of God) were the benchmark by which we verify the truth or fallacy of opinion, they dethroned the arbitrary authority of the Church, unleashing a revolution in the theory of knowledge in the area of religion. The Bible, the Word of God, became the benchmark for verifying all theological opinions. Truth was no longer held in hostage to arbitrary authority and unfounded speculations. This concept liberated men from the arbitrary authority of the Church. It set men free. In addition, the principle was soon applied to the acquisition of knowledge in the natural world. The factual events in the Book of Nature (God's second book of knowledge given to man) became the benchmark for verifying all scientific opinions and speculations.

The Reformers and early men of science (who were virtually all Christians), stated that true scientific knowledge could only be obtained by using *all* the facts of nature as the benchmark for determining the truth or fallacy of scientific opinions. From this point on, the arbitrary authority of the Scholastics elite was dethroned, and modern science was born. Henry Morris, in *Men of Science, Men of God*, wrote, "The scientific revolution really got underway with the Protestant Reformation." [1] The revolution in the theory of knowledge was caused by, and sustained by, a shift in worldviews.

You see, ladies and gentlemen of the jury, worldviews do matter. They determine the type of medicine we practice. As we change worldviews, our science and medicine gradually change to conform to the values and assumptions of the new worldview. For over one hundred years, America has been in the transition period in which the evolutionary, rationalistic worldview has gradually replaced the creationist, empirical worldview of our Founding Fathers. The harmful impact this change made to the form of our science and medicine is now being seen.

It is historically true that the rationalistic reasoning of the Dark Ages could not give birth to modern science. The Dark Ages was a period of gross superstition when unverified assumptions were passed off as knowledge. That is true because the worldview of the Dark Ages was shaped by the religious teachings of the Greek philosophers (from Pythagoras to Aristotle) about the nature of the cosmos. Stanley Jaki, a professor at Seton Hall University pointed out that in all ancient cultures, such as the Greek, Babylonian, Egyptian, Chinese, and Mayan, science suffered a stillbirth because they all shared an evolutionary and pantheistic concept of a cosmos rising and decaying in endless cycles. [2] In this pagan religious worldview, nature was animated by spirits and demigods. Nature was capricious and not under fixed laws. Where there is no concept of law regulating the form and movement of nature, science cannot come into existence, for science is the discovery of the laws implanted in nature.

Our investigation of the phenomenon of nature does not reveal random or capricious behavior; it reveals ordered movement, which we interpret as the immutable laws governing nature.

Stanley Jaki demonstrated that in one culture only, did science experience a live birth; that was in Protestant Europe. When Christian Europe repudiated the ancient pagan notion of the divinity of eternally existing heavenly bodies and accepted the Genesis account of an absolute beginning made possible by a Creator, modern science was born. [3] Professor Jaki pointed out that under the prior rationalistic worldview, the heavenly planets and stars were conceived as divine beings, which controlled the behavior of all things, by their fickle impulses. Under these conditions, there was no inclination to investigate nature for there was no conception of fixed laws governing the operations of nature. [4]

If Professor Jaki is correct that Socrates and Aristotle killed ancient Greek science, virtually strangling it in its birth clothes, [5] then it is plausible to conclude that *but for* the domination of Plato in the early Dark Ages (500–1200 AD), followed by the domination of Aristotle in the Mediaeval Dark Age period (1200–1500), European Christianity would have resulted in the flourishing of modern science long before the Reformation. It was the opinion of the eminent French physicist and historian of science, Pierre Maurice Marie Duhem, that the flame of modern science did indeed flicker and burn here and there during medieval times; it did so whenever the conviction was entertained that the universe was the rational product of a *reasonable* Creator who "disposed everything in measure, number and weight and who commissioned men to become masters and possessors of nature." [6]

Sir Francis Bacon was therefore correct when he contended that rationalism could not arrive at true knowledge, because it rested on a wrong *religious* worldview and upon a wrong *methodology* for acquiring and verifying knowledge. In his *Advancement of Learning* and *Novum Organum*, Francis Bacon consciously and deliberately established modern science on the biblical worldview of the Reformation. It is to this worldview that modern science owes all of its advances, nay, its very existence as science. Reviewing the lives of forty-eight prominent scientists, Dan Graves in *Scientists of Faith* wrote, "Christians and a Christian worldview were crucial to the formation of the early sciences. This was the electrifying thesis of both Pierre Duhem, and Stanley L. Jaki as demonstrated in *Science and Creation: The Origin of Science and the Science of its Origin*." [7] In a similar

survey of 102 scientists, Henry Morris in *Men of Science, Men of God*, came
to the same conclusion that Christianity was indispensable to the origin
of science. [8]

The biblical worldview promoted the *empirical* study of nature because
it taught that *a reasonable God had created a reasonable universe regulated by
law, and that these natural laws could be discovered by human reason.* With
few exceptions, the great names in early modern science are associated
with a Christian or biblical worldview. Abandoning the Pythagorean and
Platonic metaphysical and religious concepts that taught that matter and
the natural world were evil and could not be the source of knowledge,
these early scientists believed that the data of sense experience provided
real knowledge—and it is this biblical worldview that makes science possible. The battle that had to be won before science would arise, Jaki stressed,
was not "about the subtleties of logic" of the Schoolmen, rather the "Fight
in question was about the nature of reality and knowledge, crucial issues
for Christian or supernatural faith as for natural science." [9]

Mark this well, men had first to believe that a reasonable God made
a reasonable universe governed by fixed and unalterable laws before they
could be induced to investigate nature and discover these divine laws.
Modern science started off as the empirical study of these laws of the universe. Today a resurrected rationalism accepts the *fruits* of empirical science while it repudiates the philosophical and cultural environment that
gave rise to empirical science. As was stated previously, empirical science
taught man how to discover. Once put in motion, the art of discovery
can be sustained to a great extent by common sense and the basic human
faculty of reason. Rationalistic man, reasoning deductively and enjoying
the fruits of technology, quite easily loses sight of the fact that it was the
creationist worldview that made all of this possible. Our modern science
and medicine is living on the legacy of the Reformation and it is fast using
up that capital.

Ladies and gentlemen of the jury, I urge you to fully understand how
modern science has *abandoned* its true empirical moorings, by attaching
itself to the fallen star of ancient Scholasticism, thereby derailing modern
scientific medicine. Because we have abandoned the creationist worldview
of the Reformation and of early modern science, in favor of the rationalistic and pantheistic worldview of the Dark Ages, we must fight the
battle of the Reformation and of early modern science all over again. The
conflict is over how we discover and verify true knowledge. With your

participation, we will fight that battle during this trial. We will utilize the commonsense criteria of empirical science that incorporates an objective standard for validating all theories and medical practices by judging them by the objective facts of experience.

Count 5:

THE PLOT: SUPPRESSING SYMPTOMS WHILE REFUSING TO CURE THE DISEASE

The evidence will show the futility of treating cancer (except in emergency cases), solely by radiation, chemotherapy, and surgery—these protocols treat only the *symptoms* of this metabolic disease. This is particularly true in light of expert testimony that removal of the cancer growth by surgery *does not* mean a *cure* of the disease; [1] and in the case of radiation and chemotherapy, often result in the near total destruction of the patient's immune system and the generation of more cancer cells. [2]

Ladies and gentlemen of the jury, the evidence will show that the fundamental error in the conventional treatment of cancer is to regard the tumor as a locally limited disease. [3] Cancer is not the mass or the lump. The mass, like the tip of an iceberg, is only the *symptom* of a nutritional dysfunction resulting in a total metabolic disturbance of the entire being. [4] You will hear testimony from Dr. Max Gerson, one of the most eminent geniuses in the history of medicine who severely criticized the symptomatic treatment of cancer and other chronic degenerative diseases.

> In particular, in degenerative diseases and in cancer, we should not apply a symptomatic treatment or only one that we can fully understand; we need a treatment that will comprise the whole body as far as we know or can imagine. These thoughts were well know by the physicians of Greece and Rome; the ancient physicians knew that there are no sicknesses but only sick human beings. [5]

Dr. Max Gerson's treatment of choice for cancer and other chronic degenerative diseases was nutritional therapy.

Ladies and gentlemen of the jury, the evidence will show the folly of shunning dietary remedies and treating Type II diabetics with insulin only, when aggressive treatment with insulin causes progressive damage to the retina, often leading to total blindness. [6] You will hear testimony from researchers, such as Dr. James Anderson, one of many prominent scientists studying diet and diabetes, who demonstrate that a high-fiber, high complex carbohydrate, and low animal fat and protein diet reduces, and in many cases eliminates, the need for insulin medication. He showed that twenty-four out of twenty-five patients in a controlled study were able to dispense with their insulin medication! [7] These experts will testify through their written works, that the use of drugs or insulin to treat Type II individuals is a classic case of symptom management. The evidence will show that high blood sugar is the *symptom* of a deeper *metabolic problem* that leads to some very serious medical complications, including heart disease, blindness, and death. Treating the symptoms of high blood sugar does nothing to stop the relentless progress of the life-impairing diseases that plague diabetics.

Ladies and gentlemen, the nutritional experts will offer testimony that it is reckless to encourage the victim of osteoporosis to drink more milk to replenish calcium stores in the body; for study after study, including epidemiological evidence, show that the excessive protein in milk and animal products cause a negative calcium balance in people using these products. [8] Dr. John McDougall will also testify through his written works, that the scientific evidence demonstrates that the incidence of osteoporosis rises with the consumption of milk.

If we examine the worldwide distribution of cases of osteoporosis today, we are struck by the fact that this disease [osteoporosis] is most common in countries where dairy products and calcium supplements are consumed in the largest quantities: the United States, Sweden, Finland, and the United Kingdom. The occurrence of osteoporosis is rare in Asian and African countries where milk is not consumed because it is not available or because of a very high incidence of lactose intolerance. [9]

Ladies and gentlemen, you will discover that the scientific evidence linking high milk and protein intake to incidences of osteoporosis is over-whelming and cannot any longer be ignored, [10] but that is precisely what the medical establishment in league with the Dairy Industry has succeeded in doing.

You will hear testimony from nutritional doctors that it is futile to treat arthritis with drugs that suppress only the symptoms of this potentially crippling disease. Indicted are drugs such as indomethacin, the side effects of which are severe headaches, dizziness, rashes, and depression. [11] The hormone cortisone is also indicted, for the side effects are worse than the disease; it often causes damage to the nerves, blood, bones, other vital organs of the body, peptic ulcers, osteoporosis with spontaneous fractures, mental disturbances, psychosis, neuropathy or degeneration of the nerves, posterior subcapsular cataracts, diabetes, hypertension, disturbances in the metabolism and utilization of protein and fats, acne, and excessive hair growth in women. [12]

Ladies and gentlemen of the jury, the evidence will demonstrate that it is a betrayal of the public trust to treat non-emergency cases of heart disease with bypass surgery (at a cost of over $46,000), or angioplasty (at a cost of over $31,000), when bypass surgery and angioplasty do not address the cause of heart disease, prevent heart attacks, or extend the lives of any but the sickest heart disease patients. [13] This is particularly true in the light of studies by eminent physicians such as Drs. Caldwell Esselstyn and Dean Ornish, both of whom will testify in this trial that a whole food, plant-based diet with exercise (at an average cost of $7,000) reversed the disease in 70 to 80% of patients with established coronary diseases. [14] Moreover, they will testify that the side effects of a plant-based diet are all beneficial, while the side effects of bypass surgery include heart attack, respiratory complications, bleeding complications, infection, high blood pressure, and stroke. [15]

You will hear testimony from Dr. F Batmanghelidj, who wrote the inspiring book, *Your Body's Many Cries for Water.* He will testify that it is folly to treat the *symptoms of thirst* by medication when the simple remedy is to drink more water! [16] Dr. Batmanghelidj will state that high blood pressure is simply the result of an adaptive process to a gross body-water deficiency. [17] He criticizes the pharmaceutical approach to treating high blood pressure in these frank words:

The present way of treating hypertension is wrong to the point of *scientific absurdity.* The body is trying to retain its water volume, and we say to the design of nature in us: "No, you do not understand— you must take diuretics and get rid of water!" [18]

Ladies and gentlemen of the jury, the list of the medical and scientific absurdities of pharmaceutical medicine can go on ad infinitum and ad nauseam. The bottom line is that we must not abandon our commonsense because the medical community tells us we must subject ourselves to their endless round of drug-induced impairment, suffering, and often death. To do so would be to yield our medical freedom to a profit-making Cartel that is callous to human suffering.

In summary, ladies and gentlemen of the jury, the evidence will show that it *should* be medical malpractice and medical fraud to treat, in non-emergency cases, the *symptoms of a disease* with pharmaceutical and other high-tech remedies that only *suppress* the symptoms, while making the underlying disease worse and more expensive to treat and more life-threatening to the patient. On the other hand the evidence will show that medical science should emphasize the *nutritional remedies—including exercise, adequate water intake, and lifestyle changes.* The medical and scientific evidence will amply demonstrate that these non-injurious modalities are highly efficacious in not only preventing, but in reversing, chronic degenerative diseases.

I admonish you to mark well the testimony of Dr. T. Colin Campbell, a man in the forefront of nutritional research who holds the title of Jacob Gould Schurman Professor Emeritus of Nutritional Biochemistry at Cornell University. His China Study, made in collaboration with colleagues from Oxford University, aptly sums up his vast research, concluding that it is *irresponsible* for modern medicine to continue to ignore the *avalanche of scientific evidence* in favor of the nutritional treatment of chronic degenerative diseases.

Through all of this, I have come to see that the benefits produced by eating a plant-based diet are far more diverse and impressive than any drug or surgery used in medical practice. Heart diseases, cancers, diabetes, stroke, and hypertension, arthritis, cataracts, Alzheimer's disease, impotence and all sorts of other chronic diseases can be largely prevented. These diseases, which generally occur with aging and tissue degeneration, kill the majority of us before our time.

Additionally, impressive evidence now exists to show that advanced heart disease, relatively advanced cancers of certain types, diabetes, and a few other degenerative diseases can be reversed by diet.

I remember when my superiors were only reluctantly accepting the evidence of nutrition being able to *prevent* heart disease, for example, but vehemently denying its ability to *reverse* such a disease when already advanced. *But the evidence can no longer be ignored. Those in science or medicine who shut their minds to such an idea are being more than stubborn; they are being irresponsible.* [19] [Emphasis added.]

After hearing the evidence, ladies and gentlemen, I doubt that you will be found among those who shut their eyes to the painful truth. In fact, I believe that you will courageously hand down a verdict of guilty as charged.

OPENING STATEMENT:
Overview of the Field of Conflict

Section 1:

THE WAR ON NUTRITION

Ladies and gentlemen of the jury, you will find it beneficial to have an extended overview of the field of conflict raging in our society between nutritional medicine and pharmaceutical medicine before examining in detail the evidence relating to each of the six chronic degenerative diseases discussed in this trial. Today the health of America is at a crossroads. Epidemics of chronic degenerative diseases—like cancer, heart disease, diabetes, arthritis, and osteoporosis—are sweeping the land, killing and crippling millions. What is even more tragic is that these crippling diseases are largely, if not totally, preventable. They are the result of poor life-styles and eating habits. However, pharmaceutical medicine practiced for a profit has no incentive to inform the public of the connection between nutrition, or the lack thereof, and disease.

Historically these degenerative diseases were confined to the affluent few in rich and decadent civilizations. Today they are striking down the common man and the wealthy jet setter without distinction. The twentieth century boasts that it is history's technological and information age. However, in one area, gross darkness has settled over the land. We have lost the connection between eating and nutrition. We eat the poorest grade of food and self-deceptively call that fine dining. In addition, when we come down with degenerative diseases, we fail to reason from cause to effect.

This trial presents the case that the medical establishment, aided and abetted by the pharmaceutical and refined-food industries, is largely to blame for the present state of affairs. Obsessed with profit and the acquisition of power over the lives of the human race, they negligently and in some instances deliberately fail to educate the public as to the true relationship between proper food consumption and nutrition, and between the lack of proper nutrition and disease. In so doing, the medical establishment has forgotten the purpose of its existence.

Ladies and gentlemen, the problem is systemic. Modern medicine has forgotten the common sense injunction of Hippocrates to treat disease with proper nutrition. He clearly understood that if doctors ignore the relationship between what man eats and the diseases that befall him, they would not be able to understand these diseases and consequently be unable to adequately treat these diseases. He understood well that in the laws that govern the universe, (having being imprinted in the very fabric of nature by the Creator), effect follows cause with unvarying certainty. Since a man's diet is either the foundation of his health or the cause of his disease, nothing can be either more important or necessary for a physician to know than these things. Today doctors are taught almost nothing about nutrition. Dr. Julian Whitaker and other doctors that advocate nutritional medicine lament the fact that only a few hours in four years of medical study is devoted to the study of nutrition in medical schools. He states that in specialty training nutrition is not only ignored, it is even ridiculed. [1] The result is that most physicians disregard the role of diet in treating disease, particularly degenerative diseases such as heart disease, diabetes, and arthritis.

The evidence will show that in the spring of 1984, Dr. William P. Castelli, the medical director of the famous Framingham Heart Study, in Framingham Massachusetts observed:

It is a sad fact that for most heart attack victims, diet alone would work if we advocated diet in American medicine—but we don't. The average patient who comes out of a coronary unit or a cardiologist's office never gets hooked up to a diet program. [2]

Because the orientation of our current healthcare system is on treating, or rather, managing, disease it does little toward promoting *wellness*. We do not have a *healthcare* system; we maintain a *disease management* system, which is dependent upon people getting sick.

If more Americans discovered the preventative measures that would greatly reduce their risk of developing many common diseases the whole healthcare system as it now stands would probably collapse, because it is not fed by people who are well and healthy, but rather by people who are sick. [3]

Because of the profit that is being made by treating sick people, our entire healthcare system is focused on treating diseases rather than on promoting wellness. Focusing on intervention instead of prevention results in more sick people feeding the profits of massive industries who in turn encourage our over reliance on their drugs. John Robbins, heir of the founder of Baskin Robbins ice cream chain of stores, pointed out in his best seller, *Diet for a New America*, that a vicious cycle is thereby set up—reliance on drugs coupled with unhealthy lifestyles lead to an ever-increasing demand for the services and products of these chemical and pharmaceutical industries. [4]

The public has become pawns in a fast-pace-profit-making industry that masquerades as our healthcare system. Their health is traded for dollars. To maximize their profits the pharmaceutical-medical industry has to keep the people ignorant and dependent. The pharmaceutical-medical industry has become the new High Priesthood of the gods of medicine. Years of propaganda by the new Medical Deity has finally severed any connection between health and nutrition in the public's mind. Ignorance breeds diseases and diseases breed even more profits for the pharmaceutical industry. In frustration over the new medical darkness that has descended on America, Bob Livingston wrote in his June 1999 newsletter about the virtual 'black-out' of nutritional information:

> The nutritional relationship to health is blacked-out and erased from the public memory. *The entire medical monopoly, the sickness industry, is based on malnutrition.* Its foundation is deception and misinformation about nutrition ... Using chemicals (drugs) to heal is every bit witchcraft and superstition as was the bloodletting that killed George Washington. Yes, at one time bloodletting was "orthodox" medicine. Education itself becomes a conspiracy against health and nutrition when the learned, educated, and professional class is neutralized against common sense and objective realty. "Science" becomes a mask and charade for cover up of the medical monopoly. [5]

Nutritional doctors such as Drs. Julian Whitaker and John McDougall, stress that the key to good health is a balanced, nutritious diet with healthy lifestyles, and they are courageously trying to educate the public of this fact.

The emphasis on treating the symptoms of diseases with drugs necessarily diverts interest away from prevention and other safer medical modalities such as nutritional and natural remedies. [6] Consequently and disastrously, patients are not educated how best to preserve their health by natural and nutritional means. It is more important to build the immune system and so ward off diseases than to attempt to cure diseases by uncertain and dangerous means.

Ladies and gentlemen of the jury, this concept is at the core of the dispute between modern pharmaceutical medicine and nutritional medicine. It is a dispute with ancient roots. However, the terms of the dispute were more clearly defined by Pasteur and his contemporaries in the late eighteenth and early nineteenth centuries. While Pasteur focused on identifying infectious organisms and finding a weapon against them, his fellow Frenchman and scientist Claude Bernard contended that the state of a person's internal environment—in today's terms, his immune system—was more important in determining his susceptibility to disease. This concept is simple and very familiar to all of us. While we are all constantly exposed to viruses and other organisms, we do not always get sick. Why this is so, is of critical importance. Claude Bernard taught that a person should focus on making his internal *terrain* a very inhospitable place for infectious organisms. [7] Modern medicine has forgotten this sound advice.

The evidence will show that Bernard's work on finding ways to assist the body to heal itself influenced a Russian scientist by the name of Elie Metchnikoff, who discovered white blood cells and their role in defending the body against germs. He discovered by self-experimentation that if his immune system was sufficiently strong, he could swallow millions of cholera bacteria without coming down with the disease. His heroic efforts to reform medicine have long been forgotten. After a lifetime of fierce contention between Bernard and Pasteur regarding the relative merits of the germ theory versus the health of a person's internal terrain in fighting infectious diseases, Pasteur admitted to his colleagues on his deathbed that Bernard was right. The pathogen is nothing; the terrain is everything he conceded. This was a critical admission by one of the most influential proponents of the germ theory of disease. If it had been heeded, the whole course of nineteenth and twentieth century medicine might have been altered. The main emphasis of medicine today might have been on prevention and building the immune system through proper nutrition and exercise.

But alas, Pasteur's deathbed confession has either been forgotten or disregarded. Conventional medicine acts as though the only legacy left by Pasteur is his germ theory and the drug war against pathogens. Modern medicine has virtually forgotten the importance of keeping the terrain or immune system of the individual healthy and strong, so that the body can ward off disease and, if not compromised, heal itself.

The evidence will demonstrate that Antoine Bechamp (1816–1908), Professor of Medicine at the University of Montpellier, took up the debate between Pasteur and Bernard on the causes of disease. Bechamp considered the fundamental question to be, does the germ cause the disease, or does the disease cause the germ? Ladies and Gentlemen, please print the following concept indelibly into your minds, for the entire conflict between nutrition and pharmaceutical medicine turns on this point: *Bechamp's research convinced him that the disease causes the germ*. Bechamp discovered certain fundamental biological units, tiny living protein microorganisms that he called microzymes. His observations revealed that these tiny living protein microorganisms were the building blocks of microbes. He stated that these microbes could take on different forms, a phenomenon called pleomorphism (literally *many forms*). Normally these microbes are harmless. Their role is to assist the body's immune system. However, Bechamp discovered that when the body becomes acidic or toxic because of poor diet and other unhealthy lifestyle choices, the microzymes change into *pathogenic* microbes. Commenting on Bechamp's work, Dr. Harvey Bigelsen stated:

> Pasteur's concept that infectious disease can be caused only by external microbes was wrong. Rather, Bechamp showed microbes to be a secondary manifestation of the disease, a symptom rather than a cause ... Bechamp had solved a fundamental problem in the origin of disease. He had discovered a basic building block, essential to normal, healthy life, but which, under toxic conditions caused by chemical, environmental, emotional, or other factors, could change into pathogenic forms, including not only pathogenic bacteria, but also viruses, fungi, and molds. [8]

Bechamp's discovery of microzymes, and their alteration under toxic conditions to pathogenic disease-producing microbes, was in direct conflict with Pasteur's claim that disease stemmed from external causes. [9] With one stroke, the entire fabric of Pasteur's microbian theory of disease was destroyed. The way was now opened for medicine to strike at the root causes of diseases, both infectious and degenerative, by focusing on restoring the immune system. But to do so would have washed away the entire framework of pharmaceutical medicine that depended upon the treatment of recurring symptoms for the sake of profit. Great and strenuous efforts were made to bury this important medical and scientific breakthrough and its relationship to nutritional medicine. The petrochemical industry, the pharmaceutical industry through their control of the medical schools, and the medical establishment won and the public lost. Ladies and gentlemen of the jury, this is the wrong that you have the power to make right.

The immune system is the body's defense mechanism against disease. In doing its job, it also acts as the intelligence department. It gathers information on the germs that invade the body and on disease conditions, and reports back to the cells, organs, and glands that are part of the immune network. It then uses this information to produce specific ammunition to destroy the foreign invaders. It sends out white blood cells, specialized T-cells, and other cells to isolate, neutralize, and then destroy the enemy. [10] The body is capable of manufacturing its own drug-like substances to destroy agents of disease. Dr. Elinor Levy observed that within each of us exist the most creative and formidable array of medical tools ever conceived which makes the immune system the best defense against diseases. [11] This immune defense mechanism is kept in place by a sound nutritional diet. It is wrecked by a poor diet and unhealthy lifestyles. It is this defense mechanism that God created to protect and heal the body, which modern science seeks to duplicate by commercially manufacturing drug weapons to kill agents of disease. Unfortunately, man-made drugs can wreck the immune system making the patient even more susceptible to disease. [12]

Instead of relying upon man-made drugs to fight chronic diseases, we need to take responsibility for our own health and adopt lifestyles and diets that will boost the immune system and shield us from contracting disease. This will take a new way of thinking for each of us. This concept, if adopted, will virtually revolutionize the medical profession and reduce our national healthcare costs to a fraction of its present levels. Physicians must rediscover their ancient role. They must rediscover that their calling is to educate the public to adopt lifestyles that will promote the healing forces within themselves. If, for economic reasons, they are unwilling to perform this noble duty, then we, individually, must seize the opportunity, educate ourselves, and take charge of our own health. Let us take advantage of that body of nutritional knowledge, once virtually lost, but is now being restored by courageous nutritional physicians. Dr. Andrew Weil wrote:

> The evidence is incontrovertible that the body is capable of healing itself. By ignoring that, many doctors cut themselves off from a tremendous source of optimism about health and healing. [13]

The people must be taught from an early age that improper diet and intemperate habits can seriously injure the immune system. Research has shown that smoking, stress, and refined sugar disrupts healthy immune function. Dr. Julian Whitaker pointed out that the level of immune suppression in a person is virtually proportional to their level of stress. [14] This fact is especially important in cancer prevention and cure. It is now widely understood that our food choices can also adversely depress our immune systems. The ability of white blood cells to search out and destroy germs and viruses, such as the virus associated with cancer, is hindered by the presence of fatty acids, bile acids, cholesterol, and triglycerides in the blood stream. These unhealthy blood conditions are also linked to chronic problems such as high blood pressure, heart disease, diabetes, and various joint disorders. [15]

The evidence will demonstrate that proper nutrition is not only essential for building a vigorous immune system, it can also prevent us from contracting many of the common chronic degenerative diseases plaguing America today. This is one of the best-kept secrets of our modern society. A virtual bounty is placed on the head of those nutritional doctors who dare to either advocate or practice this concept in their treatment of patients with cancer and other chronic degenerative diseases. Our state and federal governments have become the enforcement arm of a medical, chemical, and drug cartel, which see immense profits in keeping the populace ignorant of these facts.

Undaunted, courageous nutritional doctors like Dr. John McDougall insist that diet is the primary causative factor in such systemic and degenerative diseases such as: allergies, arthritis, arteriosclerosis, diabetes, gout, gall stones, heart disease, hormone imbalances, hypertension, kidney failure, kidney stones, multiple sclerosis, obesity, osteoporosis, and strokes as well as cancers of the breast, colon, kidney, pancreas, prostate, testicle, and the body of the uterus. [16] Other habits such as smoking, immoderate use of alcohol, stress, and inactivity are *secondary* factors in causing these diseases. [17] Dr. McDougall argued that a *primary* factor must be present for the disease to develop. A secondary factor merely aggravates the disease process *after* the development has begun. [18]

Many people weaken their resolve to overcome chronic degenerative disease by buying into modern medicine's habit of blaming heredity for their chronic diseases. Nutritional doctors disagree with the official position on the role of heredity. They feel that although heredity may be a factor, it is not under our control, and so we must focus on what we can control—strengthening our immunity and lessening our susceptibility to diseases. Dr. Campbell cited a report prepared for the U.S. Congress in 1981 which conceded that heredity only accounted for a 2–3% risk of contracting disease; he contrasted this with a 10,000 % risk if you have the wrong diet! These facts, he stated, were also borne out in his China Study findings that some Chinese counties had 100 times the risk of cancer than others. [19] Heredity could not account for this variance, therefore there were obviously other factors in operation.

Do not be fooled by the genetic theory of disease that leaves us helpless victims. While many aspects of our biological makeup are recorded in our genes, disease is not primarily a result of your genetic inheritance. Our life span and the state of our health are to a great degree dependent upon the choices we make. We are poisoning ourselves with rich greasy food, nicotine, caffeine, and other poisons. Neal Barnard, John McDougall, and other nutritional doctors have insisted confidently that if we eat right, we will live longer and have a better quality of life. Dr. McDougall also emphatically stated:

> Diet and lifestyle changes are the most effective treatment for chronic forms of all these degenerative diseases ... far surpassing in results any drug or surgical therapy according to scientific and medical literature. This should not surprise you; what causes disease promotes disease. If you eliminate the cause, then the body's healing mechanisms can take over, resulting in improvement or recovery. [20]

Ladies and gentlemen of the jury, the medical and drug cartel have at their disposal millions of dollars to fashion one of their most effective propaganda tools in their war against nutrition. This tool is the myriad of so-called scientific studies that purport to *prove* that nutrition is not efficacious in preventing or reversing chronic degenerative diseases. The evidence will show that these studies are designed to fail. Nutrition gets a black eye and the people, kept in ignorance, are inclined to continue their use of pharmaceutical remedies to "manage" the symptoms of their diseases.

One example of such flawed studies is the recent study published by the American Medical Association on July 17, 2007 that "proved" that a "diet very high in fruit, vegetables and fiber in women with breast cancer did not decrease the risk of cancer recurrence." [21] What is wrong with this study? It does not tell you the whole truth; nor does it correctly represent the position of nutritional physicians or nutritional medicine. You will not hear any of the experts who will testify at this trial argue that *simply* eating a diet high in fruits, vegetable, and fiber will prevent the onset of chronic degenerative diseases. This assumption fails to acknowledge the true nature and progression of chronic degenerative diseases.

What these nutritional experts will testify is that eating a nutritious diet will *not* protect you from degenerative diseases such as cancer if you *include* harmful foods in your diet and pursue intemperate lifestyles! The simple fact is that degraded foods such as refined sugar, white rice, and white bread interfere with the digestion of even healthy foods so that the body not only fails to get adequate nutrition, but harm is done to the body. Despite an otherwise healthy diet, the excessive use of animal fat and proteins, excess sodium salt, and addictive substances like alcohol and caffeine can also lead to chronic degenerative diseases.

Ladies and gentlemen of the jury, Dr. Max Gerson will testify that despite generous portions of fruits, vegetables, and fiber, the chances are that you will come down with cancer and a cluster of degenerative diseases *if* you include excess sodium chloride [salt] in your diet. The sodium ion displaces the potassium ion inside your cells, thus impairing the function of multiple systems in the body.

> Laboratory findings reveal that in chronic diseases, sodium and calcium, both negatively charged, invade the weaker positively charged organs; accordingly, K (potassium) is lost from these organs, opening the door to further negative metabolic transformations. Here the disease starts, but not the symptoms. [22]

Dr. Gerson observed that potassium appears to play an indispensable and unique role in protein synthesis and enzymatic reactions; [23] therefore, "when unbalanced, the salts become a source of trouble for cell metabolism." [24] This mineral imbalance can lead to cancer: "Mineral imbalance becomes a question of profound importance in all discussions of the causative nature of cancerous processes." [25]

Dr. Gerson argued that in reversing cancer, eating good food is simply not enough; one must detoxify the body. [26] As reported, the UC Davis Study did not include a detoxification process for the 3,088 women in their breast cancer program, and permitted up to 20% fat in their diets. It was destined to fail, for like so many other studies, it failed to take into consideration *all the facts* about the nature and cause of cancer.

Dr. Michael Colgan will testify that although a low animal fat and high-fiber diet and the hearty consumption of organic fruits and vegetables can prevent cancer, [27], if you also eat *refined foods* like white flour and white bread, you will increase your risks of getting a variety of cancers. [28] He contended that the reason for this is that all refined foods, such as white flour, "lack the nutrients required for their metabolism in the human body." [29] He observed that even tough animals like rats, when fed on white bread, die within sixty days. [30] But, one may protest, what about "enriched" flour? Is this healthier ? Michael Colgan will testify that "enriched flour puts back only three of the essential vitamins required for metabolism, thiamin, niacin and riboflavin," [31] but human metabolism of carbohydrates requires the following vitamin and minerals: "thiamin, riboflavin, niacin, pantothenic acid, pyridoxine, phosphorus and magnesium." [32]

Ladies and gentlemen of the jury, mark this well—Dr. Michael Colgan will also testify that the *absence* of any one of these micronutrients will *prevent* the metabolism of the carbohydrate.

Even if one of these nutrients is not present in adequate amounts, the body cannot use the carbohydrate. Virtually all of the eight nutrients are lost in the processing of white flour ... So, in order to use enriched flour breads and baked goods, the body has to rob itself, depriving bones and heart of phosphorous and magnesium, and draining blood and brain of pyridoxine. In this way, high use of processed foods creates degenerative processes in the body that indirectly prepare it for cancer. [33]

Dr. T. Collin Campbell will testify through his famous China Study that even if you eat generous portions of fruits and vegetables, if your animal protein consumption is greater than 20% you will increase your risk of getting cancer, even preventing your recovery from cancer. [34] He will also testify that it is not only excessive animal protein that causes cancer, it can be caused by the consumption of excessive animal fat, and the risk is particularly high for breast cancer. [35]

However, Dr. Collin Campbell will also testify that it is not just animal fat and protein that increases the risk of cancer; *refined foods* also promote cancer. [36] He therefore emphasized that to *minimize your risk of cancer*, you also have to *avoid or minimize* your consumption of *refined foods*.

The recommendations coming from the published literature are so simple that I can state it in one sentence: eat a whole-food, plant-based diet, while minimizing the consumption of refined foods, added salt and added fats. Daily supplementations of vitamin B12, and perhaps vitamin D for people who spend most of their time indoors and/or live in the northern climates are encouraged. For vitamin D, you should not exceed RDA recommendations.

That's it. That is the diet science has found to be consistent with the greatest health and the lowest incidence of heart disease, cancer, obesity and many other Western diseases. [37]

Ladies and gentlemen of the jury, one of the great myths you will hear is that being a vegetarian will save you from cancer and other forms of degenerative disease. However, the truth is that if you persist in eating refined foods along with otherwise wholesome foods, your risk of getting cancer is greatly increased! Much less will eating generous portions of fruits and vegetables help you avoid or recover from cancer. Dr. Nancy Appleton has made this very clear and will so testify in this trial through her informative book, *Lick the Sugar Habit.*

The average person consumes 20% of his or her calories from some form of refined sugar. This makes it difficult for the body to get the nutrients it needs from the other 80 percent. Many people think that they can eat anything they want as long as they take their multivitamin and mineral pills daily. Sugar so upsets the body chemistry that it doesn't matter what else you put in your mouth, neither healthful food nor junk food will digest properly. [38]

She will testify that the reason for this is that refined sugar is so depleted of essential nutrients that they rob the ingested foods of the proper minerals and vitamins needed for the digestive enzymes to function.

> Every food we eat needs a variety of enzymes to digest and metabolize the food before it can be used by our cells. None of these enzymes will work without the proper minerals to help them out. If the usable minerals in the body decrease, as in the presence of sugar, there will not be enough of them for proper enzyme function. Therefore, when we ingest sugar, it is difficult for the body to digest anything else that is in the small intestine. [39]

Ladies and gentlemen, this is a very important point to grasp. The sweet taste of refined foods like sugar may be deceptive. The stomach may be full, but insufficient nutrition may be reaching the vital organs and tissues. To a large extent America is obese and malnourished at the same time. Without adequate nutrition, one can expose the body to degenerative diseases. However, Dr. Nancy Appleton argued that the situation is much worse; refined sugar interferes with the process of digestion. Not only does the body fail to get adequate nutrition from the healthy foods ingested along with refined sugar, it is *poisoned* by the partially digested foods.

> When protein is digested correctly, it is broken down first into polypeptides and then into amino acids, which are absorbed in the blood stream. When it does not break down completely, when the enzymes charged with the job are incapable of performing properly due to a mineral deficiency, protein can be absorbed through the intestinal wall and into the bloodstream, reaching tissue in partially digested form. The body's immune system correctly interprets this undigested or "putrefied" protein as foreign matter and goes on the attack, causing an allergic reaction ... [40]

Ladies and gentlemen, Dr. Nancy Appleton will therefore testify that the "free use of sugar will impair the immune system," [41] "and slowly but surely lead to degenerative disease." [42] The pathway to the destruction of the immune system is not difficult to understand she states. It occurs through the "combined effects of mineral imbalance, allergic reaction, and phagocytic suppression." [43] The excessive consumption of refined sugar is a key factor behind the slow but steady destruction of America's health.

Unfortunately, Dr. Nancy Appleton observed, "many people in the nutrition field have not come to the understanding that as long as sugar is eaten, nutrients will be unavailable to the body." [44] These nutritionists, she observed, are ignorant of the destructive nature of refined sugar and other refined foods because their schools have been kept in ignorance by the medical and drug cartel. They have been taught that if you simply take in the required daily allowance (RDA) of minerals and vitamins set up by the Food and Drug Administration or the governmental agencies, you will be fine. However, Dr. Nancy Appleton will argue that the RDA is not a valid measure of health, for "sugar so changes the body's chemistry that its cells fail to benefit from these minerals and vitamins." [45]

Dr. Nancy Appleton further observed that despite the fact that much of the money that goes into research on food and diseases comes from the food and pharmaceutical industries, neither will alert you to the destructive effects of refined sugar on the body. [46] It is a case of mutual collaboration for the sake of profits. The food industry relies on sugar to manufacture their processed foods and to make them palatable to the public. [47] Addiction to sugar guarantees sales; and the excess consumption of refined sugar results in disease and the subsequent use of drugs to combat theses diseases. Under these lucrative circumstances, do you thing that the pharmaceutical industry will help you preserve your health by advising you to eat healthily? Do not bet on it. Dr. Nancy Appleton contended that if people stopped eating sugar, they will not need so many drugs to manage the symptoms of impaired health. [48] It is all about the money, folks. It is not about your health.

Section 2:

THE CAUSES OF CHRONIC DEGENERATIVE DISEASES

Ladies and gentlemen, a major argument of this trial is that research in the last several decades and the recent clinical experiences of prominent nutrition-oriented physicians point clearly, consistently, and overwhelmingly to rich foods in the form of meat, dairy products, eggs, sugar, and processed and refined foods (and to lifestyle practices involving smoking, caffeine, and physical inactivity), as the major causes of death and disability in society. This same scientific research shows that these degenerative diseases can be treated more effectively by *removing* the causes than by using any of the drugs and surgical practices available today. [1] When one understands how a high-fat, high-protein, refined-carbohydrate diet can cause degenerative diseases, the knowledge to reverse these diseases comes within one's grasp. Although more fully discussed in the body of the evidence presented during this trial, the concept is simple and can be briefly stated and outlined here.

The evidence will show that, broadly speaking, there are two or three primary causes of chronic degenerative diseases. Firstly, consuming the macronutrients fats and proteins in the wrong proportions, while eating too little of natural complex carbohydrates. This is compounded by the over consumption of simple carbohydrates such as refined sugar, white rice, and white bread. We over consume fats and proteins because of ignorance and well-aimed propaganda from the meat and dairy industries. Secondly, eating too little of the micronutrients such as vitamins, minerals, enzymes, and other phytochemicals, all of which are found in complex carbohydrates such as fruits, grains, nuts, vegetables, and fruits. Thirdly, lifestyle factors such as smoking, alcohol, stress, and lack of exercise.

World-renowned sports nutritionist, Dr. Michael Colgan, will testify that we have forgotten that fats and proteins are primarily *building materials* and that the main *fuel source* for the body is complex carbohydrates. [2] Consequently, because of its overwhelming need for energy, the body was created to crave carbohydrates more than any other component of our food. Dr. John McDougall maintained that the adult human needs approximately thirty-five times more carbohydrates for energy than they need protein for growth, and about 800 times more carbohydrate for energy than fat. [3] In terms of measurable quantities, an adult requires about 700 grams of carbohydrates for energy, 20 grams of protein to maintain healthy cell replacement and repair, and 3 grams of fat for hormone and cell membrane synthesis. [4] He will state that our nutritional needs will be completely met when we eat the following proportions of carbohydrates, fats, and proteins:

Complex Carbohydrates: 75–90%
Protein: 5–15%
Fat: 5–10%

Compare this to the typical American diet, which consists of high fat, high protein, and low complex carbohydrates, with very little fiber. The typical American diet breaks down in the following proportions:

Complex Carbohydrates: 20–30%
Protein: 30–40%
Fat: 40–50%

It is not surprising our systems are clogged and we run out of energy. Dr. Julian Whitaker will also testify that this high-fat (typically saturated fat from meat and dairy), high-protein, fiberless, low-carbohydrate diet is the *genesis* of our all our generative diseases and health problems. [5] He will state that there is a link between arteriosclerosis, heart disease, high blood pressure, diabetes, and obesity. The common factor is high saturated fat, which creates high cholesterol and triglyceride levels in the blood. [6]

There is also a link between gout, arthritis, and osteoporosis. The common factor is high uric acid concentrations in the blood from too much protein. [7] Likewise, there is an inescapable link between digestive diseases and colon cancer. Here the common factor is excess refined foods and low fiber in our diets. [8] All these diseases are metabolic disorders caused by eating the wrong kinds of foods in the wrong combinations. Animal products are the primary source of excess fat and protein in the American diet.

Excess refined sugar in the diet is perhaps the worst offender, according to Dr. Nancy Appleton. She stated that by itself, an excess of refined sugar could precipitate all of the degenerative disease plaguing our society: hypoglycemia, hyperglycemia, diabetes, constipation, gas, asthma, headaches, psoriasis, cancer, arthritis, candida, obesity, heart disease, osteoporosis, tooth decay, multiple sclerosis, inflammatory bowel disease, canker sores, gallstones, and cystic fibrosis. [9] Sugar upsets the body chemistry by depleting and altering mineral levels in the body so that even healthful food cannot digest properly. [10] Depleting mineral levels in the body is extremely dangerous, because minerals are essential to many bodily functions. [11] Minerals also activate enzymes important to numerous metabolic functions. [12] When refined sugar is eaten, nutrients will be unavailable to the body. [13] Dr. Nancy Appleton emphasized that unless we stop doing the things that make us sickly and diseased, all the medicine, vitamins, and other nutritional supplements in the world will not make us well. [14]

Ladies and gentlemen of the jury, pause for one moment and consider this pivotal question: how did America become attached to this rich meat and sugar diet? The answer to this question will provide a profile of other members of the industrial Cartel preying on our health: the fast food and refined-food industries and the animal-products industry. Although pestered by infectious diseases due to ignorance of proper sanitation and hygiene, our ancestors did not have a fraction of the degenerative diseases we now have. It was usually the affluent classes of past centuries who experienced these degenerative diseases. The common factor: they ate the rich foods we now eat. [15] Dr. John McDougall pointed out that modern technology, refrigeration, and better transportation of food from the fields to the market place and then to the home allows the general population to eat the rich foods at affordable prices that were once available only to the rich and privileged. [16]

The evidence will show that although research over the last eighty years has consistently pointed to the use of rich foods, such as meat, dairy, fowl and refined sugar as the primary causes of all our diseases, lucrative industries have sprung up to produce these foods. The industries that produce these rich foods promote their products for maximum profits, not for maximum nutrition to the public. In some instances, they have misrepresented the facts regarding good nutrition. Dr. McDougall contended that in some cases, there has been a responsible party concealing the truth. [17] He stated that the meat, dairy, sugar and refined-foods industries have so interacted with the government, the scientific community, the medical community, and the public (that is the public media and advertising industry), that grossly incorrect concepts concerning our nutritional needs are propagated and accepted as fact with only a rare dissent. [18] Truth and nutritional common sense no longer motivate our food industry; the quest for greater and still greater profits does.

Few people are aware of the fact that the recommendation that we should eat a high-protein meat-based diet came from the research on the nutritional needs of rats. Yes, rats! [19] Such an assertion would seem like an absurdity to make were it not regrettably true. It would appear that the self-appointed guardians of our health and welfare have taken leave of their collective common sense. The apostle Paul states that whenever man forsakes the wisdom of God, they become fools in their imaginings, even while loudly professing to be wise (Romans chapter one). The dietary recommendations of our so-called experts have exemplified this truth.

Dr. John McDougall laughed at the absurdity of basing the diet of humans on the nutritional needs of rats. He observed that throughout nature, there are specific and narrow nutritional requirements for each plant and animal. [20] The Lord of Creation so ordained it, and we would do well to heed his counsel. Interchanging the diet for horses with that for cats would result in poor health for both. [21] Similarly interchanging the diet for humans with that of pigs or rats would result in poor health for humans. [22] Dr. John McDougall and other nutritionally oriented physicians have pointed out that research over the last several decades convincingly establish that the diet that best supports health and healing in humans is a pure vegetable diet centered on unrefined starch foods with the addition of fresh fruits and vegetables. [23]

How then did we come to establish the diet of rats for humans? John Robbins, in his remarkable and influential book *Diet for a New America*, related that in 1914, Osborne and Mendel did some studies on rats while doing research on protein requirements. They found that rats grew faster on animal protein than they did on plant proteins. [24] Before long, and without any justification or consideration for the particular needs of humans, nutritionists began to alter the dietary habits of humans. They commenced by classifying meat, egg, and dairy as *Class A* proteins and proteins of plant origin as *Class B* proteins. [25] Thus in a moment of rash insanity, so-called nutritional experts relegated to secondary status the food the Creator designed that man should consume, while exalting to priority status foods he did not provide for in man's original diet. Were these nutritionists beholden to the meat and dairy industry? The answer seems obvious.

Animal foods are the lowest grade of food because of their high saturated fat and protein content. The introduction of animal foods into the human diet appears to have been responsible for shortening man's life. Man's diet before and after Noah's flood provides ample evidence that animal foods shortened human life spans. Man's life span declined from 950 years to 170 years, then to 70 years in a relatively short time only after he began to consume animal products. [26] Our dietary habits over the last century also provide ample evidence of the harmfulness of eating excessively of animal foods. In modern times, twentieth-century man has enjoyed a greater consumption of animal products than any generation since the flood. Not surprisingly, the last century has seen the rise of chronic degenerative diseases in apocalyptic proportions.

Ladies and gentlemen, let us continue with our story about the introduction of the diet of rats to humans. In the 1940s, researchers discovered that the optimum proportion of amino acids that produced the fastest growth in rats was similar to that found in animal protein, particularly in eggs. Again, without any supporting research on the nutritional needs of humans, the assumption was then made that the proportion of amino acids that provided the most rapid growth in rats would be the optimum amount of proteins for humans as well. [27] Is this too incredible to believe? Just follow the evidence, and the dollar, folks. Today we have discovered, after untold suffering, that this is not the right combination of amino acids for humans. [28]

The leap from rats to humans was made without the least shred of scientific evidence and in blatant disregard of the most elementary biological facts about the growth patterns of human babies and baby rats. Dr. John McDougall and John Robbins both point out that baby rats need three and a half times more protein than human babies because they develop much faster, doubling their birth weight in four days compared to 180 days for human babies. [29], [30]

By the mid twentieth century, the National Egg Board began to promote eggs as the best source of protein for humans; a food source that is 98% cholesterol! How blind and misguided man can be when profit is the prime motivation! This arrogant ignorance has been responsible for untold suffering from cardiovascular disease. It was not long before the Dairy Council and Livestock and Meat Board got involved. They loudly proclaimed that animal products were the best source of protein for humans. Relying only on limited animal-based experiments, they declared to an unsuspecting public that proteins from eggs, dairy, and meat were superior food for humans. Soon this animal products cartel introduced one of their most powerful adverting tools: the famous poster depicting the *Four Basic Food Groups*. This authoritative poster was hung up in almost every classroom wall. Generations of children, soon to become parents with children of their own, were indoctrinated to believe that good eating required one to build one's meals around the meat group and the milk group of foods with fruits vegetables and cereals as secondary foods. Some of you may recall the slogan recited in our schools in the 1960s: Milk, butter, cheese and eggs for breakfast.

The recommendations, or more accurately, propaganda, of the Dairy Council and Livestock and Meat Board of the last century contributed to providing generations of Americans with false information about proper nutrition based on the nutritional needs of rats. Of course, their interest was not in maximizing the health of Americans, but in maximizing their profits through the sale of their animal products. Never before has so many generations been gulled and deceived in a matter so vital to their health. What is even more scandalous is that the original research on the diet of rats was itself flawed. Therefore, erroneous assumptions were based on false information. What the meat and dairy industries failed to tell Americans is that *the rats fed this rich, high-fat, and high-protein diet died sooner from chronic degenerative diseases than rats fed a plant-protein diet!* [31] What has been accepted as conventional wisdom for decades has now been exposed as an artfully concealed work of fraud.

Ladies and gentlemen, although the researchers were correct in their observations that the rats doubled in size under animal protein, that fact alone did not equate with good health for the rats. The results have been equally devastating for human beings: generations of Americans suffer from obesity, heart disease, arthritis, osteoporosis, diabetes, tooth decay, and constipation, to mention only a few of the degenerative diseases. It is high time that Americans woke out of their slumber and began to think for themselves in matters pertaining to their health and nutrition. The evidence will show that it is the wide spread and excessive use of animal products that is causing the epidemic of degenerative diseases sweeping America. All the evidence points to a link between the consumption of animal products and the onset of chronic degenerative diseases. Yet despite the clear scientific evidence demonstrating that the consumption of animal products can be detrimental to our health, the meat and dairy cartels continue to spew forth voluminous one-sided, profit-oriented advertisements attesting to the advantages of using their products. By their propaganda, they keep in ignorance and dependency the gullible public who continue to consume meat, eggs, and dairy products with dire consequences. [32]

In his landmark book *Reversing Heart Disease*, Dr. Julian Whitaker presented statistical and epidemiological evident that demonstrates the fact that as the percentage of animal source protein consumed increases, so does the death rate from heart disease. This is true for all cultures examined. [33] In another of his influential books, *Reversing Diabetes*, Dr. Julian Whitaker stated emphatically:

Most of the degenerative diseases in this country can be traced to our meat-based diet, and diabetes is no different. [34]

The dairy industry has become one of the most powerful and successful advertising agencies in modern times. Dr. John McDougall observed that with their well-orchestrated campaigns they have convinced dietitians, doctors and parents that milk is nature's most perfect food and that poor health will be the inevitable result of a diet that fail to provide generous amounts of dairy products. [35] He stated that the stark and inescapable truth is that dairy foods are the *most harmful* of the traditional four groups because they are high in fat, protein, and environmental contaminants while being deficient in fiber and carbohydrates. The lactose carbohydrates in animal products are mostly indigestible by humans, he stated and is the source of diarrhea, gas, and stomach cramps. [36] Dairy products, which are virtually *liquid meat*, are also the leading source of food allergies. [37]

Dr. Julian Whitaker also agreed with Dr. John McDougall's opinion on the harm generated by the use of animal products, when he wrote that contrary to the dairy industry's assertion that milk is essential to build strong bones, the naked truth is that the excessive protein in milk creates a negative calcium balance in the person consuming milk, and this leads to such bone diseases as osteoporosis. [38] He pointed out that the average American male weighing 150 pounds requires only about 35 grams of protein daily. Yet the typical American diet can provide about 100 grams or more of protein. That is about 300 to 400% more protein than needed. [39]

It is not difficult to understand how excess animal protein can do harm to the body. It is well known that the human body cannot store excess protein, nor does it use protein for energy; so it must get rid of it through the kidneys. Because the breakdown products of protein are acidic, minerals are leached out of the body; and this loss of minerals causes accelerated aging and diseases such as cardiovascular and bone diseases as well as kidney stones and kidney failure. [40]

Ladies and gentlemen of the jury, because of our daily bombardment by the propaganda of the meat and dairy industries, all of this may sound too incredible to be true. Yet the stark, naked, and brutal truth is that for the last several decades, Americans have been subjected to a campaign of misinformation about what foods provide adequate nutrition and about the relationship between animal products and disease. Millions of Americans have needlessly suffered diseases, impaired quality of life, heartache, and premature death because of their immoderate consumption of a rich diet of meat, eggs, milk, and refined sugar. In his well-researched book, *Diet for a New America*, John Robbins observed that because of enormous breakthroughs in the science of human nutrition, we are receiving irrefutable scientific evidence of how different eating patterns affect our health. Recent research in nutrition also exposed the deadly misconceptions that have been foisted on us in this century about proper nutrition.

Thousands of impeccably conducted modern research studies now reveal that traditional assumptions regarding our need for meats, dairy products and eggs have been in error. *In fact it is an excess of these very foods, which had once been thought to be the foundations of good eating habits, that is responsible for the epidemic of heart disease, cancer, osteoporosis, and many other diseases of our time.* [41]

The amount of suffering and death that has been caused by this calculated nutritional misinformation makes the holocaust look like a tempest in a teapot. The Nuremberg trials held that raw power must never again triumph over human rights and human life. Yet no sooner were these war trials over that the vast financial and industrial combination that triumphed over the German war machine perpetrated a greater holocaust upon the Western Democracies. Through its control of the medical, pharmaceutical, and processed food and animal products industries, the Cartel has profited on the death and sickness of entire nations. Surely, the quest for raw profits must never again be allowed to triumph over human rights and human health.

Section 3:

THE MEDICAL GENIUSES AND NUTRITIONAL EXPERTS YOU WILL HEAR FROM

Ladies and gentlemen of the jury, the evidence that will be presented to you will not constitute an unmitigated litany of gloom and doom. The amazing breakthroughs in nutritional health care, though forced in some respects to labor underground, will inspire you. You will also discover that there are signs that the public and some members of the medical community are beginning to wake up to the nation's plight. In the wake of the overwhelming scientific evidence that animal products, refined foods, and sugar-filled foods are at the root cause of our plagues of degenerative diseases, there arose in the latter part of the twentieth century a number of Wellness institutions. These institutions are operated by pioneering physicians who endeavore to integrate the best of modern medicine with nutritional and lifestyle changes as the primary tools to prevent and reverse (or cure) chronic degenerative diseases.

Testimony will be presented from the works of the most prominent of these pioneers of nutritional medicine. You will hear from Dr. Andrew Weil, director of the Department of Integrative Medicine at the University of Arizona in Tucson; Dr. Dean Ornish at the University of California, San Francisco Pacific Medical Center; Dr. Julian Whitaker at the Whitaker Wellness Institute in Newport Beach, California; Dr. John McDougall, formerly of St. Helena Hospital Medical Center and one of the earliest pioneers of nutritional medicine; Dr. Vernon Foster, previous director of Weimar Institute, California; Dr. Richard Schulze; Dr. Neal Bernard; Dr. Neil Nedley; Dr. Richard Passwater; Dr. James Anderson; Dr. Lynne Paige Walker; and Dr. Dharma Singh Khalsa;

You will also hear from nutritionist Dr. Nancy Appleton, whose *Lick the Sugar Habit* has rescued untold numbers from addiction and diseases; Dr. Michael Murray and James Marti; Dr. Patrick Quillin who wrote the influential work, *Beating Cancer with Nutrition;* Dr. Max Gerson, (acclaimed to have been the "most eminent genius in the history of medicine"),who made prominent the concept that cancer is not the mass or lump—those are only the symptom of an underlying metabolic dysfunction of the body. Dr. I. William Lane who opened up a new conception of cancer in his book *Sharks Don't Get Cancer;* Dr. Harvey Bigelsen who made prominent the work of Antoine Bechamp, who revolutionized our understanding of disease and germs; Drs. T. Colin Campbell and Thomas Campbell, whose exhaustive and recently published *China Study* has shaken the medical establishment. Much of the evidential material for this trial is drawn from their work.

Women with breast cancer should take particular note of the work of Dr. Lorraine Day, formerly chief of orthopedic medicine at San Francisco General Hospital, whose story of healing herself of breast cancer solely by nutritional means (including adequate hydration) is becoming well known. You will also hear from Dr. F. Batmanghelidj. As a young Oxford medical graduate he was thrown as a political prisoner into a prison camp in Iran, where he had nothing but water to treat the sick prisoners. His experiences in prison drove him to write *Your Body's Many Cries for Water*, in which he demonstrates that adequate hydration can prevent and reverse many diseases.

Although they now sleep in the dust, you will hear from such medical geniuses and scientists as Hippocrates; Paracelsus who reformed Medieval medicine; Sir Francis Bacon, physician and Father of modern science; the acclaimed German physicians Hermann Boerhaave and Samuel Hahnemann; the confidant of John Locke, Dr. Thomas Sydenham; Dr. Antoine Bechamp who revolutionized our understanding of germ theory; and Dr. Linus Pauling who was ranked with Einstein for his work in Molecular Chemistry. Their testimonies cry out to us from the grave indicting modern pharmaceutical medicine.

Nutritionists such as Drs. Colgan and Appleton have also contributed much to the understanding of the connections between improper nutrition and disease and proper nutrition and optimum health. Despite the valuable work of these professionals, it is sad to say that the revolution in health care has not been driven by the medical profession. It is being motivated and driven by pioneering nutritionists, dissenting physicians, and a growing multitude of laypersons that are demanding better answers about their health. They are sick and tired of expensive drugs and surgeries that treat the symptoms of their diseases while leaving them with broken health. They are tired of medications with side effects worse than the original disease. They are tired of being held hostage to ignorance, like helpless victims in the hands of a self-appointed Medical Deity whose failures are all too apparent. It is a shame to the medical profession that it was left to laypersons like Nathan Pritikin, John Robbins and Kevin Trudeau to demonstrate that a low-fat, low-protein, complex-carbohydrate diet is a valuable tool in preventing and reversing many chronic degenerative diseases.

During the course of this trial, you will be presented testimony on many of the major degenerative diseases that have struck and are striking down millions of Americans. The chronic diseases examined are arthritis, cancer, diabetes, heart disease, high blood pressure, and osteoporosis. Neither space nor the scope of this book permits a detailed examination of other common degenerative diseases. The reader is referred to the books written by the nutritional doctors cited. The purpose of examining these six prominent degenerative diseases is to marshal the evidence and submit it to the court of public opinion.

Ladies and gentlemen of the jury, the vast amount of evidence you will hear will be presented to you in this trial in the following manner in order to make this potentially complex subject understandable: First, the nutritional and lifestyle causes of the selected degenerative diseases are examined. Once the causes of the diseases are understood, it will be easy to intelligently determine which is the best remedy. Next, the pharmaceutical attempts to *manage* the symptoms of these diseases, while *refusing to cure* the diseases will be presented. Next the testimony of physicians practicing nutrition-based medicine, outlining their successes in preventing, and in most cases curing these selected chronic degenerative disease will be presented. At this point in the trial, you will be able to judge the effectiveness of the two major approaches to treating chronic diseases—drugs and surgical procedures, verses nutrition and life style modalities. Finally, you will hear admissions from members of the medical establishment that drugs do not cure diseases and are often more harmful than the remedy; and that they oppose nutrition-based medicine because they undermine profits generated from the sale of pharmaceutical remedies.

The testimony will show that the conventional medical approaches only deal with the *symptoms*, while nutrition and lifestyle approaches go the core of the problem and eliminate the causes of the disease. You, the jury, will then be asked to compare the results and decide for yourself which approach can best serve the public interest. The evidence is convincingly clear, ladies and gentlemen of the jury, that symptom-oriented drug therapy does not cure degenerative diseases; only proper nutrition and temperate habits do.

As a vast national jury, you must look at the evidence and render a verdict. It should be a verdict of indictment, for the evidence is overwhelming that a vast financial, industrial, and medical cartel are aware that drugs do not cure but aggravate and perpetuate the plague of chronic degenerative disease sweeping this country. The evidence is equally overwhelming that nutritional modalities and healthy lifestyle changes are the most efficacious means of halting and reversing the epidemic of chronic degenerative diseases we are suffering from today. Those responsible for this holocaust of diseases, including governmental agencies that have carried the water bucket for the profit-driven Cartel, must be brought to the bar of justice.

And so, ladies and gentlemen of the jury, as members of the court of public opinion, the appeal is made to you. You can vote with your pocket book, your ballot, and your feet. You are at a crossroads. Indeed all Western Democracy is at a crossroads. You can chose to follow along the path of total dependency on a moribund medical system that insists on defeating disease with inefficacious and dangerously potent drugs and invasive procedures. If you continue down this path, you have everything to lose—including your health and perhaps life. On the other hand, you can stand up and take full responsibility for your life and health. You can educate yourself about good nutrition and follow healthier lifestyles that will provide a happier and longer life. Moreover, you can, by your example and personal choices, demand an accounting from the medical profession.

Ladies and gentlemen, it has been over two centuries since our founding fathers "brought forth a nation conceived in Liberty and dedicated to the proposition that all men are created equal." But we are not now free. We are not now equal when a Medical Deity in collusion with governmental agencies determines what remedies are available to us. They have for too long held the power of life and death over us. Enough is enough. A grave responsibility rests on our shoulders. Will we stand up and be counted, or remain forever in ignorance and in bondage?

Physicians must be persuaded to revert to their ancient role of educating the public in the ways of health. They must remember their motto— to first do no harm. They must then promote the healing forces within the patient by administering proper nutritional modalities and the least invasive and harmful procedures. The proper role of a physician is to help us become healthier; therefore, their goal should be to take us off medications—to make us less dependent on medication, not more dependant. As Dr. John McDougall stated, a drug-free state is the natural state for the healthy human body. [1] Because physicians are taught next to nothing about nutrition in medical school, they have lost sight of this ancient tradition. We can become their teachers.

Section 4:

FOODS THAT HEAL: ONE WOMAN'S JOURNEY INTO HEALTH

Ladies and gentlemen of the jury, I wish to present to you the testimony of my wife Nancy Jean. Nancy is a good example of how a layperson can teach physicians about the healing power of the body when fortified with good nutrition. She stumbled upon a nutritional cure for advanced gum disease that doctors told her could not be reversed. Here is her story in brief. In August 1995 her father, Bill Adams, passed away after fighting leukemia for six weeks. She was rudely introduced to the grim reaper of souls for the first time in her life. It was up close and personal. She was astonished that modern medical science was unable to do anything to cure this disease. She was rudely introduced to the dark side of modern medicine. Identifying with her father, she felt a helpless victim. But Nancy Jean is a determined fighter. Before long, she was reading everything she could about cancer and alternative forms of treatment. She learned that the dairy products that her father richly consumed were a prime source for the cancer virus. She also discovered that people had successfully beaten the cancer germ through nutritional approaches.

Timidly at first, she took a firm step on the long journey into vibrant health. She began to read widely. Nancy Jean was encouraged by the experience of Dr. Lorraine Day, former chief of orthopedic surgery at San Francisco General Hospital who cured herself of breast cancer. She read of macrobiotic diets and of the necessity of cutting out refined sugar and other refined foods from one's diet. All this new information came too late to be of benefit to her father, but after his death, she decided to go on a liver-cleansing diet as outlined by Dr. Nancy Appleton in her book, *Lick the Sugar Habit.* After several months on a diet that consisted of a variety of beans with brown rice and fresh vegetables, both raw and cooked, and generous servings of fruit, she discovered something that both amazed her and emancipated her from her victim-like dependency on the medical cartel.

Before her father's death in 1995, she had consulted an oral surgeon at the recommendation of her dentist, a friend of the family. She had begun to suffer from gum problems despite an otherwise seemingly normal state of health. The periodontal probing measured the pockets in her gums at eights and nines, and her dentist felt she would require dental surgery. The expert who examined her was of the same opinion, and tentative arrangements were being made for gum surgery when her father's illness intervened and prevented her from going through with the surgery. While grieving for her father, she gave no thought about her need for gum surgery. After several months on the liver-cleansing diet that excluded meat, dairy, and eggs as well as sugar, she went in for a dental cleaning appointment. After examining her gums, her dentist asked in amazement, what did you do to your gums? She replied, why nothing. I have not yet made the surgical appointment with the oral surgeon. He then told her that the pockets in her gums were ones and twos. Her gums had healed themselves!

Nancy Jean then remembered that she was on the liver and colon cleansing diet. A nutritional diet that excluded animal products and refined sugar had provided her body with the nutrients to heal itself. Freed from the impediments of high fat, high protein, and sugar that is typical of the American diet, her immune system had kicked in and restored her health. Dr. Nancy Appleton is right—give the body back the minerals and other nutrients it needs and it will heal itself. [1] Dr. Richard Schulze healed himself and thousands of others using this concept, coupled with a rigorous detoxification and cleansing of the body. [2] Some physicians unacquainted with Nancy Jean to whom she has told her story have responded with incredulity—a sad commentary on the poor nutritional education of the medical profession. But it is a good testimonial to the wisdom of the Creator in carefully selecting the diet for his earthly children.

Ladies and gentlemen of the jury, mark this well, *knowledge is power.* Arm yourselves with the truth about the nutritional needs of your body and you will acquire the power to live a healthier life and enjoy keener mental faculties. One of the great tragedies of the nutritional misinformation we have been fed for decades is the damage that a rich diet of meat, dairy, and sugar has done not only to our bodies, but also to our brains. For example, cheese and other sources of saturated fat causes the red blood cells to clump together, thereby reducing the amount of blood as well as the oxygen and nutrients available to our brains and other vital organs. [3] The result is decreased brainpower, in addition to increased risk of cardiovascular disease. What is harmful to the heart is also harmful to the brain. Dr. Dharma Singh Khalsa, notable brain nutritionist, stated that saturated fat literally rots the brain. [4] In his remarkable book, *Brain Longevity*, Dr. Dharma Singh Khalsa pointed out that because of improper care of our brains, 20% of our brain cells die over the course of our lives. The size of our brains shrivels and brainpower diminishes. He felt that many hard-driving people experience neurological burnout long before they are able to achieve their goals in life. [5] This is a tragedy.

Our bodies are the most wonderful and delicate *living* machinery ever created. Our brains are the most powerful and complex biological computers created. We treat puny, inferior man-made machines with more regard, being careful to follow the operating manual so that they function properly. Yet when it comes to the awesome machinery of our bodies and minds, we wreck them by ignoring or disregarding their operational needs. The good news is that this damage can be repaired with timely intervention. Dr. Khalsa stated that if we eat a low fat, primarily vegetarian diet composed of grains, vegetables, and fruits, with plenty of soy and adequate supplements, we can not only boost our brain power, but our immune system se well. This diet cuts our risk of cancer by at least half, of cardiovascular disease by 70%, and it greatly reduces our risk of other degenerative diseases. [6]

What is good for the body is good for the brain. Proper nutrition is the key. This fact is graphically illustrated by the account of the examination of Albert Einstein's brain. In the mid-1980s Dr. Marian Diamond, renowned brain researcher at the Lawrence Hall of Science at UC Berkeley, dissected Einstein's brain. The decision was made to dissect his brain to help answer an age-old question, are the brains of geniuses physically different from those of average people? [7] What Dr. Marian Diamond discovered is truly remarkable and helps thrown light on the importance of nutrition to every cell and organ of the body. Examination of the superior prefrontal and inferior parietal lobes—the location where abstract reasoning and imagery is processed—revealed that there was no physically discernable difference between Einstein's brain and that of the average person; except for one notable exception—Einstein's brain had significantly more of a certain type of cell in the part of his brain responsible for reasoning, abstract imagery, memory, letter recognition, and calculations. [8]

The type of cell that was more plentiful in Einstein's brain was the glial cell, *a housekeeping* cell. The glial cell is not a *thinking* cell. It is responsible for supporting the metabolism of the *thinking* cell. [9] Although Einstein had the same number and size of thinking cells as the average person, his *thinking* cells had twice as many *housekeeping* cells supplying nutrients to them! [10] Einstein's *thinking* cells needed a lot of nutritional support because of the amount of hard thinking he did. His genius was probably due not only to what he had done with his brain, but also to what nutrients he fed it. Einstein was, wisely, a vegetarian. So also, incidentally, was Sir Isaac Newton, perhaps the most eminent scientist that ever lived. [11]

Ladies and gentlemen of the jury, as you listen to the evidence presented in the course of this trial, exercise the *thinking* cells of your brain and ponder your medical destiny. Throw off the old misconceptions that were forged to enslave and impoverish us. Examine the causes of the popular degenerative diseases and consider how you can best avoid them. If perchance you now suffer from any of these degenerative diseases, consider how you can best reverse them and regain vibrant health. You *must* assume responsibility for your health. It is too precious a commodity to blindly entrust into another's care. A revolution in health care is taking place. Lay people everywhere are emancipating themselves from the profit-making mills of the medical and pharmaceutical cartel. You can join this revolution and recapture your health.

Section 5:

RECAPTURING MEDICAL FREEDOM

Ladies and gentlemen of the jury, we lost medical freedom in a century—1850 to 1950. [1] We have been under medical bondage for all of the twentieth century. The victors—the petrochemical industry and their sycophants in the medical and governmental agencies—wrote the laws that now govern our medical destinies and our legal remedies. And if the history of the Dark Ages throws any light on the future, we may not regain medical freedom for another ten centuries, unless each one of us stands up to be counted. Are you willing to tell the Medical Deity and Pharmaceutical High Priests who now rule over us, enough is enough? Do you have the courage to bring back a verdict of guilty?

Ladies and gentlemen, as you hear, read, and ponder the evidence set forth, ask yourself which branch of medicine better treats and prevents chronic degenerative diseases—symptom oriented Allopathic medicine or nutritional medicine? The testimonial evidence is convincingly clear. Act on your decision. A majority of your peers, John Q. Public, has already returned a verdict—and they are seeking alternative medical remedies in increasing numbers. The choice is yours.

In 1994, Dr. Patrick Quillin wrote in *Beating Cancer with Nutrition:*

If 50% of cancer patients this year will seek alternative cancer care, which is non-reimbursable, imagine the stampede toward alternative cancer treatment if people could choose their own therapies. [2]

Let the stampede come. Our destiny is or should be in our hands. In his enlightening and daring book *World Without Cancer*, G. Edward Griffin

issued the following challenge to every American living in the closing
years of the last century.

> There are more human beings alive right now than the sum total
> of all those born from the beginning of time to the beginning of
> this century ... if we fail to realize that medical freedom is just as
> important as the other freedoms guaranteed by the Bill of Rights;
> then, before this century is over, more human beings will have died
> of cancer than the total of all men who have lived on this earth
> prior to that time. And this will happen in a century during which
> the solution was *known* and written in the scientific record.

> In the days ahead, the controversy over medical freedom will
> intensify. Let it come ...

> It is maddening but it cannot be helped, for the battle is not of our
> choosing. Our only alternatives are to resist or not to resist—to
> fight back with all we have or to surrender and perish. Yes, the
> battle is grim, but the stakes are high. We must not be intimidated
> by the strength of the opposition and, above all, we must not fail.
> Someone has to stand up against the bureaucracy. And we are the
> ones who must do it! [3]

Let us take decisive action to reclaim our God-given freedom from the
pharmaceutical and industrial tyrants who now rule over us and corrupt
our medicine. We can topple the bureaucratic edifice and medical establishment that now dominates our healthcare options by voting with our
feet and our pocket books.

Ladies and gentlemen, you are not alone in this fight. It may be that you
have now become a majority fighting against the Goliath of established
medicine. Harris Coulter asserted that for the first time in the history
of modern medicine, the number of patients seeking alternative, natural
medical care outstripped those seeking conventional medical remedies; he
stated that in 1990 there were 425 million medical visits to alternative
practitioners, as opposed to 388 million visits to conventional drug-based
medicine. [4]

Of course, the medical establishment and their allies still hold the medical reigns. They possess all the power of big government and the wealth of their industrial allies—the petro-chemical industry, the fast-food industry, and the dairy and meat industries. They have the power to saturate the media and public opinion with disinformation. Serious matters are being weighed in the balance. The health and economic soundness of our country is at stake. Regardless of the numbers, you are in a majority. Anyone who stands with the Creator of the natural laws that government our health and well-being *is* in a majority, regardless of how popular the false medical therapeutics appears to be. If it is any additional comfort to you, know that when you stand with the great Hippocrates who taught that diet should be the first and foremost means of preventing and treating diseases, [5] you are in good company and on the right side of true medicine.

Finally, ladies and gentlemen of the jury, as you consider the merits of drug therapy as compared and contrasted with the benefits of nutritional modalities in the treatment of selected chronic degenerative diseases, remember that the testimony you will hear is not intended to constitute the practice of medicine. This trial transcript is not a medical treatise. It is an indictment of modern conventional medicine. You are required as a vast national jury to judge between two historically competing therapeutics in the treatment of chronic degenerative disease. These two medical approaches are based upon polar opposite concepts of science. In rationalistic science, which seeks to enslave you and make you dependent upon the whim and authority of an elite, opinion rules. In empirical science, which seeks to liberate you and empower you, facts are king. It is the great leveler and liberates you from the dominance of the elite. The evidence is overwhelming. The choice is yours.

The testimony you will hear during this trial should not be construed as medical advice for the treatment of any one specific illness. Whether you chose to consult an Allopathic doctor who uses drugs or a nutritional doctor who uses nutrition is a decision you have to make for yourself. The trial testimony is not designed for application to any one patient's condition. That should be reserved for consultation with a physician of your choice.

This trial is designed to present to you the expert testimony of nutritional physicians at the cutting edge of modern medical science. In one sense this is a battle between competing experts; it reflects the civil war raging within the medical profession. In another sense, it is not. You, the jury and members of the public as the sole judges of the facts, have the right and power to judge the experts. You are invited to draw your own conclusions, and after examining the evidence, render a judgment for or against indictment on the commonsense of the matter.

Ladies and gentlemen of the jury, America now stands at a crossroads. And you, ladies and gentlemen of the jury, have the *power* to alter its course—but only if you have the *will* and the *courage* to do so. If you, the jury, cannot discern the truth, what hope is there for justice? Or for the recovery of medical freedom in America? Ponder these words as you hear the evidence.

THE EVIDENCE

Arthritis

A Nutritional and Metabolic Disease

Section 1

WHY AFRICANS DON'T GET ARTHRITIS

Ladies and gentlemen of the jury, the first chronic degenerative disease you will consider today is arthritis. In referencing their published works, you will hear from a number of experts in the field.

Did you know that Arthritis is rare among Africans? Yet millions of Americans live with this crippling degenerative disease. Did you know that there is a cure for arthritis? That it is but a nutritional and metabolic disease. In conventional medical circles, these are un-welcomed comments. Two much money is riding on the hope that arthritis is incurable. Millions of suffering Americans are condemned to a lifetime of drugs and finally to surgery when their major joints completely collapse and must be replaced with artificial ones. Official medicine and the Arthritis Foundation assure us that there is no cure for arthritis. [1] The typical doctor will put you on pain medication, and then tell you that there is nothing more he can do for you. [2] The Arthritis Foundation publishes and distributes a pamphlet entitled, *The Truth about Diet & Arthritis*. This paper unabashedly states in bold print:

> There is *no* special diet for arthritis. No specific food has anything to do with causing it. No specific diet will cure it. [3]

Now ladies and gentlemen, many of the nutritional physicians whose evidence will be presented to you consider this statement a result of either gross ignorance or cunning deception. The only ones who gain from such a position are the drug companies and the physicians who treat their patients for the duration of their pain-wrecked lifetimes. Drug companies take in billions by selling the victim arthritic medication to manage the symptoms of this crippling disease. Because of the colossal amounts of money spent in suppressing the symptoms of arthritis, this degenerative disease provides a good test case for exploring the general merits of treating symptoms versus removing the underlying causes of the diseases and so curing the patient.

What exactly is arthritis? Arthritis is a general term used to describe the signs and symptoms of inflammation and pain in any joint of the body. It is characterized by pain, swelling, redness, or stiffness in the joints, which can become deformed. [4] Although it is not a big killer like heart disease, arthritis is the most crippling and agonizing of all degenerative diseases, causing more pain and suffering to more people than any other single disease. [5] There are many forms of arthritis. Osteoarthritis (involving the bones and joints) and rheumatoid arthritis are the most common forms of the disease. Gout or arthritis of the big toe is also often seen. About 50 million Americans have osteoarthritis and about 2 million suffer from rheumatoid arthritis. [6]

Most people think of joint pain when arthritis is mentioned. But joint pain is only a part of a much larger problem. Arthritis is merely one symptom or manifestation of a disease process that is crippling other tissues and organs of the body. [7] Like other degenerative diseases, arthritis is the result of a metabolic disorder or dysfunction caused by ingesting excessive amounts of certain nutrients such as proteins, fats, and cholesterol. [8] In her fascinating book *Lick the Sugar Habit*, Dr. Nancy Appleton argued that mineral imbalances due to the ingestion of refined sugar can also lead to arthritis by leaving the body helpless against the development of allergy induced immune complexes that cause tissue damage and inflammation.

In simple language, we are eating certain foods and nutrients in the wrong proportions, and they are upsetting the chemical balance of our bodies and disease is the result. This is a sad state of affairs. By our eating habits, we are bringing disease upon ourselves. We are digging our graves with our spoons. We are not helpless victims of strange diseases; we are victimizing ourselves. We eat for momentary pleasure and not for nutrition. This is not rational. We do not behave this way in other aspects of life. We treat our pets far better than we treat our bodies.

The human body is the most sophisticated mechanism ever created. It operates on delicate chemical balances. It needs to be fueled and maintained like any other machinery and more so. Food is just the Creator's way of providing us with pleasure while supplying the machinery of the human frame with the chemical supplies it needs for proper operation. We do not put junk fuel or incorrect portions of gas and oil into our automobiles, because we know they will dysfunction. So why should it be any different with our bodies? Therefore, to avoid dysfunction and disease we need to pay attention to how we gas up our bodies.

Now when our automobiles malfunction, we do not treat the symptoms. We get to the root of the problem. When we run out of oil, a warning light comes on. The warning light is not the problem. By analogy it is the symptom of a deeper problem—the lack of oil. If we ignore the red light *symptom*, we ruin our engines. If we suppress the red light *symptom* by cutting the wire or removing the bulb, we may get rid of the symptom, but the underlying problem of insufficient oil in the engine is still there and if we continue to run the automobile, we will ruin the engine.

In much the same way, the arthritic signal of pain in the joints is merely a symptom of a deeper problem. We may suppress the pain symptom by taking pain medication that will not cure the problem. The pain medication merely gives us a false sense of well being while we continue to run the engines of our bodies until the joints wear out, making our doctors rich by performing knee or hip joint replacements. Nutritional doctors are emphatic that arthritic drugs merely cover up the symptoms while the disease rages on underneath. [9] In this sense, drug medicine is the big *cover-up* of the true causes of chronic degenerative diseases.

What are the facts about arthritis and can nutritional therapy reverse it? We will first examine in greater depth the causes of arthritis, then armed with this knowledge we will explore ways of eliminating the causes, thus curing the disease. We can approach this task with confidence for the truth is that there are entire societies and cultures that are almost entirely free from this crippling and most painful disease. In parts of Africa, hardworking people are essentially free from osteoarthritis, even though they carry heavy loads and do hard work every day. [10] The major difference between Western cultures and these hardy Africans is in their respective diets. By diet, we refer to the types and portions of foods we eat on a daily basis. Those Africans not yet converted to the Western way of eating consume a low-fat, low-cholesterol, low-protein, starch-based diet. Animal products are eaten very little, if at all. Consequently, Dr. John McDougall stated, arthritis and its companion disease osteoporosis are rarely seen in Africans not on the Western diet. [11]

Gout is a form of arthritis that can provide us with a clear understanding of the cause and effect relationship between a chemical imbalance in our bodies and the development of arthritis. From our foods, we obtain carbohydrates, fats, proteins, calcium, phosphorus, and other trace minerals and vitamins that provide nourishment for our bones and joints. These nutrients are generally found in the right health-generating proportions in natural foods such as fruits, vegetables, greens and grains. When the protein and purine elements in our food are increased to an excessive level, gouty arthritis can develop. [12]

Purines are nitrogenous compounds. They are part of the building blocks of DNA and RNA. Animal products such as shellfish, fish, fowl, and red meat are rich in proteins and purines. When these concentrated sources of protein are eaten along with other plant-based foods, which contain all the protein we need, the result is an excess of protein ingested. Protein cannot be stored in the body like fats or carbohydrates. The excess is broken down and discarded by the body. The liver breaks down purines and proteins into uric acid and other acidic by-products. The amount of protein in the diet directly affects how much uric acid is produced. [13]

When uric acid levels in the blood become excessive, the uric acid crystallizes out into the tissue in the form of tiny needle-like crystals. When these are deposited in the joints, they cause the sudden and severe pain, redness, and swelling we recognize as gout. [14] The big toe is usually the unfortunate recipient of this form of gouty arthritis. Sometimes when an overweight person losses weight too rapidly, the uric acid stored in the body tissues may pass out of the tissues in such quantity that some of it is deposited in the joints, precipitating the attack of gout. Doctors utilize a variety of medications to lower the uric levels in the body and relieve the condition. [15]

Osteoarthritis is the most common form of arthritis. Today over 50 million Americans are afflicted with this preventable and curable disease. [16] By the age of thirty, as much as 35% of Americans get osteoarthritis in their knees. By age seventy, an amazing 85% of Americans are afflicted with arthritis. [17] How is osteoarthritis caused? Osteoarthritis literally means *bone joint inflammation*—bone from the Greek *osteo*, joint from *arthro*, and inflammation from *itis*. In reality, it is joint pain, as inflammation is rarely seen with osteoarthritis. It involves the degeneration of the cartilage at the end of the joint. But the subchondral bone to which the cartilage is attached, as well as the capsules that surround the joint and the muscles adjacent to the joint, may all be affected. [18]

Ladies and gentlemen of the jury, conventional doctors often relate this disease to the excessive wear and tear of joints. They note that people engaged in repetitive labor or hard physical labor like carpenters, tailors, and woodcutters often complain of osteoarthritis in their joints. Obese people often abuse the joints of the knee and ankle as well as the hips and vertebrae. Although the excessive exercise engaged in by football players, joggers, and tennis players can injure joints and precipitate osteoarthritis, wear and tear is not a sufficient or sole explanation for this disease. Dr. John McDougall argued persuasively that the fact that hard working people in Africa, who primarily eat a plant-based diet, do not seem to come down with osteoarthritis, suggests that there is a nutritional connection to the disease. [19]

Dr. Jason Theodosakis cited three well-used misconceptions about osteoarthritis:

1. That it is a normal part of aging.

2. That it is a wear and tear disease.

3. And that nothing can be done about it. [20]

Dr. Theodosakis contended that osteoarthritis is not inevitable. He found that the examination of aged joints and arthritic joints reveals a vast difference. While aged joints show some bone loss in the non-weight bearing areas of the joint, they show little or no destruction of the cartilage. Arthritic joints reveal extensive erosion of the weight bearing areas of the joint, as well as extensive destruction of the cartilage. [21] Dr. Theodosakis also pointed out that primary arthritis is not caused by the wear and tear of the body due to strenuous exercise. Rather the opposite is true. Scientific studies demonstrate that vigorous exercise actually *increases* the functional status of people with osteoarthritis. [22] Nutritional minded doctors such as Jason Theodosakis, John McDougall, and Paavo Airola all affirm that there is a nutritional cure for arthritis despite the claims of official medicine.

The evidence shows that arthritis is caused by an improper diet and that it can be reversed by a well-balanced diet. Osteoarthritis is facilitated by the osteoporosis of the bones at the joints, and there is a well-established connection between high-protein intake and calcium loss from the bones, which gives rise to osteoporosis. Osteoporosis literally means porous bones. The connection between osteoarthritis and osteoporosis cannot be seriously disputed. Osteoporosis weakens the bones around the joint and leads to tiny fissures or fractures. Osteoarthritic joints show these tiny fractures when closely examined. The body's attempt to heal these fractures is interfered with by the ongoing process of osteoporosis and physical abuse of the joints. The result is degeneration of the cartilage, which we call osteoarthritis. [23]

Ladies and gentlemen of the jury, the role of saturated fat and cholesterol in the development of arthritis is significant. Anything that interferes with the supply of blood and nutrients to the bone underlying the cartilage surfaces can also contribute to the weakening and degeneration of the cartilage. The blood vessels that supply the bone are very small, and they can be damaged by cholesterol in the blood stream. This impairs the circulation of blood to the bone. Excessive fat in the blood stream can cause sludging of the blood, which consequently carries less oxygen and nutrients to the tissues, including the bone. The sludging may be so severe that blood cannot efficiently pass though these small capillaries to get to the bone underlying the cartilage. The result is degeneration of the cartilage and the manifestation of osteoarthritis. [24] Thus, it is not so much the excessive wear on the joints that give rise to arthritis but the inability of bony joints, weakened by osteoporosis and undernourished by lack of oxygen and nutrients, to sustain the stress placed on them.

When the metabolic dysfunctions from excessive protein and cholesterol weaken the bone and cartilage, the physical use or abuse of the joints produces what is known as primary and secondary arthritis. In primary arthritis, there is a slow, progressive deterioration of the weight-bearing joints of the knees and hips and often of the lower back, neck, and fingers. This primary arthritis usually manifests after age forty-five. [25]

Dr. Theodosakis stated that the famous Framingham Heart Study also investigated the origin of osteoarthritis and not just the causes of heart disease. That study demonstrated a conclusive link between obesity and osteoarthritis, the disease appearing less frequently among slim people under the same cultural setting. [26] The weight-bearing joints of the body can experience loads of between two and ten times a person's weight. Hence, if you are 200 pounds, your knee joints can experience a ton of pressure as you walk; and considerably more if you run. [27]

Secondary arthritis is different from primary arthritis. It appears before age forty and can be caused by a variety of factors: trauma, injury, joint infection, joint surgery, and metabolic imbalances. [28] Trauma is the main culprit. It can be acute, as from a sudden accident or injury, or the trauma can be chronic or repetitive such as created by the repeated use of the arm by a baseball pitcher. Over time, these repeated motions damage the cartilage and adjacent bone, and the result is osteoarthritis. [29]

Ladies and gentlemen of the jury, while rheumatoid arthritis afflicts over two million Americans it is rare in societies that consume a mostly plant-based diet. [30] This form of arthritis is really a species of immune disorder. [31] Again, high fat and cholesterol play a major role in precipitating this immune disorder. The improper nutrition that initiates the metabolic disorder causes the body's elaborate immune defense mechanism to break down as the body tries to deal with the high fat and cholesterol levels in the blood. Here is how it works. When antigens—such as bacteria, viruses, or certain food proteins—invade the body, the immune system produces antibodies that attack and neutralize the invading antigens. Piles of dead antibody-antigen complexes collect in the blood vessels at the site of the invasion. [32] Normally, the body's scavenger cells engulf these complexes and clear them from the blood stream. However, when there is excessive fat and cholesterol in the blood, this part of the immune function is impaired and these antibody-antigen complexes accumulate in the blood vessels causing inflammation. When these complexes are deposited in the joints, pain, swelling, redness, and stiffness are the results. We call this process rheumatoid arthritis, and it can result in the destruction of the joints and permanent deformity. [33]

These antibody-antigen complexes can also form in the joint tissues that are injured by inadequate supplies of oxygen and nutrients to the joint tissues. [34] Fats and cholesterol can degrade the blood vessels by initiating the process of arteriosclerosis in which the blood vessels are first narrowed by deposits of fats and cholesterol. These fatty deposits impair the circulation of blood to the tiny capillaries that feed the joint tissues, thus causing them to become inflamed. This inflammation process contributes to the formation of antibody-antigen complexes in the joints. [35] While a variety of antigens can give rise to the antibody-antigen complexes, certain foods are implicated in the frequent occurrence of this condition. Dairy foods are the most frequent source of the dietary antigens that cause a variety of food allergies. [36] Eggs and beef are a close second and third cause of the formation of antibody-antigen complexes. Investigators at Wayne State University Medical School observed that dietary fats in the amounts normally eaten in the American diet caused inflammatory joint changes seen in rheumatoid arthritis. [37] Some people can also be allergic to wheat, corn, and other common foods that can create the antibody-antigen complexes. Excess refined sugar can cause food allergies, which then become the triggering cause for the buildup of antibody-antigen complexes. [38]

Lupus erythematosus is another serious form of arthritis that is caused by the antibody-antigen immune dysfunction. It mostly affects women. [39] Proteins from beef and dairy products have been found in the blood of patients with lupus and are thus thought to be a causative factor in creating the disease. [40]

Ankylosing spondylitis is a form of arthritis that has characteristics similar to rheumatoid arthritis and is generally restricted to the hips and backbone. [41] The antibody-antigen complexes often move into the skin, lungs, brain, and kidneys where they cause similar damage to these tissues. [42] Psoriasis is a skin disease. But patients with psoriasis often experience joint pain and deformation. Psoriatic arthritis can be caused by a high-fat diet. [43]

Ladies and gentlemen of the jury, the evidence is clear that a poor diet, consisting mainly of saturated fat, cholesterol, and refined foods and sugars, is the primary factor in causing arthritis. This fact should provide the physician with a good clue about the appropriate remedy. Yet the astonishing fact is that the doctors practicing conventional Allopathic medicine virtually ignore the part that diet plays in the development of this chronic degenerative disease. And what is even more inexcusable, they grossly fail to educate their patients on how to prevent the onset of this avoidable disease.

Ladies and gentlemen of the jury, now that you have a working knowledge of what arthritis is and its primary causes, you can judge for yourselves, which is the best and proper treatment for this chronic degenerative disease. The next two sections compares and contrasts the ineffectual pharmaceutical remedies with the nutritional healing of arthritis.

Section 2

DRUG THERAPY: A FALSE HOPE FOR THE ARTHRITIC

Ladies and gentlemen of the jury, now that we have some idea as to the cause of arthritis, let us now consider what is or should be the proper course of treatment. There have been two general approaches—that of conventional medicine, which only suppresses the symptoms of the disease, and that of nutritional medicine, which seeks to eliminate the underlying causes of the disease. In this section, we shall consider the pharmaceutical remedies of conventional medicine.

A few decades ago, Dr. Paavo Airola, N.D., that the average practitioner of orthodox medicine did not have a clear understanding of the basic cause and effect relationship between diet and arthritis. Their treatments and remedies are therefore understandably based on symptom management in which the isolated symptoms of the disease and not the disease itself are being treated. [1] He stated that injections and oral medications are used to suppress the superficial symptoms of a deeper metabolic disorder. The result is that these drugs cause more damage to the system and aggravate the condition instead of improving it. [2] Moreover, the side effects of these drugs can ruin your health permanently. The hapless patient therefore sustains a twofold insult to their system: the original disease is worsened by drugs and the side effects of the drugs cause them additional harm.

It is a sad fact that each year thousands of people die from the adverse effects of both the anti-inflammatory and steroid drugs used in the treatment (or rather the symptom management) of arthritis. [3] Yet most arthritis-related research dollars are spent on testing high-profit drug therapies. [4] The justification for this, Dr. John McDougall stated, is that the medical profession views arthritis as an inherited disease for which diet can do nothing. For example in the case of gouty arthritis, the Arthritis Foundation stated:

Gout is a special kind of arthritis, caused by an inherited defect in body chemistry, not by high living. [5]

Ladies and gentlemen of the jury, this faulty presumption not only *blinds* the physician to the obvious cause and effect relationship between dietary habits and arthritis, it *guarantees* that the wrong remedy will be applied. For example, when you develop high levels of uric acid in your blood from eating too much of protein-rich foods, the response of the medical profession is to prescribe drug therapies to reduce the levels of uric acid. This is an expensive and harmful method of addressing the problem. The more inexpensive and commonsense approach would be to reduce the amount of protein consumed at mealtime. Unfortunately, conventional medicine, being controlled by the pharmaceutical industry, will not point you to the simple and inexpensive way of avoiding the buildup of uric acid in your body because it cuts into their bottom line. But their profits are made at the patient's expense, for all drugs have side effects, and gout medication is no exception. In 1981, Dr. W. Duffy did a risk/benefit analysis of medication to lower uric acid levels in the blood. His conclusion was that people were better off not taking medications to lower uric acid levels because the side effects of the drugs prescribed can be serious. [6]

Aspirin is perhaps the simplest, cheapest, and most common remedy used by millions of arthritic suffers. It belongs to a class of drugs called salicylates that were first derived from the bark of the willow tree. [7] Aspirin's chemical name is acetylsalicylic acid, and it has been used for over a hundred years to treat arthritic symptoms. It is readily available over the counter, and it appears to relieve pain without creating any additional problems. In 1968, Americans used 18 million pounds of aspirin a year, that is 15 tons a day, most of which was probably for arthritic pain. [8]

But is aspirin harmless? Not really. There used to be general agreement among medical practitioners that aspirin is a toxic chemical that can cause poisoning and damage to the brain, liver, and kidneys. [9] This information is now either suppressed or conveniently ignored. With prolonged use, acetylsalicylic acid can depress the immune system and undermine the body's healing powers. [10] It is suspected that aspirin's negative effect on the immune system is due in part to the fact that aspirin is a vitamin antagonist and destroys large amounts of vitamin C in the tissues. [11]

Today we hear a lot about how aspirin helps to prevent heart attacks by thinning the blood. But this very virtue can be a risk factor: it enhances a tendency to bleed. As early as 1911, *The Journal of American Medical Association* reported that even small doses of aspirin can cause cardiac weakness with excessive pulse rate, edematous swelling of the mucus membranes, irregular pulse, and albumin in the urine. [12] In some individuals, aspirin can also precipitate delirium, restlessness, confusion, and a state of incoherency. [13]

Aspirin may not be as user friendly as everyone makes out. The potential hidden harm it can do outweighs the only real benefit it provides to the arthritic patient: it masks the symptoms of the disease while leaving the underlying disease to become progressively chronic, moving the patient toward crippling disability in their old age. One of the suggestions coming out of a Workshop on Prevention of Disability from Arthritis, which was convened by a former Surgeon General of the United States, was that the medical profession and drug companies should attempt to curtail the advertising claims of salicylate derivatives so commonly heard on radio and television. [14] There are other salicylate derivatives beside aspirin (Bayer or Bufferin) that are commonly used to mask the symptoms of pain and to reduce the inflammatory process in arthritis. The most common are: Choline magnesium tri-salicylate (Trilisate), Diflunisal (Dolobid), Magnesium salicylate (Magan), and Salicylsalicylic acid (Disalcid or Mono-Gesic). Dr. Theodosakis provided us with a list of many of the more modern drugs, along with their serious side effects, that are used to treat arthritis. I've detailed some of the most popular below.

Phenylbutazone, which was first marketed in 1952, and Oxyphenbutazone, which came out in 1961. Their use has since been restricted due to their tendencies to cause two fatal blood diseases: agranulocytosis and aplastic anemia. These arthritic drugs are suspected of causing a lupus-like disease; they also promote water retention and rapid weight gain. [15]

Indomethacin (Indocin) is generally used to relieve hip pain and bursitis of the shoulder. Its side effects include peptic ulcers, gastrointestinal upset, severe headaches, dizziness, rashes, ringing in the ears, and depression. [16]

Ibuprofen is a favorite of many rheumatoid arthritis sufferers, as well as those suffering with osteoarthritis. The side effects of Ibuprofen include gastrointestinal problems, nausea, vomiting, dizziness, and skin rash. Fenoprophen calcium is similar to Ibuprofen and Naproxen in its chemical makeup, and has similar side effects to those listed for Ibuprofen. [17]

Tolmetin sodium is used to treat rheumatoid arthritis, but it has the unpleasant side effect of promoting kidney failure. Likewise, Meclofenamate sodium is effective with rheumatoid arthritis as well as acute and chronic osteoarthritis, but can produce severe nausea, diarrhea, and stomach pain. [18]

Piroxicam has been successful in treating osteoarthritis, rheumatoid arthritis, gout, and ankylosing spondylitis but at the expense of gastrointestinal distress and sun rash. [19]

Ladies and gentlemen of the jury, the problem with these drugs, as with the salicylates, is of course that they do not cure the underlying metabolic problem of arthritis. While they may relieve pain, swelling, and inflammation, they do so at the cost of varying degrees of insults to the body due to their side effects. [20]

Cortisone was at one time hailed as the panacea for arthritic suffers. When introduced in the 1950s, it was considered a milestone achievement by medical science. Claims were made that it would conquer arthritis. But as is common, not too many years later this miracle drug was suspected to be a *remedy worse than the disease* when the dangerous side effects of the drug become apparent. [21] Cortisone is a hormone secreted by the adrenal glands. Like other related hormones such as prednisone and prednisolone, it can be manufactured synthetically.

What is the rationale behind the use of cortisone? Medical research revealed that the dysfunction of the cortisone-producing adrenal glands contributed to the development of arthritis, so medical scientists introduced cortisone into the system in an attempt to correct the results of this glandular dysfunction. [22] But this attempt was merely trying to fix one symptom of a general metabolic problem. As usual, no one bothered to determine why the cortisone-producing adrenal glands were dysfunctioning. Artificially introducing cortisone into the human body proved a mixed blessing. The side effects of cortisone are truly scary. It can damage the liver, kidneys, the blood, the nerves, and the bones, as well as other vital organs of the body. [23]

Dr. Airola provided a partial list of the side effects of cortisone: peptic ulcers, osteoporosis with spontaneous fractures, mental disturbances, psychosis, neuropathy or degeneration of the nerves, posterior sub-capsular cataracts, diabetes, hypertension, disturbance in the metabolism and utilization of protein and fats, acne, and excessive hair growth in women. [24] These serious and potentially lethal side effects are unexplainably *acceptable* to the FDA while that regulatory body *strains* to find phantom dangers lurking in the use of nutritional modalities in the treatment of chronic degenerative diseases.

Perhaps the most serious aspect of cortisone therapy is its tendency to destroy the body's own healing mechanisms. [25] It disturbs the entire biochemical stability of the arthritic patient. It can cause the adrenal glands to atrophy. It can also cause the tissues of the joints to deteriorate. [26] Corticosteroids can wreck havoc on the body's nutrient status. They are known to decrease absorption of vitamin D and to increase excretion of zinc, potassium, and vitamin C. [27] Thus, like other pharmaceutical medicines, corticosteroids are a mixed blessing. They are sometimes necessary but can be a real threat to the health of the body by degrading its nutrient status.

And what does the patient get for all these serious side effects? Momentary freedom from arthritic pain and discomfort during the short period of time that the arthritic symptoms are suppressed by the drug. That is all. However, when the effect of the drug wears off, the patient feels worse than ever. The patient can also become addicted to cortisone and experience painful withdrawal symptoms. [28]

Although animal fats are implicated in the cause of osteoarthritis and rheumatoid arthritis, one fat does seem to relieve the condition of rheumatoid arthritis. A ploy-unsaturated fat found in marine fish called eicosapentaenoic acid (or EPA), has been shown to reduce the inflammation when taken in drug-level doses. It does this by decreasing the production of prostaglandin hormones and by suppressing the activity of the white blood cells that are part of the inflammatory process. [29] Fish oil capsules are good sources of this fat. But using EPA does not remove the cause of the arthritis, and because of the high fat content, fish oil may contribute to obesity and may increase the risk of gall bladder disease and certain types of cancer. [30] Using food substances as *silver-bullets* to target individual symptoms is not a solution in treating metabolic diseases.

Gold injections were once popularized as one of the most effective remedies for arthritis. It has never been clear how they work to suppress

the symptoms of arthritis. They are, however, highly toxic and may produce many diseases and complications. Liver and kidney damage can be
experienced by using gold injections. [31] Dr. Max Warmbrand, N.D.,
D.O., listed some other serious side effects of gold injections in *The
Encyclopedia of Natural Health*, which include stomach disorders, deafness,
anemia, hemorrhages under the skin, neuritis, headache, eye impairments,
and ulcerations of the mouth and gums. [32] Does a risk/benefit analysis
justify the use of gold injections? The conclusion is obvious, but you will
be the judge at the end of this trial.

Ladies and gentlemen of the jury, the pharmaceutical industry constantly produce new drugs in their search for a miracle cure for arthritis.
Powerful drugs like D-penicillamine, corticosteroid, and cancer chemotherapy agents have been tried. But all such drugs will only provide temporary relief, because drugs do not go to the bottom of the problem. Dr.
John McDougall considers drug therapy at this level of toxicity to be far
from ideal because they provide only temporary relief, while not eliminating the disease. [33] The drugs do not reverse the causes of arthritis; they
merely suppress the symptoms of the disease. Ladies and gentlemen, it
is unconscionable to practice medicine in this fashion. It offers only the
illusion of well-being to the patient. The patient's health is sacrificed on
the altar of mammon. A day of reckoning will come. Because arthritis
is a metabolic disorder, effective treatment must aim at restoring proper
metabolic functioning of the body. This is where nutritional therapy plays
a vital role.

Section 3

REVERSING ARTHRITIS WITH NUTRITION

Ladies and gentlemen of the jury, the link between improper nutrition and arthritis has been clearly established by expert testimony for all those who care to consider the evidence. It is the excessive use of refined white sugar, as well as the excessive intake of saturated fats and proteins so readily available in animal products, that are the primary contributing factors. Together they orchestrate the metabolic dysfunction that gives rise to the symptoms of arthritic pain and discomfort. This relationship has been admitted by some candid members of the medical profession. [1] For example since the eighteenth century it has been common knowledge that the rich foods of the affluent classes played a causative role in the development of gout. While some doctors have recognized this, many still adhere to the idea that heredity is the primary, if not sole, cause of gout. [2]

Although heredity is a factor, it is not the ultimate cause. The harmful effects of the improper diets of our ancestors can of course be passed on to us. It is well recognized that metabolic rates differ among individuals. Some people convert purine into uric acid faster than others and eliminate them from the body slower than others, thus predisposing them to the development of gouty arthritis. [3] But Dr. John McDougall rightly pointed out that Filipinos who excrete uric acid slower than other ethnic groups do not develop arthritis when they maintain their native diet of low-protein, low-purine, and starch-based diets. Filipinos who follow a Western diet develop this metabolic disorder. [4] Dr. John McDougall emphatically stated that gout is easily stopped if you eat foods that are low in purines and proteins. [5] He advised that in most cases the medication to lower uric acid levels can be abruptly stopped once the patient starts a low purine, low protein diet. In serious cases of the disease, the medication may be continued on a decreasing basis after the diet has been commenced. The patient should periodically check their uric acid levels to make sure they are being maintained at low levels. As the patient recovers, checks can be done on a monthly basis, then annually, to monitor their uric acid levels. [6]

In the case of osteoarthritis, some conventional doctors have reached the conclusion that this disease can also be arrested and even reversed. This finding was the subject of an article by Dr. J. Bland in the *American Journal of Medicine* in 1983 entitled *The Reversibility of Osteoarthritis: A Review*. [7] Thus Dr. McDougall has advocated a low-protein, low-fat, no-cholesterol diet along with rest of the joints from vigorous activity as the best approach to achieving a reversal of the osteoarthritic condition. [8]

It has also been demonstrated that rheumatoid arthritis can be reversed by diet. Researchers at Wayne State University Medical School fed a select group of patients a fat-free diet and obtained complete remission of rheumatoid arthritis within seven weeks. [9] The link between diet and rheumatoid arthritis was reinforced by the observation that the symptoms recurred within seventy-two hours of the patients returning to a high fat diet. Implicated were chicken, beef, cheese, coconut oil, and safflower oil. [10] Dr. McDougall's recommended diet for treating and preventing arthritic disease is:

1. 5 to 10 % of calories from fats

2. 5 to 10% of calories from protein.

3. Majority of calories from starches, vegetables, and fruits.

4. Restriction of foods high in protein such as legumes: beans, peas, and lentils.

5. Restriction of foods high in fat such as avocados, nuts, seeds, olives, soybean products, and vegetable oils.

6. Avoiding foods with food additives. [11]

A low-fat, animal-product free diet has been shown to improve lupus ery-thematosus. [12] Dr. McDougall also recommended an *elimination diet* to discover foods that one is allergic to and that can cause rheumatoid arthritis. The *elimination diet* begins by eating those foods that people are least allergic to for one to three weeks. This diet typically consists of a starch-based diet centered on foods such as sweet potatoes, brown rice, winter squashes, and taro. One can add one's favorite green and yellow vegetables and cooked non-citrus fruits. If the arthritic pains decrease, then it is safe to conclude that one or more foods in your regular diet are causing allergic reactions. [13] Next, one adds every two days one new food to this basic diet, eating considerable more of this added food item to see if an allergic reaction occurs. When such symptoms as headache, muscle pains, and fatigue reoccur, you can then identify the food that gave rise to these allergic reactions. [14]

An alternative form of the *elimination diet* is to simply cease consuming all animal products, especially dairy and eggs. [15] Impressive studies exist to support this sensible but seemingly radical approach. In 1981, the *British Medical Journal* reported a dramatic improvement in arthritis by the elimination of *all* dairy products from a patient's diet. [16] The strong link between dairy products and arthritis is because the protein molecule found in cow's milk can readily pass through the intestinal wall and initiate the antibody-antigen complex inflammatory process, which starts the arthritic process. [17]

Ladies and gentlemen of the jury, in addition to a proper nutritional diet other modalities assist in preventing and reversing of arthritis. In the case of osteoarthritis, Dr. Jason Theodosakis stated that researchers in the famous Framingham Heart Study found that obese middle-aged women could greatly reduce their risk of developing osteoarthritis by simply losing weight. [18], [19] There are also nutritional supplements that can be purchased over the counter that can help rebuild the damaged cartilage in osteoarthritis. Dr. Jason Theodosakis stated that doctors in Europe have been using glucosamine sulfate in conjunction with chondroitin sulfates with remarkable success to rebuild the degraded cartilage of people suffering from osteoarthritis. [20] The bodies of people with this form of arthritis do not produce proteoglycans and collagen fast enough to repair the damage to the cartilage. Proteoglycans and collagen are the building blocks of cartilage. Additionally the body's dysfunction may cause carti-lage-destroying enzymes to degrade the cartilage. Working together, glu-cosamine and chondroitin sulfates stimulate the synthesis of new cartilage while at the same time keeping the destructive enzymes under control. [21]

Some physicians feel that damage to cartilage tissue by free radicals may contribute to osteoarthritis. Free radicals are unstable molecules with either insufficient electrons or additional electrons. These unstable mol-ecules either steal or add electrons to the molecules of the body's tissue, thereby inflicting tissue damage. The antioxidant vitamins and minerals combat free radical activity and prevent tissue damage. Antioxidants are therefore important in preventing and treating osteoarthritis. [22]

The important antioxidants are beta-carotene (precursor to vitamin A), vitamin C, vitamin E, and Selenium. These antioxidants act synergis-tically, assisting each other metabolically. The best sources of these anti-oxidants are natural foods, especially greens. However, soil depletion may require supplementation. [23] Dr. Jason Theodosakis recommended the following dosages of these vital antioxidants in treating and preventing arthritis:

Vitamin A . . . . .5,000 IU
Vitamin C . . . . 500 to 4,000 mg.
Vitamin E. . . . . 100 to 400 IU
Selenium. . . . . 55 to 200 mcg

Bioflavonoids are another group of nutrients important for the arthritic patient. They are found in virtually all foods and are essential for build-ing and maintaining healthy capillary walls and connective tissue. [24] They also assist in the metabolism of vitamin C. They can help in treating osteoarthritis by reinforcing the ability of collagen to form strong matrix. Bioflavonoids also prevent collagen from being destroyed by the inflam-mation process, prevent free-radical damage, and slow down the inflam-mation process. [25]

Boron is another nutrient that has been linked to the prevention of osteoarthritis. It helps maintain healthy joints and suppresses free radical activity. [26] Osteoarthritis is more prevalent in geographic areas where boron intake is low and less prevalent in areas where boron intake is high. 3 mg daily is recommended. [27]

Dr. Jason Theodosakis recommended the use of other antioxidants such as pycnogenol at 30 to 100 mg; curcumin at 100 to 500 mg; garlic at 100 to 500 mg; cysteine at 250 to 1,000 mg; and coenzyme Q10 at 10 to 100 mg. [28] Dr. Jason Theodosakis' recommendations for preventing arthritis are simple, sensible and can be followed by most everyone.

1. Eat a healthful, joint-building diet.

2. Maintain your ideal weight.

3. Exercise regularly.

4. Prevent injuries.

5. Ensure proper recovery if you are injured.

6. Optimize your biomechanics to counteract stress to your joints.

7. Consider the use of glucosamine and chondroitin sulfates prophylactically.

Ladies and gentlemen of the jury, let us consider in closing, testimony relating to the importance of exercise in the treatment and prevention of arthritis. For a long time conventional doctors believed that exercise either caused or aggravated osteoarthritis. And hence, they advised against it. In this case, they were dead wrong to the detriment of their patients. Today we know that exercise is one of the best medicines for osteoarthritis. [29] This bad advice has had other long-term detriments, for lack of exercise contributes greatly to the development of other diseases such as high blood pressure, obesity, diabetes, and heart disease. Dr. Jason Theodosakis stated that the sedentary lifestyle is second only to smoking as the most common cause of disease and death in the United States. [30]

Vigorous exercise not only greatly increases the functional status of people who are suffering from primary osteoarthritis, it can help prevent the disease in the first place. In fact, vigorous movement of any kind—

whether walking, running, lifting weights, or swimming—is now widely accepted as important modalities in the treatment of arthritis. [31] Water exercise is especially helpful as it takes weight off the affected joints while providing the needed conditioning of the diseased tissues.

A study of the effects of walking and water aquatics on osteoarthritis by the University of Missouri demonstrated the benefits of exercise. In this study, eighty arthritic patients were randomly assigned to two groups. One group did aerobic walking or aerobic pool aquatics. The other group did non-aerobic range of motion exercises. The study lasted twelve weeks and consisted of three one-hour sessions per week. The results were impressive. In contrast to the non-aerobic group, the aerobic group of exercisers demonstrated significant gains in aerobic and physical capacity levels. [32] Exercise also helps one lose weight, a plus for the arthritic, and it improves the immune system—just what the arthritic needs to help rebuild health.

Exercise increases the amount of synovial fluid going in and out of the cartilage. This physiological activity lubricates and nourishes the cartilage. The constant movement of liquid into and out of the spongy cartilage keeps the cartilage moist, healthy, and well nourished. [33] Thus with the proper nourishment and supplements, exercise can maximize the rebuilding of damaged cartilage.

Cancer

The Most Exploited Disease

Section 1

THE PROFILE OF A KILLER EPIDEMIC

Cancer! Ladies and gentlemen of the jury, the very word inspires fear. It is one of mankind's most horrible of diseases. At the turn of the century, it struck down one in twenty Americans. Today cancer strikes one in three Americans and kills one in four. [1] After heart disease, cancer is the second leading cause of death. Within a few years, it will become the leading cause of all deaths in the United States. It is the most expensive disease in America. Dr. Scott Gottlieb, the Deputy Commissioner for the FDA's Medical and Scientific Affairs, stated on March 7, 2006, that the price tag was $156.76 billion in 2001, the latest year for which he had completed analysis.[2] Annually there are over 50 million cancer-related medical visits to the doctor. This includes one million cancer surgeries and 750,000 radiation treatments. [3] Clearly, this disease has reached epidemic proportions. Joining a swelling chorus of protesting voices, Dr. Patrick Quillin scathingly pointed out that although President Richard Nixon confidently launched a national *War on Cancer* on December 23, 1971, assuring the American people that we would have a cure for cancer within five years, two decades later, and with over 35 billion dollars spent on research, one trillion spent on therapy, and 7 million casualties, there is no cure or relief in sight for cancer from conventional therapies. It is patently obvious, Dr. Patrick Quillin stated, that the time has come for us to re-examine some discarded options in cancer prevention and treatment. [4]

Ladies and gentlemen of the jury, the testimony will show that despite repeated assurances of impending breakthroughs, the medical establishment's war on cancer has failed. What are the facts supporting this assertion? In 1991, a group of sixty prominent physicians and scientists charged that the cancer establishment—as represented by the American Cancer Society, the National Cancer Society, and the American Medical Association—were confusing the public with repeated claims that they were winning the war on cancer. The truth is, they asserted, our ability to treat and cure most cancers have not materially improved since the war on cancer began in 1971. [5]

In support of their claim that they were winning the war on cancer, the National Cancer Institute contended that the five-year survival rate from discovery to death increased from 20% in 1930 to 53% in 1994. But Dr. Patrick Quillin rebutted this assertion. The real facts he stated, are truly disturbing.

* Living five years after discovery of the cancer has nothing to do with curing the disease. More efficient methods, resulting in earlier detection, can certainly account for the longer survival rate.

* The average cancer patient has a 50/50 chance of living five years after discovery—same odds as in 1971.

* The number of new cases of cancer is increasing every year.

* Since 1950, the overall cancer incidence has increased 44%.

* Over 2.5 million Americans are currently being treated for cancer and another 1.3 million cases are diagnosed every year.

* In 1950, one in twenty women got breast cancer. By 1994, it was one in nine.

* Deaths from cancer are increasing.[6]

Dr. James Anderson provided additional evidence that we are losing the war against cancer. He noted that since 1950:

* Breast cancer rates have increased 60%

* Colon cancer rates have increased 60%

* Prostate cancer rates have doubled

* Lung cancer rates have increased 262%, while cigarette smoking has decreased from 50 to 25% [7]

Dr. Michael Colgan, Ph. D., world-renowned scientist and nutritionist, wrote in *Prevent Cancer Now* (a book that was once selected as the *Health Book of the Year*), that the war on cancer is a *bloody rout.*

> Ever since then [1971, the year Nixon declared war on cancer] the U.S. National Cancer Institute has claimed enormous progress. As we enter the 1990s, it has become obvious that many of these claims are false ... The sad truth is, cancer patients die in America today, at a faster rate than they did in the "pre-war" days of the fifties and sixties ... *We are not only losing the war against cancer, it's a bloody rout.* [8] [Emphasis added.]

A decade after President Nixon declared war on cancer, Dr. Linus Pauling, two-time Nobel Prize winner, declared:

> Everyone should know that the war on cancer is largely a fraud. [9]

Ladies and gentlemen, like his war in Vietnam, President Nixon's war on cancer was a *no win war.* The medical establishment that defined the terms of engagement in the war on cancer never intended to hand us a victory. There was too much profit to be made in *managing* the symptoms of this most expensive of diseases. Again, as it was with Vietnam, the American people were betrayed, fleeced, and their ranks decimated by the 7 million cancer victims since 1971. Why has the war on cancer failed? What *was* our tax dollars spent on? What portion of our research dollars was spent on methods of treatment, on prevention, and on curing the disease? Who were the beneficiaries of the billions that have been spent on cancer research and treatment? The American taxpayer deserves answers to these questions. These answers may provide us with the clue why modern medicine's war on cancer is failing.

In 1976, Senator George McGovern convened a meeting of the United
States Select Committee on Nutrition and Human Needs. Responding to
a question from Senator McGovern, Dr. Arthur Upton, director of the
National Cancer Institute, testified that as much as 50% of cancers are
caused by diet. Dumbfounded, Senator McGovern retorted how can you
assert the vital relationship between diet and cancer and then submit a
preliminary budget that only allocates a little more than 1% of NCI funds
to this problem. Mr. Upton could not provide an answer to the Senator's
question. He lamely responded that he too was concerned about the dis-
parity. [10]

John Robbins asserted that organizations like the National Cancer
Institute are not motivated to focus much attention on preventing cancer
through dietary means because there is vastly more money to be made in
treating the symptoms of the disease. Furthermore, he charged, those food
industries whose products are implicated in causing cancer—like the meat,
dairy, and refined food industrial giants—apply immense pressure on government and public health organizations to keep them from informing the
public on what is known about dietary prevention. [11] While nutritional
approaches to prevention and treatment are discouraged or neglected, the
standard *cut, burn, and poison* approach to cancer treatment has become
big business for the medical and pharmaceutical industries. In the mid
1990s when John Robbins and Dr. Patrick Quillin were making these
charges, the treatment of cancer by surgery, radiation, and chemotherapy
was a $110 billion dollar a year industry. [12]

Ladies and gentlemen of the jury, over the past one hundred years a
war has been raging between the medical establishment and practitioners
of alternative medicine over the best approach to cancer treatment, prevention, and cure. The only *cancer war* the medical establishment has won
has been the war against nutritional and other alternative cancer cures.
The international pharmaceutical companies fund much of the cancer
research and most of the medical schools, therefore the only methods for
controlling cancer approved by the medical establishment, the National
Cancer Institute, and the American Cancer Society are the three-prong
approach of surgery, radiation, and chemotherapy. Donald McAlvany, editor of the *McAlvany Intelligence Report*, observed that with the help of
the Food and Drug Administration (FDA) the managers of the cancer
lobby successfully keep out of the main stream of medicine all nutritional
and other alternative cures for cancer. [13] Donald McAlvany stated that

every approach to cancer treatment that is not Allopathic (drug-based and symptom-orientated) is labeled as quackery or medical fraud with dire consequences to anyone attempting to implement these unapproved methods.

In California, laws have been passed making it a criminal offense (even for medical doctors) to treat cancer with any therapy but surgery, chemotherapy, or radiation—even though many alternative therapies have proven very successful. All across America dozens of clinics practicing alternative medicine have been raided by the FDA police—equipment, records, and bank accounts have been seized, and practitioners have been taken to court, jailed, or financially ruined. [14]

What has been the result of this medical monopoly? The tragic death of thousands and the untold suffering of millions of Americans. Dr. John Bailar of Harvard University and a former editor of the *Journal of the National Cancer Institute* admitted that we are losing the war against cancer. After carefully analyzing the figures on what the Institute's war on cancer had and had not accomplished, Dr. Bailar reported his findings in the May 8, 1986 issue of the *New England Journal of Medicine*.

We are losing—losing more patients than ever, losing this medical Vietnam, a war in which we lack the vision we need to win. [15]

Endorsing sentiments such as those expressed by Dr. John Bailar and other physicians, Dr. Patrick Quillin stated that is has become:

... blatantly obvious that our current cancer treatment methods are inadequate and incomplete and that we need to examine some options—like nutrition. [16]

Ladies and gentlemen of the jury, the testimony will show that the nutritional approach to curing cancer is based upon the concept that many cancers are caused by a buildup of toxins or poisons in the body, which a depressed and shattered immune system cannot eliminate. Thus most alternative remedies stress detoxification of the body and strengthening the immune system so that the body can heal itself. In contrast, conventional medicine primarily treats the symptoms of cancer with chemicals that further toxify and poison the body while doing further damage to the immune system. [17] Which of these two approaches to cancer treatment is more effective? Whom can we trust to provide us truthful and life-saving information—the mainstream medical establishment and cancer associations who are manipulated by the profit-seeking pharmaceutical industry, or the minority of physicians and nutritionists who are restoring people to health, courageously doing so in the face of severe criticism and harassment?

The answer may appear to be blatantly obvious. Nevertheless, the blind stranglehold that traditional medicine has upon the public mind demands an objective demonstration of which method of dealing with the cancer epidemic is more effective. To determine which is the best treatment for cancer, we must understand what cancer is and what causes it. Unless we discover what cancer is, we will remain powerless against it. The rest of the testimony in this segment will be devoted to this issue; succeeding presentations will compare and contrast the relative merits of the *cut, burn, and poison* method with the *alternative and nutritional* approaches to the prevention and cure of cancer.

Ladies and gentlemen of the jury, the most critical concept we must grasp at the outset is that cancer is not merely a lump of runaway, multi-plying cells as conventional medicine would have us believe. These visible cells are merely the *outward* manifestations of a far more serious prob-lem. By focusing on this superficial symptom only, conventional medicine applies the wrong remedies. On the other hand, nutritional doctors like Andrew Weil contend that cancer is a systemic disease that represents a failure of the healing system. [18] According to Dr. Max Gerson, who was one of the most eminent geniuses in the history of medicine (that was the opinion of Nobel laureate Dr. Albert Schweitzer), cancer is a chronic degenerative disease that develops in a body that has more or less lost the normal functions of metabolism due to a chronic daily poisoning, espe-cially of the liver. [19] Cancer is a metabolic disease and once it develops, the cancer works to bring about a derangement of total metabolism in the human body. [20] As a result of this poisoning and subsequent breakdown of cellular metabolism, normal cells become chemically altered mutations and they begin to reproduce in an uncontrolled manner growing into vis-ible tumors, often spreading and invading healthy tissue. [21]

Normally it is the function of the body's immune system to search out and destroy foreign invaders and mutant cells. This task of the immune system is actually assisted by the malignant cancer cells, which display certain antigens on the surface of their membranes, thus actually assisting in their detection and removal. Dr. Andrew Weil believes that the continuous surveillance of the body by the immune mechanism in order to weed out malignant cells is a key function of the healing system and it is the best defense against cancer. [22] But because of self-poisoning through an improper diet and other means, the body's immune system becomes so depressed that it is unable to remove these mutant cells fast enough. This view of cancer correctly points to the strengthening of the immune system along with detoxification of the body as the keys to cancer therapy.

The folly of focusing on the external lump is further seen by the fact that cancer can exist in the body for years before it is large enough to be detected. Dr. John McDougall explained that cancerous cells multiply at different rates depending on the type and location of the cancer. [23] For example, a breast cancer cell will double in one hundred days. In two hundred days, these two cells will double into four. At the end of one year, the original cells will grow into twelve cells. At the end of six years one million cells about the size of a pencil point will be formed. In ten years, the cancer would have grown into the size of the eraser of a common pencil, represents a colony of one billion cells, and is now detectable. [24] In agreement with Dr. John McDougall is world-famous sports nutritionist Dr. Michael Colgan. He observed that breast cancer is usually a slow growing cancer that can take 10–15 years to become obvious, and often 20 years to kill. [25]

Dr. Andrew Weil stated that by the time a cancer lump is noticed, the failure of the healing mechanism and of the immune system has already become a fixed pattern.

> In order for a transformed cell to give rise to a detectable tumor, it must have escaped immune destruction, undergone many divisions, and produced countless generations of daughter cells, all without interference ... [26]

Dr. Max Gerson also argued that a body's normal defensive mechanism must first be reduced to a state of ineffectiveness before cancer can grow freely.

> A normal body also has additional reserves to suppress and destroy malignancies. It does not act in that manner in cancer patients, where the cancer grew from the smallest cellular unit freely,

without encountering any resistance. What forces can suppress such a development? My answer is that this can be accomplished by the oxidizing enzymes and the conditions which maintain their activity. [27]

The systemic nature of cancer disease was also emphasized by the International Congress for Totality-Treatment in Malignant Disease, held in Stuttgart in 1953. The participants recognized that:

... before the [cancerous] growth starts, the function of the organism must have been abnormal ... This is a real blow to the conception that the tumor is a locally limited disease. [28]

Dr. Andrew Weil also pointed out that those mutations in DNA, even if they become malignant, do not necessarily give rise to cancer. The body recognizes these abnormal cells and eliminates them—that is the function of the immune system.

For a mutant cell to persist and give rise to a detectable tumor, a failure of immunity must occur, a failure of the body's defense system. [29]

Dr. James Anderson and Maury Breecher, Ph.D., presented a very clear picture of the initiation and growth of cancer cells in their book, *Dr. Anderson's Antioxidant, Antiaging Health Program.* They pointed out that there are at least three phases to the development of cancer: an *initiation phase*, a *promotion phase*, and a *progression phase.* [30]

The initiation phase of cancer begins when the DNA, the control and command center of the cell, is damaged by a free radical, toxic chemical, virus, or by radiation penetrating the cell membrane. In 1865, over a hundred years before medical science realized the relationship between chemical drugs and cancer, Ellen White, well-known religious and health author, wrote in *Health and How to Live,* that physician-prescribed drugs such as calomel, when taken by the patient can manifest itself in tumors, ulcers, and cancers, years after it has been introduced into the system. [31] Then in 1905, she linked cancer to germs (or viruses) from animal foods.

Flesh was never the best food; its use is now doubly objectionable, since disease in animals is so rapidly increasing ... People are continually eating flesh that is filled with tuberculous and cancerous germs. Tuberculous, cancer, and other diseases are thus communicated. [32]

Protecting the cell membrane from these toxins and germs becomes a first line of defense. Antioxidants like beta-carotene and vitamins E and C work synergistically to protect the cell membrane from damage, or they can repair the damage to the cell once it occurs. [33] The average cell is bombarded by 10,000 free radicals every day, and each hit can lead to mutations and consequent changes in cell memory and possibly cancer. Normally this damage is repaired by enzymatic activity, by antioxidants and other phyto-chemicals (*phyto* means plant, hence literally, plant chemicals). [34]

A damaged cell can remain in a dormant, non-cancerous state for a long period. This dormant state allows the immune system time to intervene. If a damaged cell is not repaired by enzymes or destroyed by the body's immune system, it can move into the *promotion phase* in which the initiated cell becomes precancerous. This is accomplished by the activity of tumor promoters such as toxic chemicals or hormones. [35] If these damaged, precancerous cells sustain further damage to their chromosomes, resulting in loss of cell regulation, then the cell commences a period of uncontrolled growth and tumor formation. If our immune system is functioning well, our bodies can develop anti-bodies to attack and destroy these runaway cancer cells. Certain phyto-chemicals such as soy isoflavones can also inhibit cell growth by limiting new blood-vessel formation or stimulating the enzyme machinery that limits cell growth. [36]

Ladies and gentlemen of the jury, I wish to erase from your minds the fear and mystery about this dreaded disease we call cancer. As long ago as 1902, Dr. John Beard, a professor of embryology at the University of Edinburgh in Scotland, discovered the nature of these mutant cancer cells. His findings revolutionized the treatment of cancer for a while, but was finally rejected and suppressed by the profit-oriented cancer establishment. In a paper published in *Lancet,* the prestigious *Journal of the British Medical Society*, he stated that there was no difference between mutant cancer cells and certain pre-embryonic cells known as trophoblast cells that are normal to the early stages of pregnancy. In short, cancer cells *are* trophoblast cells. [37] Cancer is in fact rapidly dividing trophoblast cells that the body can no longer restrain due to metabolic dysfunction.

The trophoblast cell is generated by the diploid totipotent cell, which is a cell basic to the development of life. These cells are found plentifully in the ovaries and testes and sparsely in other parts of the body. The diploid totipotent cell has the total capacity to evolve into any organ or tissue and into a complete embryo. It is therefore often called the *total life cell*. This *total life cell* plays an important part in pregnancy and in the healing mechanism. [38]

During pregnancy, the *total life cell* generates trophoblast cells at a rapid rate in the presence of the female hormone estrogen, thus causing the embryo to grow rapidly until the eight week, when certain mechanisms in the body suddenly stop this growth of trophoblast cells. [39] The rapid growth of trophoblast cells from *total life cells* that were previously generated by the fertilized egg results in the mass development of the placenta, the umbilical cord, and other tissue, by the eighth week of life. Trophoblast cells, like the total life cells, play a vital part in the development of life. They also play a vital role in the healing mechanism. When the body of an adult is injured, the hormone estrogen and other steroids are released into the blood stream, and they promote the proliferation of trophoblast cells as part of the healing process. But when the metabolism is dysfunctional due to improper diet and other causes that poison the system, the natural healing mechanism also dysfunctions and the healing process is not turned off. The result is an uncontrolled proliferation of trophoblast cells in the body, which we call cancer. [40] The critical concept to grasp is that any trauma that causes damage to the body can cause cancer *if* the body's healing processes are not functioning properly. [41] Dr. Steward M. Jones of Palo Alto California has stated:

Whenever a trophoblast cell appears in the body outside of pregnancy, the natural forces that control it on a normal pregnancy may be absent and, in this case, it begins uncontrolled proliferation, invasion, extension, and metastasis. When this happens, it is initiated by an organizer substance, usually estrogen, the presence of which further promotes the trophoblast activity. This is the beginning of cancer. [42]

The uncontrolled growth of trophoblast cells eventually show up as a lump, which we characteristically call cancer. But the lump or tumor is not 100% trophoblast cells. The body tries to contain the trophoblast cells by surrounding them with local tissue in an effort to contain the growth. Dr. Steward Jones observed:

In order to counteract the estrogenic action on the trophoblast, the body floods the areas of the trophoblast in a sea of beta-glucuronidase (BG) which inactivates all estrogen upon contact. At the same time, the cells of the tissues being invaded by the trophoblasts defensively multiply in an effort at local containment.

Usually the efforts of the body to control the nidus of trophoblast are successful, the trophoblast dies, and a benign polyp or other benign tumor remains as a monument to the victory of the body over cancer. [43]

The evidence is so clear, that cancer is simply trophoblast cells out of control, members of the medical establishment have finally admitted that cancer cells and trophoblast cells are identical. On October 15, 1995, ninety-three years after Dr. John Beard published his findings, a study written up in the journal *Cancer* conceded, "After 93 years, Beard has been proved to be conceptually correct [about the nature and growth of cancer]." [44]

Ladies and gentlemen of the jury, another important fact to grasp is that there are not different types of cancer. This only *appears* to be so, because tumors in different locations of the body consist of trophoblast cells and *local tissue cells* in different proportions. As the lump approaches total malignancy, the ratio of trophoblast cells to tissue cells change, with the trophoblast becoming dominant. The active malignancy of the cancer is not the tumor but the cancerous or runaway trophoblast cells within the tumor. The fact that cancer is runaway trophoblast cells permits its detection without invasive biopsies. Biopsies can spread the cancer by cutting into the tumor. Non-surgical detection is possible because all trophoblast cells give out a distinctive hormone called chorionic gonadotrophic hormone, or CGH, which no other cells produce. CGH is easily detected in the urine. So if a urine test is positive, the person is either pregnant or has cancer. If the patient is male, he obviously has cancer. It is that simple. This urine test is 95 to 100% accurate. [45]

One of the fatal and erroneous assumptions being made by conventional cancer researchers is that cancer is *foreign* to the body and therefore can be identified and attacked by some magic bullet. This type of research will continue to produce dead-end trails. Ladies and gentlemen, the truth is that the cancer cell is a *normal part* of the life cycle of pregnancy and healing and is *not* foreign to the body. For this reason, it is not identified as a *foreign* invader by the body's immune system. Although the trophoblast cell is a normal cell, the body's natural healing mechanism, when functioning properly, controls the proliferation of these trophoblast cells, thus preventing cancer from developing. This subject will be further discussed in the section on nutritional remedies.

Because cancer is a metabolic dysfunction, there are common causes of cancer and other chronic degenerative diseases. Many diseases appear in cluster form. For example gall-bladder diseases, often combined with liver dysfunctions, appear together with myocardial changes and cirrhosis of the liver. [46] Diabetes and cancer both alike result from metabolic dysfunctions of the body. [47] Whatever disrupts the metabolism of the body is capable of causing a myriad of diseases. Chronic degenerative diseases are all metabolic diseases, and cancer is no exception. [48]

What is distinctive about cancer is that it is a metabolic dysfunction of the *healing system*. This dysfunction is precipitated by a more general metabolic dysfunction of the body. Dr. Max Gerson observed that a combination of several degenerative diseases—such as osteo-arthritis, high blood pressure, heart disease, and diabetes—frequently occur in the cancer patient. [49]

Ladies and gentlemen of the jury, I wish to draw your attention to a vital piece of evidence. In 1982, the National Research Council released a technical report called *Diet, Nutrition, and Cancer*. The report stated that diet was probably the greatest single factor in the epidemic of cancer, especially cancers of the breast, colon, and prostate. [50] Thus, the role of an improper diet in precipitating cancer by interfering with the metabolic processes of the body must be examined if we are interested in understanding the cause of cancer and its proper treatment. A definition of terms will help us understand the role diet plays in the proper functioning of the body.

The term metabolism refers to all of the chemical processes occurring in the body that support life. [51] This chemical activity is facilitated by enzymes, vitamins, minerals, and hormones. Hormones give individuality to tissues and cells and are the primary regulators of metabolism. But hormonal control is ineffective without the proper balance of minerals and vitamins. [52] Enzymes assist in bringing about all metabolic activity. Vitamins are organic nutrients whose main function is the regulation of physiological processes, thereby helping metabolic differentiation and vitality. [53] Minerals are inorganic substances such as sodium and potassium and are carriers of electrical potentials in the cells. Minerals enable the hormones, vitamins, and enzymes to function properly. [54], [55]

Ladies and gentlemen of the jury, mark this well, in the *absence* of minerals all metabolic life will cease and the organism will die. [56] Two of the minerals essential to life are potassium, a positive or anodic ion, designated by the symbol K , and sodium, a negative or cathodic ion, designated by the symbol Na. Potassium and other anodic minerals are predominant *within the cells* of the organs and tissues such as the liver, muscles, brain, heart, kidneys, etc. Sodium and other cathodic minerals function *outside the cells* in the fluids such as serum and lymph, but also in such tissues as connective tissue, thyroid, bile ducts, etc. [57] About 60% of the body tissues belong to the K-group and 30% to the Na-group, with 10% on the borderline. [58] Dr. Patrick Quillin stated that the ideal ratio of potassium (K) to sodium (Na) should be 4 to 1, but our dietary habits have reversed this ideal health-sustaining ration.

Our modern American diet reverses this ration from an ideal of 4 to 1 (potassium to sodium) to our current 1 to 4, a full 16-fold deterioration in this crucial balance of electrolytes. All of your cells are bathed in a salty ocean water, higher concentrations of potassium inside the cell to create the battery of life. [59]

This imbalance of potassium to sodium, often due to excess salt intake, is a significant step in the metabolic dysfunction of the human organism. Hormones, enzymes, and vitamins also divide themselves into an anodic or positive group and a cathodic or negative group. The anodic hormones, enzymes, and vitamins function *within* the cell, intracellularly, and are dependent upon the intracellular minerals such as potassium to properly perform their metabolic functions. [60] The cathodic hormones, enzymes, and vitamins function *outside* of the cell, extracellularly, and are dependent upon the extracellular minerals such as sodium to perform their metabolic duties. [61] Dr. Max Gerson stated that *almost all acute and chronic sicknesses begin with an invasion by sodium chloride and water into the anodic organs, displacing potassium and other anodic minerals in the cells of the heart, pancreas, liver, and other organs.* [62] Normally, during daily activities, some sodium penetrates the potassium tissues, and this is followed by chloride and water, a process which brings on fatigue, a feeling of heaviness, and swelling. At night, the sodium is reabsorbed, and in the morning, it is eliminated in the urine and the person feels refreshed. [63] If the ratio of potassium to sodium is disrupted, metabolic function is impaired and the hormones, enzymes, and vitamins do not function properly. [64] When unbalanced, the potassium and sodium salts, particularly the sodium salts, become a source of trouble for cell metabolism. [65]

Dr. Birger Jansson, Ph.D., of the University of Texas; Dr. Stephen Thompson, Ph.D., researcher at the University of California San Diego; and Dr. Maryce Jacobs, Ph.D., former research director of the American Institute of Cancer, have all written on the link between the dietary sodium to potassium ratio and cancer onset. [66] Dr. Stephen Thompson observed that increasing the sodium content in animals accelerates the metastasis of colon cancer. [67]

Ladies and gentlemen of the jury, let us for a moment consider the role of white sugar and other refined foods in cancer onset and proliferation. Dr. Nancy Appleton maintains that one sure way to turn normal cells into cancerous cells is to continually upset the body's chemistry by altering its mineral balance. She believes the primary way of upsetting the mineral balance of the body is by the consumption of refined sugar and other harmful foods. [68] During normal cell metabolism (that is, chemical activity), the cell produces harmful free radicals such as peroxide, hydroxyl group, and superoxide. Enzymes in our bodies engage these free radicals and turn them back into useful products; but in order to do so, the enzymes must have adequate supplies of the right minerals and in the right combinations. [69], [70] Refined sugar depletes the body of essential minerals; this results in inadequate enzymatic activity and the consequent build up of free radicals in the tissues. Excessive free radicals interfere with the oxygenation process, and when the oxygen deprivation of cells reaches 35%, the cell turns cancerous. In 1920 Dr. Otto Walberg demonstrated this when he took human cells and removed 35% of the oxygen from the cells and the cells turned cancerous. [71]

Dr. Otto Walberg also observed that in normal human cells, metabolism is based upon the process of oxygenation, whereas in malignant tissue, the cells rely on anaerobic glycolysis or fermentation to sustain life. [72] In other words, because of genetic changes abnormal cells are forced to switch over from the use of oxygen to the use of fermentation. Dr. George Medes reported to the American Chemical Society in 1955 that changes in the chemistry of the cells have been observed in rats when cancer strikes. He found that cancer cells lose the ability to synthesize and oxidize fats while they can easily utilize glucose. [73] Dr. Max Gerson stated that in all experiments except one that he was aware of, it was found that cancer cells cannot be stimulated to change back from the use of fermentation to the use of oxygen. Consequently, they have to be killed by the immune system and reabsorbed by the body. [74]

Dr. Patrick Quillin maintained that tumors are primarily *sugar feeders*; they are fueled mainly by glucose and not by fats or proteins. Hence, he believes that the American diet, which provides as much as 20% of its calories from refined sugar, is a primary cause of the high incidence of cancer in our society. [75] Ignorance of this fact can kill us. We must think for ourselves. We cannot rely on the assurances of others, not even public institutions. Are our hospitals safe havens for their patients? Is hospital food contributing to the onset of diseases and inhibiting patient recovery? Dr. Quillin thought so. He cited recent research that shows that the standard high sugar hospital diet given to cancer patients actually promotes tumor growth whereas a low sugar diet selectively starves the cancer. [76] Thus through ignorance of proper nutrition, hospitals are actually injuring the patients they are supposed to be helping.

Ladies and gentlemen of the jury, we begin now a line of testimony that is of vital concern to our wives, mothers, daughters, and sisters. The subject is breast cancer, and we must take a sober look at the evidence. Let us first consider the expert testimony on the role of estrogen in cancers of the breast. The evidence is ample that upsetting the body chemistry with refined sugar can increase one's metabolic rate and produce an excess of free radicals, which can result in the buildup of excessive estrogen around the cells. Of course, other emotional and lifestyle factors such as stress, distress, anger, and rage can also result in the buildup of excessive estrogen around the cells. Excessive estrogen can turn these cells into cancerous cells. [77] Because of the prominent role estrogen plays in a woman's metabolism, breast cancer is 100 times more common in women than men. Breast cancer is the single most common form of cancer found in middle aged to older women. [78] But neither breast cancer nor any other kind of cancer is genetic. While one's genetic blueprint can *predispose* one to the development of cancer, it does not *cause* cancer. The genetic blueprint merely determines what disease will develop out of unbalanced body chemistry. [79] Dr. John McDougall argued that the incidence of breast cancer in families from generation to generation can be explained on the basis that daughters learn from their mothers what foods to like and cook. Therefore, if a particular dietary pattern is linked to cancer, that eating habit is passed on as well as the metabolic fallout from the use of those foods. [80]

The more estrogen a woman produces to stimulate her breast tissue, the more likely it is that cancer will develop, especially if her metabolism and immune system is in dysfunction. [81] Estrogen stimulates cells to divide and proliferate, making them vulnerable to mutagenic activity. [82] When cells divide, their DNA uncoils so that their genetic information can be copied. But in its separated state, DNA is most susceptible to injury from radiation, or from mutagenic chemicals, as well as from random accidents in the cell division process. [83]

There is a natural affinity between cancer cells and estrogen. Research has discovered that cancer cells have receptors to which estrogen molecules attach. [84] Hence, whatever promotes the buildup of estrogen increases the risk and progression of cancer. For example, taking estrogen pills increases the likelihood of developing cancer. Likewise, the ingestion of the hormones fed to poultry and beef increases the risk of cancer in women. [85] Birth control pills are toxic and increase the risk of cancer because of their high estrogen content. Hormone replacement given after menopause also increases the risk of cancer because of their high estrogen content. [86]

Estrogen is produced in the ovaries, adrenal glands, and adipose tissue. It is important to understand that estrogen is not itself the problem. It is an imbalanced diet and a dysfunctional metabolism that is the problem. Normally the body controls the level of estrogen by eliminating excessive amounts it. Excess estrogen bonds with non-absorbable substances in the liver and are sent to the colon to be excreted. Excessive fat in the diet can interfere with this estrogen control mechanism. [87] Dr. John McDougall states that fats can promote the growth of certain bacteria in the colon. These bacteria have the ability to break the bond between estrogen and the liver substances, thereby freeing the estrogen for reabsorption through the bowel wall into the blood stream where it is transported back to the cells. The result is higher levels of estrogen in women who eat rich foods high in animal fats. [88] The four primary factors that increase the risk of breast cancer in women are all interrelated: obesity, cholesterol, and the levels of the hormones, estrogen and prolactin. [89]

Since estrogen is also produced in the adipose tissue—that is, the fat cells—the amount of estrogen is increased by obesity. Hence controlling obesity can help control estrogen levels and thus reduce the risk of breast cancer. Not surprisingly high blood sugar levels can cripple these built-in mechanisms for controlling estrogen levels. [90] High estrogen levels in obese women also results from the conversion of the male hormone androgen in females into estrogen. Older women are more efficient at converting androgen into estrogen, hence the greater risk of cancer in older women. [91]

Ladies and gentlemen of the jury, the evidence is overwhelming and clearly convincing that breast cancer is related to diet. In the United States one in ten women will get breast cancer, whereas women living in societies with low-fat diets, especially diets low in animal saturated fats, have a much lower incidence of breast cancer. [92] Women who are meat eaters have 50% more estrogen-related cancers than women who do not eat meat. [93] A major study by Drs. Bruce Armstrong and Richard Doll compared countries with varying diets and found a strong correlation between the per capita consumption of fat and the breast cancer rate. Dr. Oliver Alabaster noted that Japanese women have the lowest breast cancer rates in the world. He concluded that it is their low-fat diet, and not genetics that determined this.

Many Japanese women have migrated to Hawaii and the U.S. mainland. While marrying within their own community and keeping the population relatively unchanged genetically, they shifted their diet toward a more Western, higher fat diet, and their breast cancer rate steadily climbed. Within one generation, it approximated that of Caucasian women living around them. This is very dramatic evidence that cancer is mainly environmentally induced, rather than genetically inherited. [94]

In his illuminating book *The Power of Your Plate*, Dr. Neil Barnard pointed out that within Japan itself, women of high socio-economic strata who eat meat daily have more than eight times the risk of breast cancer compared to poorer women who rarely eat meat. He feels the culprit is the fat in the high meat diet. [95] Fat acts to promote cancer in a variety of ways. High fat diets are usually low in fiber. The high-fiber diet in mostly vegetarian diets acts as a barrier to the reabsorption of estrogen. [96] Also the type of bacteria found in the colons of people on a low-fat diet do not convert much of the excreted estrogen into the absorbable form, therefore more is eliminated in the stool. [97]

Dr. Neil Barnard pointed out that after a high-fat meal the gall bladder releases bile acids into the intestines to absorb these fats. He noted, however, that excess bile acids could be a factor in causing cancer.

Bacteria in the intestines turn these bile acids into cancer-promoting substances called secondary bile acids. And this is where fiber comes in, as Dr. Burkett points out: Fiber in the diet alters the bacteria in the intestines and reduces the breakdown of primary into secondary bile acids. In addition, fiber absorbs these bile acids the same way that blotting paper absorbs spilled ink. It gets them out of the way. It also dilutes them into a large stool instead of a small stool. So they are reduced, absorbed, and diluted. So in a nutshell, fat would seem to be promotive, and fiber would be protective. [98]

Too much saturated fat in the diet will also depress the immune system, thereby reducing one's defenses against cancer. Oxidized cholesterol is especially immunosuppressive. [99] Depressing the immune system impairs its ability to attack and destroy cancer cells. A high-saturated fat and cholesterol diet will also increase the risk of other types of cancers. For example, colon cancer, which affects 20% to 30% of American families, is caused by a high fat and cholesterol and low-fiber diet. [100], [101] Dr. Julian Whitaker stated that while a diet high in fat has been strongly linked to cancer and other diseases, on closer examination the culprit is not fat in general, but *saturated* fat, predominantly all *animal* fats. [102] He noted that a diet low in saturated fat but high in unsaturated fat has actually been shown to exert a protective effect against cancer. [103]

Men are also made vulnerable to cancer by a high fatty diet. In his highly informative book *Eat Right Live Longer*, Dr. Neal Barnard stated that countries such as the U.S. and Western Europe, with high fatty meat diets, have higher incidences of prostate cancer than countries such as Asia and Latin America. For example, a Swedish male is eight times more likely to die of prostate cancer than a man in Hong Kong. And by age fifty,

40% of Americans get cancer of the prostate. [104] Young males between the ages of thirty and forty examined after accidental fatalities have shown cancer in the prostate. [105] Testosterone and related hormones stimulate prostate cancer. A high fat and meat diet boosts testosterone's effects and thus increases the rate of prostate cancer. [106]

A high intake of animal fat is not the only villain in causing cancer. The evidence is clear, that it is not only saturated animal fat that is linked to cancer; animal protein has been implicated as well. Our way of life is related to our way of death. [107] Dr. Andrew Weil decisively linked animal protein to cancer. In *Natural Health, Natural Medicine* he wrote:

> Cancer of the colon, one of the major killers in our society, sometimes runs in families, but it also correlates well with diet, particularly with high consumption of fat, animal protein and refined starch and low consumption of vegetables and fiber. [108]

In his groundbreaking work in treating cancer victims, Dr. Max Gerson also made frequent reference to the damaging influence of animal proteins. When he reduced the amount of animal protein in his cancer patients' diets, they responded much better to treatment. [109] He found that the harmful and toxic end products of protein metabolism, namely nitrogen urea and uric acid, can be eliminated in greater amounts if less animal protein is ingested. Dr. Neil Barnard has also noted the link between high protein intake and cancer. He observed that foods high in protein, such as beef, are also high in fat and low in fiber, known factors in cancer causation. But protein itself is an independent cause of cancer. Dr. Barnard cited statements from the National Research Council in support of his opinion:

> ... evidence from epidemiological and laboratory studies suggest that high protein intake may be associated with an increased risk of cancers at certain sites. [110]

Diets that are too high in protein have been generally linked to cancers of the breast, colon, rectum, pancreas, uterus, and prostate. But on closer examination, the primary culprit seems to be animal protein and not plant-based protein. [111] Commenting on his experience with cancer patients and different dietary regimes, Dr. Max Gerson noted the harmful effects of animal protein:

I observed that almost all patients with a higher protein intake could not be saved. In some cases, I observed a much quicker growth of the cancer or metastasis. [112]

Ladies and gentlemen, Dr. Max Gerson's insight regarding the role of animal protein and cancer was recently and dramatically confirmed by the epochal and groundbreaking *The China Study* by Drs. T. Colin Campbell and Thomas Campbell. We have introduced you to these experts before. Let us now tell you what they found regarding high animal protein intake and the onset of cancer. Earlier in his career, Dr. Colin Campbell, like other cancer experts, realized that there are three stages in cancer manifestation. First there is the initiation phase in which a carcinogen or other virus enters the cell. These are metabolized by enzymes within the cell to form carcinogen-DNA complex compounds. Unless destroyed by the cell, these complex compounds then damage the DNA of the cell. When this damaged cell divides or reproduces, daughter cancer cells, also genetically damaged, are formed. These daughter cells now create the potential for cancer formation in the body. [113] The whole process takes only minutes. UV light, carcinogens, and viruses strike all of us daily, creating genetically damaged cells.

The promotion phase occurs when these daughter cells begin to multiply. But like seeds in the soil, these initial cancer cells will not grow and multiply unless the right conditions are met. [114] And it is at this point that we can control our risk of developing cancer. By our dietary habits and our lifestyles, we can determine whether a genetically damaged cell starts to grow within us in a cancerous fashion, remain dormant, or are destroyed and removed by the body's internal defense mechanism. Discussing the need for the right conditions to occur before cancer cells begin to multiple, Dr. Colin Campbell wrote:

This is one of the most profound features of promotion. Promotion is reversible, depending on whether the early cancer growth is given the right conditions in which to grow. This is where certain dietary factors become so important. These dietary factors, called promoters, feed cancer growth. Other dietary factors, called anti-promoters, slow cancer growth. [115]

If the right conditions are met, the genetically damaged cells begin to grow in the promotion phase, and as they multiply out of control, the

progression phase is initiated and the cancer cells begin to do their damage. Dr. Colin Campbell discovered that the amount of protein eaten
determines whether cancer is initiated and whether, after initiation, it is
promoted. The reason for this is that enzyme activity within the cell is
affected by the amount of protein we eat. Decreasing protein intake from
20% to 5% reduces enzyme activity by 76%, thereby frustrating cancer
initiation within the cell. Furthermore, by decreasing protein intake there
is a 72% decrease in carcinogen binding to DNA components in the cell, a
68% decrease in Chromatin binding, and a 66% decrease in protein binding to nucleus components in the cell. [116]

Dr. Colin Campbell found that a low protein diet of 5% also retarded
or frustrated the promotion phase of cancer. Moreover, the multiplica-
tion of the cancer cells was entirely dependent upon how much protein
we consumed, regardless of the amount of carcinogen we are exposed to.
[117] He found that there were no cancer clusters in the promotion phase
when the protein intake was between 5 and 10%. Above that, the growth
of cancer cells began. [118] If we consume more than the 12% of protein
needed to satisfy our needs, cancer formation in genetically damaged cells
is promoted. [119]

Astonishingly, Dr. Colin Campbell discovered that we can turn cancer off and on by the amount of protein we consume! He demonstrated
that after cancer promotion commenced at 20% protein intake, if the protein consumption was reduced to 5%, the growth stopped. When protein
intake was again increased the cancerous cells began to grow once more.
[120] This finding is vital to our standing of how diet is related to the
onset and promotion of cancer. But it is also vital to our ability to prevent
or reverse cancer. When the experiment was repeated, allowing the tumors
to advance to the proliferation stage, the results were very astonishing.

The effects of protein feeding on tumor development were
nothing less than spectacular. Rats generally live for about two
years, thus the study was 100 weeks in length. All animals that
were administered aflatoxin and fed the regular 20% levels of
casein (animal protein from cow's milk) were dead or near death
from liver tumors at 100 weeks. All animals administered the same
level of aflatoxin but fed the low 5% protein diet were alive, active
and thrifty, with sleek hair coats at 100 weeks. This was virtually

a 100 to 0 score, something almost never seen in research and almost identical to the original research in India. [121]

Moreover, ladies and gentlemen of the jury, Dr. Colin Campbell found that not all proteins have the same effect on the body. Plant-based protein and animal-based proteins are very different in their affect on cancer initiation and promotion. Rats fed 20% plant-based proteins did not reveal any cancer initiation or promotion formation, despite exposure to carcinogens. [122] If animal protein was kept below 5%, there was little to no cancer growth. The implication is clear; the over-consumption of animal products may have made our Western society particularly vulnerable to cancer.

In the 1970s, Dr. Colin Campbell had the opportunity to confirm his earlier cancer experiments using rats in a study of cancer growth among a large cross section of the Chinese population. He assembled an excellent scientific team from America and Oxford University, England, and took them to China. In collaboration with Chinese scientists, his team took blood tests and administered questionnaires about their dietary habits, to 6,500 Chinese in sixty-five different semi-rural counties in China. They gathered data on 367 variables. The study assembled more than 8,000 statistically significant associations between lifestyle, diet, and disease variables. The *New York Times* called the study the Grand Prix of epidemiology. [123]

The findings of this landmark China Study created seismic waves throughout the medical and nutritional world. He found that as blood cholesterol in rural China rose in certain counties, the incident of Western diseases such as cancer and heart disease increased. [124] In the West the average cholesterol is around 170 to 290mg/dl, and we consider 150mg/dl as normal. But in China, the average cholesterol level is as low as 94 mg/dl!

As blood cholesterol levels decreased from 170 mg/dl to 90 mg/dl. Cancers of the liver, rectum, colon, male lung, female lung, breast, childhood leukemia, adult leukemia, childhood brain, adult brain, stomach and esophagus (throat) decreased. [125]

How does this relate to protein and cancer? Dr. Colin Campbell found that consuming animal-based protein increased blood cholesterol levels, and hence increased the incidence of cancer. [126]

The finding: Casein and very likely all animal proteins may be the most relevant cancer-causing substances that we consume. Adjusting the amount of dietary casein has the power to turn on and turn off cancer growth. [127]

He also found that the high-fiber diets of rural Chinese was linked to lower blood cholesterol and lower rates of cancers of the rectum and colon. [128] The study also showed that high vitamin C intake in the form of fresh fruits was linked to lower levels of cancers of the esophageal, breast, stomach, liver, leukemia, colon, and lung. [129] Reducing dietary fat from 24% to 6% was linked to lower breast cancer rates. [130] In the context of cancer prevention, Dr. Colin Campbell had discovered what Hippocrates knew 2,500 years ago—that food is the best medicine.

Our most powerful weapon against cancer is the food we eat every day. [131]

Of course, the harmful effects of animal products go beyond their saturated fat and protein content. Meat cooked rare may transmit certain viruses suspected of playing a role in causing cancer. [132] Although cooking may kill these viruses, it will not remove the toxins and contaminants in meat that also cause cancer.

What about other animal products such as dairy foods? Are they linked to high cancer rates too? Dr. Neil Barnard thinks so. He noted that there is preliminary evidence that dairy products may contribute to cancer of the ovary. The culprit this time is a breakdown product of milk sugar, lactose. Lactose itself is further broken down into another sugar called galactose, which in turn is broken down by enzymes. Dr. Bernard cited a study done by Dr. Daniel Cramer at Harvard demonstrating that when dairy product consumption exceeds a woman's enzyme capacity to break down galactose, there is a buildup of galactose in the blood, which adversely affects a woman's ovaries. Women who have low levels of this galactose-digesting enzyme, and who consume dairy products on a regular basis, can triple their risk of developing ovarian cancer. [133]

Other environmental factors, including those related to diet, play an important role in the causation of cancer. Research shows that replacing saturated fat in the diet with polyunsaturated fats may lower blood cholesterol, but may have risks of their own. Dr. Andrew Weil pointed out that the molecular points of unsaturation in fatty acid chains are unstable and vulnerable to attack by oxygen if left standing or heated in the presence of air. These oxidized polyunsaturated fats can damage DNA and lead to an increased risk of cancer. [134]

Stress, a familiar factor in our social environment, can also increase one's risk of cancer. Dr. Patrick Quillin related that in his years of experience, 90% of his patients have had major trauma in their lives one to two years before developing cancer. This is especially true for breast cancer according to the medical textbook, *Stress and Breast Cancer*. [135] The mechanism is not always clear. Stress and depression can lead to a suppression of the immune system and therefore reduces our ability to resist cancer. The mind is a powerful thing. It can help you eliminate disease or leave you vulnerable to disease, as Dr. Patrick Quillin observed:

Helplessness and hopelessness are just as lethal weapons as cigarettes and bullets. [136]

Ladies and gentlemen of the jury, let us focus briefly on other environmental causes of cancer. X-rays are a standard diagnostic tool in modern medicine. It is used all too frequently in mammography tests for cancer in women. It is also a hazardous by product of our nuclear age. The evidence shows that radiation creates a twofold threat in the development of cancer. It can directly damage the DNA of cells, transforming them into cancerous cells, and it can damage the immune system, weakening our natural defense against cancer. [137] Radiologists are known to have a shorter life span due to their frequent exposure to radiation. Ultra-violet light can damage DNA in the cells of fair-skinned people. [138] Only a small percentage of known chemicals are carcinogenic, but they are responsible for more incidences of cancer than radiation. Some of the chemicals contained in coal tar and tobacco smoke can react directly with the DNA in the cells, damaging them and causing the cells to become malignant. [139]

As we have seen, chemical carcinogens work in two steps. An initiation stage results from rapid alterations in the DNA on exposure to the carcinogen. If these mutated cells are not eliminated by the immune defense, repeated exposure to the carcinogen transforms these mutated cells into malignant cancerous cells. The chemicals themselves can weaken the immune system, thereby increasing the chance that stage two malignancies will develop. [140] These chemicals can also damage the liver, which bears the burden of metabolizing and detoxifying the harmful substances that enter the body. The liver is an important ally of the immune system. [141]

Dr. Andrew Weil observed that tobacco smoke is the single most important cause of cancer in the environment. It is full of carcinogens as well as radioactive particles. Cigarette smoking is the principle cause of lung cancer. One-fifth of all lung cancer deaths are due to smoking. By the time the cancer is discovered in the lungs, it usually has already spread to other parts of the body. [142] Dr. Julian Whitaker wrote that smoking not only promotes cancer, it will also increase the incidence of almost all degenerative diseases. [143]

Alcohol has also been implicated in the risk of developing cancer. Dr. Neil Barnard stated that even one drink a day can increase breast cancer risks by up to 50%, compared to non-drinkers. [144] Heavy drinkers are at greater risk of developing cancers of the mouth, throat, esophagus, stomach, and liver because alcohol irritates these tissues directly. The danger is compounded if the person also smokes. [145]

Damage to the liver by alcohol use puts one at an extremely greater risk for developing cancer because the liver is the primary detoxifying organ of the body. Dr. Max Gerson and others contend that the appearance of cancer is preceded by the deterioration of the liver and the progression of the cancer is accompanied by further poisoning and destruction of liver function. [146] He recognized three stages in liver impairment and cancer growth. In the first stage, the liver has begun to dysfunction due to poisoning. At this stage, the liver has lost potassium and other anodic minerals so that the oxidizing enzymes can no longer be deoxidized in sufficient quantities to control cell growth. This first stage sees the development and the appearance of the cancer. [147]

During the second stage, the tumor grows and spreads with colonies appearing in the glands. [148] At this time, one can palpate an enlarged liver, evidence of its rapid deterioration. As the healing mechanism of the body decreases, the activity of the cancer correspondingly increases. [149] In the third stage the cancer has gained supremacy; rapid poisoning and destruction of the liver and other essential organs sets in. There is an acute and rapid loss of muscle and liver substance since very little is left of the body's immune defenses. [150] In this stage, poisoning from the cancer further impairs liver function. Several authors have shown that if an abdominal tumor is surgically removed, the liver is the first organ to recover. [151]

Ladies and gentlemen of the jury, it is important for you to understand that all of the body's metabolic processes work together. They are dependent upon one another and are deranged and impaired in varying degrees with each other. Metabolism is concentrated in the liver, so the health of the body is bound up with the state of health of the liver. This relationship of liver metabolism and cancer growth was first observed in 1861 by Dr. Theodor Frerichs (1819-1885), author of *Diseases of the Liver*, and later recognized by many other German physicians. [152] In light of the relationship between liver impairment and cancer onset, Dr. Max Gerson repeatedly emphasized that in fighting cancer the focus should be on the liver and its restoration and not on the symptoms of cancer.

The metabolism and its concentration in the liver should be put in the foreground, not the cancer as a *symptom*. There [in the liver], the outcome of the cancer is determined as the clinical favorable results, failures and autopsies clearly demonstrate. There, the sentence will be passed—whether the tumors can be killed, dissolved, absorbed, eliminated and, finally, whether the body can be restored. [153]

Other physicians and researchers have recognized the central role the liver plays in the onset and course of degenerative diseases. Dr. Kasper Blond has written:

In the liver, we have tried to show that cirrhosis of the liver is not a disease *sui generis*, but only a sign of a disorder of metabolism which causes a chain of events leading to many conditions which the medical generation of today considers to be disorders *sui generis*. The whole syndrome of metabolic disorders which we call oesophagitis, gastritis, duodenitis, gastric and duodenal ulcer, cholecystitis, cholangitis, pancreatitis, proctitis, and others are considered only stages of a dynamic process, starting with liver failure and portal hypertension, and resulting in cirrhosis of the liver tissue and in cancer. Cancer is a mutation of somatic tissues caused by chronic damage of the liver. The structural changes of the somatic tissues are the *result*, not the *cause* of the metabolic disorders. [154]

Dr. Max Gerson observed that Dr. Kasper Blond studied the role of the liver in cancer initiation and progression as early as 1928 and came to the conclusion that we can solve most degenerative diseases, including cancer, if we study the physiology of man as a whole, rather than individual cells, isolated structures, or single organs. In that respect, his opinion runs contrary to most modern cancer doctors who, Dr. Gerson stated, emphasize a study of the site of the malignancy itself despite the fact that 98% of all patients with cancers of the internal organs succumb not to the cancer but to the liver disorder. [155] Dr. Michael Spellberg in *Diseases of the Liver* noted the relationship between the deterioration of the liver and onset of liver cancer:

> Primary cancer of the liver occurs so much more frequently in the cirrhotic liver as compared with the normal liver that cirrhosis has been referred to as a precancerous lesion. [156]

The function of the liver cells is so vital to the health of the body that they have been compared to the chlorophyll of plants. The liver has been called the balance wheel of life. [157] Michael Spellberg emphasized the importance of restoring the health of the liver through proper nutrition:

> There is no dispute that an adequate diet is essential in the treatment of liver diseases. [158]

Ladies and gentlemen of the jury, some of this very compelling evidence concerning the dietary causes of cancer is beginning to make inroads in conventional medicine. While the medical establishment and cancer associations have not yet embraced the role of diet in *curing* cancer, they have come to recognize the pivotal role diet plays in *causing* cancer. Dr. Gio B. Gori, Deputy Director of the National Cancer Institute, Division of Cancer Cause and Prevention, and Director of the Division of Nutrition and Cancer Program, testified to a Senate Select Committee that it was not chemicals, preservatives, or artificial food additives, but meat and fat intake that were the primary dietary factors in the cause of cancer.

> Until recently many eyebrows would have been raised by suggesting that an imbalance of normal dietary components could lead to cancer and cardiovascular disease ... Today, the accumulation of ... evidence ... make this notion not only possible but certain ...

[The] dietary factors responsible [are] principally *meat and fat intake.* [159] [Emphasis added.]

Other voices are now being heard linking cancer with the rich American diet of meat and fat. Dr. Mark Hegsted testified before the Federal Trade Commission that the American diet is responsible for a multitude of cancers.

I think it is clear that the American diet is *indicted* as a cause of coronary heart disease. And it is pertinent, I think, to point out the same diet is now found [guilty] in terms of many forms of cancer: breast cancer, cancer of the colon, and others. [160]

An article in the prestigious *Advance in Cancer Research* journal concluded:

At present, we have overwhelming evidence ... [that] none of the risk factors for cancer is ... more significant than diet and nutrition. [161]

But old prejudices die hard. Dr. Max Gerson sarcastically pointed out that animal fodder is more carefully supervised than human nutrition. He observed that when rats are fed food from organically grown soil, they have perfectly healthy organs through many generations. However, rats fed a typical Western diet developed the same degenerative diseases we experience, including cancer.

Other groups of rats, living on ordinary food in the United States and Britain developed, within one generation, all the degenerative disease and pathology known in human beings ... Other experiments showed that rats susceptible to cancer showed a decline in incidence of cancer when given proper nutrition from the time of their birth. [162]

This is very compelling evidence and it indicts the typical American diet. Dr. Max Gerson did, however, point out that we should not focus on any one single dietary factor as the *cause* of cancer. We should see the big picture. We should no more look for a single cause of cancer as for a single magic-bullet cure. It is the many damaging food items, together with other environmental factors, that derange the body's metabolism and its organs, eventually resulting in various degenerative diseases including cancer. [163] Nevertheless, dietary causes of cancer are not equally weighted. Dr. Nancy Appleton noted the powerful degenerative effect that excess refined sugar has on the body, while other epidemiological studies show the powerful carcinogenic effect of high meat intake.

John Robbins, author of *A Diet for a New America*, observed that there is not a single population in the world with a high meat intake that does not have a high rate of colon cancer. He stated that even the conservative *Journal of the Association for the Advancement of Science* has now come to admit this fact. An article in the *Journal* reported:

> Populations on a high-meat, high-fat diet are more likely to develop colon cancer than individuals on a vegetarian or similar low-meat diet. [164]

The meat industry was thoroughly frightened by the financial implications of these admissions linking meat and cancer. Their typical response was to invoke the hereditary factor, blaming genetic factors for America's high cancer rate and the low cancer rate of the Japanese. However, Dr. John Berg and his colleagues at the National Cancer Institute debunked this theory. In a massive study of Japanese who immigrated to America and adopted the typical American diet, they found that colon cancer rates among Japanese immigrants had risen to match the colon cancer rates of their American neighbors. [165]

Dr. John Berg's research correlates well with one of the many conclusions Dr. Campbell drew from his study of the Chinese diet: a high risk of cancer is associated with the lack of fiber in a diet built around animal products. There is virtually no fiber in animal products. Ladies and gentlemen, the evidence is indisputable: the more fiber ingested the less the colon cancer rate; the less fiber eaten the greater is the colon cancer rate. [166] Fiber binds to cholesterol in the intestines and eliminates it, thereby reducing one important risk factor for cancer. [167] Fiber also acts like a broom, sweeping the bowel walls clean. [168] Fiber promotes stool formation and elimination. Low fiber diets are associated with constipation and the build-up of poisons in the colon due to the longer transit rates of waste in the colon. [169] These poisonous wastes are reabsorbed through the bowel wall into the blood stream and taken to other parts of the body, poisoning the cells. Fiber binds to harmful chemicals and carcinogens in the bowel and eliminates them. [170], [171] Fat clogs up the walls of the intestines like grease clogs up drains. [172]

But merely adding fiber to one's meat diet will not substantially solve the problem. [173] The digestion of meat produces strong carcinogens that poison the body. To digest meat the liver is stimulated to produce strong bile acids such as deoxycholic acid. But deoxycholic acid is converted by intestinal bacteria into powerful carcinogens that toxify the system. Of course, the situation is compounded and the chance of self-poisoning increased if there is a lack of fiber in the diet. [174]

After comparing the mortality rates from colon cancer and heart disease among various societies, John Robbins pointed out that the death rates from colon cancer and heart disease are almost identical and are matched to the per capita consumption of meat in each country. Some people who get colon cancer may show a low level of blood cholesterol due to a peculiar design of their metabolism that sends most of the excessive cholesterol to the bowels instead of pumping it into their blood stream. They avoid clogging up their arteries but are at risk for colon cancer. Thus *low blood cholesterol* can be *consistent* with a high incidence of colon cancer and is not the *cause* of colon cancer as the meat industry would have you believe. [175]

Famous last words can often provide a pause for much needed reflection. The link between meat consumption and colon cancer provides the framework for the following famous last words. In the face of studies linking colon cancer with meat eating, John Morgan, president of the Riverside Meat Packers, announced on May 7, 1976:

We shouldn't jump to any conclusions and do something foolish just because some study seems to say something that we know from common sense isn't true. Beef is the backbone of the American diet and it always has been. To think that meat of all things causes cancer is ridiculous. [176]

As fate would have it, on March 13, 1982, John Morgan died of cancer of the colon. The last word should be given to the most prolific woman author America, and indeed the world, has known. Ever ahead of her times in health reform and disease prevention, Ellen White wrote in 1909 of the link between meat consumption and cancer.

We do not mark out any precise line to be followed in diet; but we do say that in countries where there are fruits, grains, and nuts in abundance, flesh food is not the right food for God's people. I have been instructed that flesh food has a tendency to animalize the nature, to rob men and women of that love and sympathy which they should feel for everyone, and give the lower passions control over the higher powers of the being. If meat eating were ever healthful, it is not safe now. *Cancers, tumors, and pulmonary diseases are largely caused by meat eating.* [177] [Emphasis added.]

In correlating cancer with meat consumption, Ellen White was fifty years ahead of her time. One method by which meat eating causes cancer is by acidifying the blood. Dr. Gunther Enderlein, M.D., Ph. D. (1872–1968), found that blood acidity was a primary cause of the production of pathogenic microorganisms in the pleomorphic cycle of organisms associated with cancer. [178] Pleomorphism is the concept that many microorganisms such as bacteria can take on multiple life forms within a single life cycle. The concept that cancer can have a pleomorphic origin brings us to one of the most important recent advances in cancer research and cure. Dr. Harvey Bigelsen is the leading advocate today of curing cancer through nutritional and other related remedies based on the pleomorphic nature of cancer. To fully understand this concept, one must go back to the nineteenth century and review the debate between Drs. Louis Pasteur and Claude Bernard about the nature and causes of disease.

Dr. Louis Pasteur popularized the Galenic concept that diseases are caused by *external agents* that can be identified and destroyed. His ideas have become the fundamental doctrine of infectious disease medicine, which dominates the cancer research today. [179] His *modus operandi* was identifying the antigen or invading microbe and eliminating it by pharmaceutical weapons. He also developed and popularized the prevention of disease by vaccination. On the other hand the physiologist Dr. Claude Bernard contended that it is more important to emphasize strengthening the internal environment (the *milieu interieur* or *terrain* as he called it) as the most effective way of preventing disease. [180] He argued that if the immune system is healthy and strong, the invading microbe is powerless to bring on disease. He dramatically made his point by safely drinking a glass of water containing a large quantity of the deadly cholera germs before a French medical society gathering. [181] It was only on his death bed that Dr. Pasteur admitted that Dr. Bernard was right. He admitted in his dying breath: "Bernard is right ... the terrain is everything! The microbe is nothing." [182] Dr. Pasteur's death bed confession, repudiating his overemphasis on the external antigens as the cause of disease and the proper target for fighting it, has however been lost to modern Allopathic medicine.

Dr. Antoine Bechamp (1816–1908), a Professor of Medicine on the Medical Faculty at the University of Montpellier in France, took Dr. Bernard's ideas several leagues further. In so doing he re-defined the concept of disease. He discovered certain living protein entities he called microzymes, which played useful metabolic roles in the body, but which, under toxic conditions, could be transform into harmful microbes. Dr. Bigelsen emphasized the importance of this finding; arguing that it disproved Dr. Pasteur's concept that disease can only be caused by eternal agents.

> If Bernard provided the concept that it was the internal terrain that was important, Bechamp provided the mechanism that determines health or disease, and he showed how the system works. The fundamental question being argued was really, does the germ cause the disease, or does the disease cause the germ? Bechamp showed that the latter is generally the case, and he showed how. He identified fundamental biological units, which he called *microzymes*, which are the building blocks of microbes as well as other cells and which are today considered the precursors of DNA. When the body becomes toxic, the microzymes survive by changing into pathogenic microbes. Pasteur's concept that infectious disease can be caused only by external microbes was wrong. Rather, *Bechamp showed microbes to be secondary manifestation of the disease, a symptom rather than a cause.* [183] [Emphasis added.]

Ladies and gentlemen of the jury, mark this point well—if microbes are the secondary manifestations of disease, if they are merely the symptoms of disease, then attacking and destroying the microbes is really treating the *symptoms* of the underlying disease. Treating the symptom, for example the cancerous mass, is not focusing on the heart of the problem or disease. The real problem is the toxic condition of the body and the depressed immune system. Thus Dr. Bigelsen stated:

> Today we recognize that if the immune system is not healthy, a

number of acute infectious diseases can be caused by external, transmitted microbes. However, as Bernard so dramatically demonstrated, the healthy immune system is normally able to destroy external germs with no symptoms ever appearing. Most of us walk around constantly carrying germs that, given a weak immune system, would be associated with disease. On the other hand, if our immune system is damaged, both disease symptoms and appropriate microbes will appear ... If the immune system damage becomes long-standing, acute disease symptoms having been suppressed with medications, in time chronic degenerative disease will appear. If the immune system damage is severe enough, that disease is likely to be cancer. [184]

Ladies and gentlemen, if Dr. Bechamp was correct, the implications for the treatment of cancer and other chronic diseases are enormous. If Dr. Bechamp was indeed correct, then the proper approach for treating and preventing all degenerative disease, including cancer, is to strengthen the immune system, detoxify the body, and eliminate high acid-forming foods such as excess protein, refined sugar, and other refined carbohydrates. The cancer lump, and indeed the cancer virus, is merely the symptom of a deeper metabolic disease. Understanding the pleomorphic (a word that simply means *many forms*) nature of microorganisms and their healthy and pathogenic phases is the key to selecting the right remedy. Detoxification and nutritional modalities become the primary means of curing disease, including cancer. Bigelsen concluded:

If one can restore the immune system, and in particular the microzymes, to health, the cause of the disease will disappear and the body will become healthy once again. [185]

The pleomorphic nature of cancer was confirmed by the work of other researchers who followed Dr. Bechamp. The bacteriologist, microscopist, and engineer Dr. Royal Raymond Rife made significant discoveries about the nature of cancer in the 1920s and 1930s. [186] He invented a high-resolution darkfield microscope with which he was able to identify Bechamp's cancer-causing microorganisms. The microbes he identified with cancer had four forms.

A virus BX, associated with carcinoma;

A virus BY, associated with sarcoma and larger than BX;

A monococcoid form, found in the monocytes of the blood of more than 90% of cancer patients; and

Crytomyces pleomorphic fungi, identical morphologically to that of the orchid and the mushroom. [187]

Rife performed over 300 identical experiments. He repeatedly demonstrated that anyone of these microbial forms can change back into the BX form within thirty-six hours. He showed that these pathogens could produce a typical cancerous tumor in experimental animals. [188]

Rife had demonstrated pleomorphism, confirming the work of Bechamp and the other microbiologists who had found pleomorphic changes in organisms. He had also shown that, under appropriate conditions, a fungus which converts to a cancer causing "virus" could change back into a common and harmless bacterium. [189]

Ladies and gentlemen of the jury, you can be sure that the implications of Dr. Rife's work for the conventional treatment of cancer was not lost on the lucrative cancer industry. The American Medical Association immediately went to work to blacklist and shut down Dr. Rife and his research. Dr. Rife was brought to trial by the AMA on false charges. He was vindicated, but was ruined financially and his reputation tarnished in the eyes of an unsuspecting public. His work, which had great implications for the successful and economical treatment of cancer, faded from memory and his microscope discarded. [190] The experience of Dr. Rife and so many other nutritional scientists is a warning to anyone who thinks we have medical freedom in this country. Just introduce a procedure that undercuts the profits of the financial and industrial cartel who control medicine and see what happens.

Contemporaneous with Dr. Rife and continuing beyond him into the 1960s, the German doctor and bacteriologist Dr. Gunther Enderlein (1872–1968) did extensive work on the life cycle of bacteria. He published extensively on the subject in scientific journals and books. [191] Using the darkfield microscope he found tiny particles he called *protits* in the blood and body fluids. These *protits* normally appear in healthy forms but can develop into pathogenic forms, depending on the internal environment of the human body. [192] When the body is healthy these life forms work with the cells of the body in a symbiotic relationship to assist the immune system in its function. When, however, poor nutrition, emotional stress, and other harmful practices, like smoking, causes a change in the pH balance of the blood, these microbial life forms change into pathogenic forms that cause disease. [193] These discoveries led Dr. Enderlein to develop biological remedies that could rid the body of these harmful organism by changing them back into useful forms. Dr. Bigelsen stated:

> Building upon his research into the life cycles of the protits, Enderlein in the 1940s and 1950s developed biological remedies, plant medicines or fungal extracts, that are capable of changing the disease-producing endobionts back into harmless forms, restoring the body's symbiosis, correcting the tissue's acid-base balance, bolstering the body's immune system, and helping it restore the patient to health. [194]

The French scientist Dr. Gaston Naessens, later a Canadian citizen, perfected the high-resolution light microscope, which he used to identify minute entities in the blood. He named these entities *somatids*. He discovered that they were also pleomorphic in nature. In their pathogenic forms these somatids are associated with a variety of degenerative diseases, including cancer. [195] Ladies and gentlemen, Dr. Naessens' research also proved the folly of conventional medicine in attacking the symptom of cancer, the cancer lump. He demonstrated that only immunosupportive treatment modalities can remove the real cause of cancer: *an impaired immune system caused by a toxic internal environment*. Dr. Bigelsen summed up Dr. Naessens's life work in two succinct statements.

> Naessens' studies showed once and again both that (1) there are important pleomorphic microorganisms in our blood, and (2) cancer, as well as other degenerative diseases, and diseases previously thought to stem from independent, external causes (infectious diseases), are in fact caused by the internal bodily response to a toxic lifestyle and environment. [196]

Dr. Gaston Naessens' work was endorsed and furthered by the painstaking work of Dr. Virginia Livingston-Wheeler, who demonstrated the role of pleomorphic bacteria in cancer. She developed important techniques using immunological protocols in treating cancer patients. [197]

Ladies and gentlemen of the jury, in closing this segment of testimony, I ask you to ponder well the pivotal question, if cancer is truly a systemic disease and not a localized malignancy, what is the best approach to both curing it and preventing it? As with other degenerative diseases, modern medicine offers only symptomatic remedies designed to cut out, burn out, or poison out the outward symptom of this disease. They doggedly follow this approach despite its manifest failures. They follow this hapless course because of financial incentives and because, as Dr. Julian Whitaker contended:

They mistakenly assume the body's own immune system cannot be galvanized to heal itself. [198]

Alternative medicine offers various nutritional and detoxification approaches designed to get at the root of the matter. Dr. Whitaker contended that cancer can be beaten by harnessing the body's immune system's awesome healing power. [199] Although the medical establishment has a medical monopoly on the symptomatic treatment of cancer, fully 50% of cancer victims eventually vote with their feet and seek out practitioners of alternative medicine. [200] There is no doubt which approach has shown better results. In the next section you will hear testimony regarding the pharmaceutical treatment of cancer. In the third segment you will be presented evidence on the efficacy of nutritional approaches to cancer treatment.

Section 2

CUT, BURN & POISON: CAPITALIZING ON THE POLITICS OF DEATH

There is a way that seems right to a man
But its end is the way of death.

Proverbs 16: 25.

Ladies and gentlemen of the jury, knowing the cause of cancer, common sense would dictate that its prevention and cure should involve eliminating the root cause of this metabolic dysfunction. Ordinarily this is the way it should be. However, as in the case of other degenerative diseases, the rational remedy that should be pursued in treating cancer has been derailed by the hailstorm of political and medical correctness that has been and is presently deluging America. In 1971, when the war being waged by the American Medical association, the American Cancer Society, the National Cancer Institute, and the Food and Drug Administration against the practitioners of alternative cancer medicine was at its height, Grant Leake, Chief of the fraud section of California's Food and Drug Bureau, solemnly and pontifically announced:

> We are going to protect them [that is, the public] even if some
> of them don't want to be protected [he was referring to patients
> seeking alternative forms of cancer treatment] [1]

This declaration would prove to be a death sentence to millions of

Americans who were subsequently deprived of a choice of remedies in the treatment of cancer.

In the treatment of cancer, conventional medicine primarily relies on surgery, radiation, and chemotherapy, often characterized as the cut, burn, and poison modalities. Conventional medicine is not interested in *curing* the cancer, despite claims to the contrary. Nor is conventional medicine a strong advocate in preventing cancer. By contrast alternative therapies include nutrition, nutritional supplements, enzymes, detoxification, change in lifestyle, and stress control to prevent and reverse the cancer. We should pause to ask ourselves, which is the best, safest, and most effective approach to curing cancer. A person's answer to these critical questions depends upon their view of the nature of cancer and what causes it.

To sum up the previous testimony presented to you, conventional medicine views cancer as a *local problem*, focuses on the *mass of malignant cells*, and tries to cut them out, burn them out by radiation, or poison them with chemical drugs. The radiation and chemotherapy modalities depend for their success on killing off the cancer cells before destroying too many healthy cells. They hope to eliminate the *symptom of cancer* before the patient is destroyed. [2] Generally the symptoms of cancer, not its causes, have become the focus of cancer research, clinical work, and therapy. [3] Unfortunately, these remedies often compound the problem. Often the cancer is made to spread by cutting into it. [4] Radiation and chemotherapy further suppress an already weakened immune system, undermining the body's ability to defend itself from the cancer and secondary infections. Chemotherapy toxifies and poisons an already poisoned system, which was a contributing factor in the development of the cancer in the first place. Most cancer patients die from chemotherapeutic poisoning and not from the cancer itself. Donald McAlvany compares the draconian remedy of chemotherapy to the use of a .44 Magnum to perform surgery.

Chemotherapy is a little like taking a wart off your toe with a .44 magnum. It is guaranteed to get the wart every time—but, alas, the toe disappears as well. Chemotherapy kills the good (including the immune system) and the bad, and leaves the body with very little to fight back with. The long-term survival rate for those cancer patients receiving chemotherapy is about five percent. [5]

Ladies and gentlemen, Dr. John McDougall contended that the use of surgery and radiation in breast cancer is based on the incorrect view that cancer is a localized disease.

Surgery and radiation techniques are based on the erroneous belief that breast cancer is a disease confined to the breast at the time of diagnosis and that removing the tumor in the breast will halt the disease ...

Studies show that before the tumor is discovered in the breast, when the cancer is still virtually microscopic in size, cancer cells are entering the blood stream ...

The dietary factors, as well as other factors, that are involved in the cause of breast cancer affect all the breast tissues. Breast cancer, therefore, develops not just as a disease of the one detected site but as a disease that affects all breast tissues ... When the opposite breast is examined in women diagnosed as having breast cancer, in almost 100 percent of the cases various stages from precancerous changes to actually cancerous lumps are found here too. [6]

Alternative medicine advocates view cancer as a symptom of extreme toxicity, especially of the liver, which interferes with cellular metabolism and depresses the immune system. Hence they stress detoxification of the body and strengthening of the immune system to enhance the natural healing mechanisms of the body. [7] Dr. Max Gerson reasoned that cancer is not a single cellular problem, or a specific illness, but a chronic degenerative disease that eventually involves all the essential organs of the body. [8] This systemic view of cancer suggests the correct approach to treatment.

What is essential is not the growth itself or the visible symptoms; it is the damage of the whole metabolism, including the loss of defense, immunity and healing power. [9]

The metabolism and its concentration in the liver should be put in the foreground, not the cancer as a symptom. There, the outcome of the cancer is determined as the clinical favorable results, failures and autopsies clearly demonstrate. There, the sentence will be passed—whether the tumors can be killed, dissolved, absorbed, eliminated and finally, whether the body can be restored. [10]

Conventional medical practitioners have for a long time held that cancer is incurable. [11] In contrast, practitioners of alternative remedies believe cancer is reversible or curable through detoxification, proper nutrition, and supplements. Drs. Quillin and Gerson have written that:

> Cancer growth can both be slowed and even reversed in the right conditions. [12] [13]

In recent decades the cancer establishment has appeared to change its position on the curability of cancer. They now hold that cancer is curable *if* detected early enough and *before* it metastasizes or spreads to other parts of the body. However, *their definition of cure relates only to the removal of the mass by surgery, radiation, or drugs.* In the nutritional approach, a cure is complete only when the cancerous mass is eliminated, the metabolic dysfunction is corrected, and the immune system strengthened to insure that the cancer does not recur.

Notice how Dr. Ralph Weilerstein, speaking on behalf of the California Department of Public Health in 1972, related the cure of cancer only to surgery or radiation.

> The use of laetrile in early cancer cases to the exclusion of conventional treatment might well be dangerous since treatment with acceptable, modern curative methods—surgery or radiation— would thereby be delayed potentially until such time as metastases had occurred and the cancer, therefore, might no longer be curable. [14]

On December 18, 1972, Mabel Burnett, writing on behalf of the American Cancer Society (ACS) to G. Edward Griffin, confined proven cancer cures to conventional forms of treatment only.

> Thank you for your note. There are proven cures—if detected in time—surgery and/or radiation and, more and more, chemotherapy is playing its part. [15]

Notice again the caveat, if detected in time, in the statement by the ACS.

The cancer establishment publically and repeatedly acknowledges that they have no cure if metastasis has set in.

A patient who has clinically detectable distant metastases when first seen has virtually a hopeless prognosis, as do patients who were apparently free of distant metastasis at that time but who subsequently returned with distant metastases. [16]

While conventional medicine admits its hopelessness in the face of metastasized cancer, nutritional therapists such as Dr. Patrick Quillin and Dr. Max Gerson have amply demonstrated that end stage metastasized cancers are not a problem for alternative therapy; so long as a vital organ (such as the liver) has not yet been completely destroyed by the cancer, and the immune system has not been completely shattered by the harmful effects of the proven cures of radiation and chemotherapy.

But, ladies and gentlemen of the jury, does the cancer establishment really *cure* cancer in its early stages by surgery, radiation, or chemotherapy? That depends on their definition of *cure* and their view of the nature of cancer. Removal of the cancer tumor is not the same thing as ridding the body of cancer. Nutritional practitioners point out that metabolic dysfunction due to toxicity in the body is continually creating new cancer cells, which are not detectable until years later. Conventional medicine falsely equates cancer cure with the removal of the *visible sign* of cancer, while ignoring the *invisible* yet steadily growing cancer tumors. Their view of cancer is that it is a malignant cell dividing without check. Hence if the tumor mass can be cut out, blasted out of existence by radiation, or killed by poison, they have cured the patient. Conventional medicine believes that if the patient lives five years after treatment without a recurrence, a cure has taken place.

However, surviving five years after surgery, radiation, or chemotherapy is no proof that one is cured of cancer. By the time a cancerous lump has grown to the size it can be detected (it takes ten to fourteen years or more), the cancer has already spread to other parts of the body; it is only a matter of time for these new cancer colonies to become visible. So removing the lump does not and cannot cure the patient of cancer. Merely removing the lump may eradicate cancer from the one visible site, but it does not remove cancer from other sites not yet detectable. Cancer patients need to be informed that since cancer takes ten to fourteen years or more to manifest as a visible tumor, surviving five years after removable of the visible mass, does not mean that they were cured of cancer. Dr. John McDougall made this point well.

Because the metastatic cancer cells are slow-growing and hidden in vital areas of the body, some people are fooled into believing that a cure has been achieved by the initial surgery. Usually these microscopic tumors produce no symptoms until near the time of death. The largely silent nature of the disease, combined with the fact that in up to 90 percent of cases the ultimate cause of death will be cancer of the breast, shows why five-year survival rates don't represent anything close to a cure.

Medical professionals and representatives of cancer organizations who use such short term survival statistics to support the success of present day therapy are seriously misrepresenting to the public the actual course and outcome of breast cancer. [17]

Doctors of alternative medicine vainly point out that because cancer is a systemic degenerative disease, in which the patient's metabolism and immune system is in disarray, removing one visible symptom of the disease does not by any stretch of the imagination constitute a cure. Removing the visible symptom only shifts the fight to the invisible systemic nature of cancer. Dr. Patrick Quillin stated:

We have also made the erroneous assumption that "no detectable cancer" means "no cancer." A million cancer cells are undetectable by even the most sensitive medical equipment. A billion cancer cells become a tiny and nearly undetectable "lump." When the surgeon says, "We think we got it all"—that is when the war on cancer must become an invisible battle involving the patient's well-nourished immune system. [18]

Ladies and gentlemen of the jury, the evidence proves repeatedly that conventional medicine vainly treats only the system of the disease but never the cause of the disease. This great gulf divides the medical establishment from the minority of physicians courageously trying to educate the public as to the true nature of cancer and the viability of alternative remedies.

Normally this difference of opinion would generate healthy competition in research and practice, providing the patient with an enlightened choice of remedies. Unfortunately, the medical establishment and the cancer associations such as the American Cancer Association and the National Cancer Institute have enlisted the brute force of government on their side. They have enlisted the naked force of the law to help them set up medical monopolies in the treatment of cancer. They have branded alternative cancer therapies as unproven, questionable, dubious, quackery, and fraudulent; [19] when the truth is, it is they who are deceiving the public.

The medical establishment and the FDA have shamelessly called Dr. Linus Pauling, the two-time recipient of the Nobel Prize—whose shoes they cannot even begin to fill—a *quack* because of his work with vitamin C in cancer treatment. He incurred their wrath by demonstrating that vitamin C can improve the quality and quantity of the life of cancer patients. [20] [21]

Thus, ladies and gentlemen of the jury, the *war on cancer* has not been a war against the *disease of cancer*, but in reality a war between the medical establishment and the practitioners of alternative medicine. In getting the long arm of the government to mandate that no form of cancer treatment but the standard *cut, burn, and poison* methods should be practiced in America, the medical establishment has unconstitutionally deprived every man, woman, and child in America who has fallen victim to this killer disease of the right to choose and their right to life. In protest of this government-sponsored monopoly of cancer treatment, Dr. Patrick Quillin wrote:

It is unconstitutional to think that protecting the end-stage and otherwise un-treatable cancer patient from inexpensive and non-toxic therapies is a government obligation ... to quote Hippocrates, the father of modern medicine, 2400 years ago: "Extreme diseases call for extreme measures." Nutrition therapy, surely, is no more extreme than chemotherapy, radiation therapy or surgery. [22]

An examination of the record of accomplishment of the cut, burn, and poison method of cancer treatment will demonstrate which treatment approach is indeed unproven, questionable and dangerous. Let us look first at the surgical treatment of cancer.

Breast cancer was the first form of cancer that physicians tried to remove by surgical means. [23] Surgery is still the first treatment of choice for about 67% of cancer patients. [24] It is much higher for breast cancer. Radical mastectomy was introduced by Dr. William Halstead of John Hopkins University Medical School at the end of the nineteenth century. [25] Radical mastectomy involves removing the entire breast, lymph nodes in the axilla (arm pit), and underlying chest muscles. It has been the standard by which to judge other surgical procedures for breast cancer. Dr. John McDougall listed the following range of surgical procedures that have been used to treat breast cancer.

* Lumpectomy—removal of the entire tumor without adjoining tissue.

* Partial or segmental mastectomy—removal of a large section of breast with tumor and surrounding tissues.

* Simple mastectomy—removal of the entire breast.

* Modified radical mastectomy—removal of the entire breast as well as adjacent nodes in the axilla or arm pit.

* Radical mastectomy—removal of the entire breast, lymph nodes in the arm pit and underlying chest muscles.

* Extended radical mastectomy—removal of the entire breast, lymph nodes in the arm pit, underlying chest muscle, and lymph nodes next to the sternum or breast bone. [26]

In 1985, Dr. John McDougall contended that no significant advantage of one surgical procedure over another has been found, judging by the survival rates after surgery. Incredibly, despite improved modern surgical techniques combined with radiation and chemotherapy, the death rate from breast cancer did not improve during the seventy-year period prior to 1985, the year Dr. McDougall completed his investigation. [27] Consider the thousands of women subjected to unnecessary mutilation, disfigurement, and shame, only to die in the end!

Dr. Andrew Weil observed as early as 1983 that the evidence was clear that the more radical forms of breast surgery were no more effective than the simple Lumpectomy, yet surgeons were still performing these extensive and mutilating surgeries.

> Surgery that is too expensive is as destructive as surgery that is unnecessary. Radical mastectomy, a horribly mutilating procedure that leaves severe psychological as well as physical scars, is no more effective at preventing recurrences of breast cancer than simple "Lumpectomy" or simple mastectomy followed by radiation and other supporting treatment. Despite this fact, surgeons who believe in cutting drastically have been reluctant to abandon the radical mastectomy or listen to the good arguments against it. [28]

Dr. John McDougall concurred with the argument that removal of the breast in an attempt to cure cancer is an unnecessary and mutilating procedure that creates psychological damage to the woman.

> For most women, removal of the breast is an unnecessary form of mutilation that can destroy self-esteem and sexual identity and often results in severe psychological depression. Every day physicians and patients are recognizing that the less surgery a woman receives in order to remove the obvious tumor, the better off she will be in every respect. [29]

After analyzing data from the cancer Registry at Syracuse, New York, on 3,558 women with breast cancer over a nineteen-year period, Dr. C. Barber Mueller, head of the department of Surgery at McMaster University in Ontario, concluded:

> Age, stage, or type of growth, operative therapy, or time at risk, do not determine the time of death or alter the 90 percent certainty that death will be due to cancer of the breast. [30]

Dr. John McDougall argued that it was folly to rely primarily on surgery to treat breast cancer. He stated that when the cancer is large enough to be detected, it has in most cases already spread throughout the body. [31] So surgery as a remedy of first choice is like doing too little too late. Dr. McDougall further pointed out:

When metastatic lesions appear two years or so after a small breast tumor was found, the spread through the bloodstream probably occurred about two years after the original cell in the breast became cancerous, or eight years before diagnosis! [32]

Ladies and gentlemen of the jury, the evidence is convincingly clear that surgery is not a cure for breast cancer. It does nothing to reverse the cause of the disease. Long term studies show that at least 75% of the women diagnosed as having breast cancer will die with evidence of active disease in their bodies. Dr. McDougall contended that the death rate is higher; he stated that twenty years after diagnosis, 80% of women with breast cancer will be dead and 88% of these deaths will be due to breast cancer. [33]

Twenty-five years ago, the surgery most routinely used for breast cancer was radical mastectomy. Since then new methods favor a Lumpectomy or removal of the lump, followed by radiation and/or chemotherapy. [34] Despite this less invasive approach, we are still losing the war against breast cancer. Since 1950 breast cancer has increase by 60%, despite the war on cancer and the legion of breast surgeries performed. [35] Breast cancer struck one in twenty women in 1950, and by 1990 it was striking one in nine women. [36] Clearly breast cancer is increasing faster than we can remove it surgically. It is time we put more emphasis on *preventing* breast cancer. Yet only 5% of the $1.8 billion annual budget for the National Cancer Institute is spent on prevention! [37]

Surgery for breast cancer and other forms of cancer may have its place, but it should not be a first choice. In light of the fact that detoxification and nutritional therapy is much more effective in curing cancer, the risks of surgery must carefully be considered. It should be understood that it is the risks of *surgery as a sole therapy for cancer*, not emergency surgery followed by nutritional therapy that poses serious complications. Some nutritionists follow Dr. Patrick Quillin's lead and combine nutritional therapy with traditional remedies such as surgery, especially where the tumor has been encapsulated and can be removed without bursting its collagen envelope.

Comprehensive cancer treatment uses traditional cancer therapies to reduce the tumor burden, while concurrently building up the "terrain" of the cancer patient to fight the cancer on a microscopic level. This is the "one-two punch" that will eventually bring the Predator of cancer to its knees. [38]

Notice what he said about building up the *terrain* and fighting cancer at the *microscopic level* after the surgery. He recognized that cancer is not a regionalized lump, therefore removing one visible symptom of the disease, the cancerous lump, is not a cure. Dr. Patrick Quillin fully understood the systemic nature of cancer.

> Cancer is a degenerative disease of abnormal metabolism throughout the body—not just a regionalized lump or bump. [39]

One recognized complication of surgery is that cutting into to a cancer tumor may facilitate its spread through the body. Even a biopsy can result in a spread of the cancer. [40] Surgery can also create scar tissue around the cancer, thus insulating it from the immune system and the pancreatic enzymes that can destroy it. [41] The greatest drawback of surgery alone (in the absence of nutritional modalities) is that its effectiveness in curing cancer or prolonging survival time after surgery has not been effectively demonstrated. Mr. G. Edward Griffin, after reviewing the evidence, contended:

> Perhaps the greatest indictment against surgery is the fact that, statistically, there is no solid evidence that patients who submit to surgery have any greater life expectancy, on the average, than who do not. [42]

Mr. Griffin stated that the first statistical analysis of the benefits of surgery were performed in France by Dr. Leroy d' Etoilles in 1844, and published by the French Academy of Science. Over a period of thirty years, the histories of 2,781 cancer patients were submitted by a broad spectrum of physicians (174 in all); it was found that surgery prolonged post-surgical survival by only one year and five months—about the same average today, over 150 years later. [43] An even more ominous and frightening finding was that surgery may have *shortened* the life of the cancer patients. Dr. Leroy d' Etoilles found that patients who *refused surgery* lived longer than surgical cancer patients.

> The net effect of surgery was in prolonging life two months for men and six months for women. But that was only in the first few years after the initial diagnosis. After that period, those who had

not accepted treatment [surgery] had the greater survival potential by about fifty percent. [44]

That was in 1844. What about today? Modern research reveals the same thing. There is not much difference between surgical and non-surgical patients as far as survival time is concerned. Rather, many physicians have found that non-surgical cases live longer than surgical cases! Dr. Hardin Jones, Ph.D., former professor of medical physics and physiology at the University of Berkeley, declared after years of careful analysis of the data:

> Life tables truly representative of untreated cancer patients must be adjusted for the fact that the inherently longer-lived cases are more likely to be transferred to the "treated" category than to remain in the "untreated until death."

> The apparent life expectancy of untreated cases [non-surgical cases] of cancer after such adjustment in the table seems to be greater than that of the treated [surgical] cases. [45]

About 16% of breast-cancer patients will survive five years or more after surgery. For lung cancer patients the survival rate is 5 to 10%. [46]

While the course of breast cancer in America is tragic, despite the widespread use of proven methods, the history of prostate cancer is even worse. There are no good early screening methods for prostate cancer, so by the time it is detected, in 85% of the cases, it has already spread beyond the prostate gland. Moreover Dr. Patrick Quillin noted that there is no essential difference in survival rates between surgical and non-surgical cases of prostate cancer. [47]

We must consider imagining the unthinkable. Could there be a profit motive behind these extensive and unnecessary surgical procedures? In *Death by Medicine*, Gary Null, Ph.D. and Carolyn Dean, MD, stated that in 1974 the U.S. Congressional House Subcommittee Oversight Investigation found that there were 17.6% (2.4 million) unnecessary surgeries performed that year; and following up on that finding, they estimated that there were 7.5 million unnecessary surgeries in 2001.[48] Does the profit motive also lead to unnecessary cancer surgeries? Award winning author and journalist, Kenny Ausubel, thinks so. In his highly acclaimed book, *When Healing Becomes A Crime: The Amazing Story of the*

Hoxsey Cancer Clinics and the Return of Alternative Therapies, published in 2000, he documented the admission of Dr. Paul Hawley, past director of the American College of Surgeons, that *money* was behind the amount of unnecessary surgeries that are performed. In reference to cancer surgeries Kenny Ausubel observed:

> Surgery is similarly a vastly lucrative practice, acting as the third financial mooring in the tripod of cancer treatments. The more radical the operation the more costly. Since surgeons are rewarded monetarily for the magnitude of their handiwork, excess becomes a pervasive incentive for success. The amount of unnecessary surgery is high. [49]

Ladies and gentlemen of the jury, the track record of radiation therapy is even more dismal than that of surgery. Radiation therapy is given to about 60% of all cancer patients. The logic behind radiation therapy is similar to that of surgery. Surgery is an attempt to remove the outward visible symptom of cancer by *cutting* out the mass, while the goal of radiation treatment is to *burn* it out. Neither approach tries to reverse the cause of the cancer. Radiation therapy is dangerous because it not only often increases the malignancy of the existing cancer, but it often causes cancer itself. Consider how radiation sometimes increases the malignancy of the tumor. The average tumor is composed of cancerous and not-cancerous cells. The non-cancerous cells are more vulnerable to radiation than the cancer cells. The net effect of radiation is to reduce the size of the tumor by killing non-cancerous cells, while leaving a concentrated residue of cancerous cells! Dr. John Richardson conceded this fact.

> Radiation and/or radiomimetic poisons will reduce palpable gross or measurable tumefaction. Often this reduction may amount to seventy-five percent or more of the mass of the growth. These agents have a selective effect—radiation and poisons. They selectively kill everything except the definitively neoplastic [cancer] cells. [50]

The smaller, highly potent residual mass of cancer left after radiation therapy, is more life threatening to the patient because it is more malignant and promotes metastasis.

As all experienced clinicians know—or at least should know—

after radiation or poisons have reduced the gross tumefaction of the lesion the patient's general well-being does not substantially improve. To the contrary, there is often an explosive or fulminating increase in the biological malignancy of his lesion. This is marked by the appearance of diffuse metastasis and a rapid deterioration in the general vitality followed shortly by death. [51]

Radiation after mastectomy has had widespread use, but a more conservative approach of radiation after simple Lumpectomy was first recommended in 1954. Sometimes radiation is the only form of therapy employed after a small portion of the tumor is removed for diagnosis. Although the recurrence of cancer is only 10% when radiation is prescribed after mastectomy or Lumpectomy, Dr. John McDougall has expressed concern with such frequent use of radiation therapy because of the terrible side effects and the destructive effects on the immune system. Side effects include radiation sickness, depression, loss of appetite, breast deformity, rib fractures, and inflammation in the lungs. [52] Dr. Patrick Quillin listed two additional side effects of radiation therapy in the long term: birth defects and infertility. In the short term he listed: mouth sores and oral ulcers (which can interfere with the ability to eat), rectal sores, fistulas, bladder ulcers, diarrhea, and colitis. [53]

What are the benefits of this deadly remedy? Do the benefits outweigh the very serious and sometimes fatal side effects? Research accomplished by the National Adjuvant Breast Project on the effects of radiation on cancer patients show that there is no discernable benefit to the patient in terms of increased survival.

From the data available it would seem that the use of post-operative irradiation has provided no discernable advantage to patients so treated in terms of increasing the proportion who were free of disease for as long as five years. [54]

A very serious concern for the public upon whom this deadly remedy is being foisted as a proven cure, is the fact that studies have demonstrated that women receiving radiation after mastectomy have died *sooner* than those not receiving radiation. Dr. McDougall agreed with Dr. Quillin, stating:

Women receiving radiation after mastectomy have been shown to die sooner than those for whom this additional therapy was not prescribed. [55]

The drain on the immune system after major surgery, coupled with the additional damage to the immune system by the radiation therapy, is felt to be a major contributing factor for these early deaths. [56] Radiation kills lymphocytes, which are important to the body's immune defenses. The resulting depression of the immune system increases the risk of metastatic disease. Depression of the immune system worsens women's survival rate after radiation therapy. [57]

For fear of talking themselves right out of a job, radiologists do not generally discuss or acknowledge the harm that radiation does to the patient. Nor do they generally question the value of radiation as a medical modality. Yet there have been exceptions. Dr. William Powers, Director of the Division of Radiation Therapy at Washington University School of Medicine, lamented the increased morbidity that results from radiation therapy.

> Although preoperative and postoperative radiation therapy have been used extensively and for decades, it is still not possible to prove unequivocal clinical benefit from this combined treatment ... Even if the rate of cure does improve with a combination of radiation and therapy, it is necessary to establish the cost in increased morbidity which may occur in patients without favorable response to the additional therapy. [58]

Another well-respected radiologist, Dr. Phillip Rubin, Chief of the Division of Radiotherapy at the University of Rochester Medical School, also admitted in an article in the *Journal of the American Medical Association* that the statistics show no increase in survival time from radiation treatment.

> The clinical evidence and statistical data in numerous reviews are cited to illustrate that no increase in survival has been achieved by the addition of irradiation. [59]

Moreover, the evidence is convincing that radiation can cause the development of other types of cancer in the cancer patient. How wise it is to treat a disease with a procedure that spreads the disease simultaneously with treatment? Dr. Patrick Quillin cited a study involving 400,000 cancer patients who were treated either with chemotherapy or radiation. Those treated with radiation had an increased risk for a certain type of leukemia. [60] The fact that x-rays induce cancer has been well known to the medical community for many years. In 1971 a research team headed by Dr. Robert W. Gibson at the University of Buffalo reported that less than a dozen routine medical x-rays to the same part of the body increases the risk of leukemia in males by at least 60%. [61]

Radiation also weakens the immune system, resulting in death from a multitude of secondary causes. Post-radiation death from heart attack, pulmonary pneumonia, or respiratory failure should really be listed as *death from cancer treatment*. Dr. John Richardson made this point in 1972:

I have seen patients who have been paralyzed by cobalt spine radiation, and after vitamin treatment their HCG test is faintly positive. We got their cancer, but the radiogenic manipulation is such that they can't walk ... It's the cobalt that will kill not the cancer. [62]

A study of breast cancer treatments at Oxford University noted that many women who received radiation died of heart attacks because their hearts had been weakened by the radiation treatments. [63] Increased morbidity from radiation is not generally discussed. Doing so would expose the inefficacy of this so-called *proven* cancer cure to public scrutiny.

Ladies and gentlemen of the jury, chemotherapy is, in the opinion of some, perhaps the most deadly of the methods used in conventional medicine for fighting cancer. It is now given to 75% of all American cancer patients. [64] Chemotherapy is a spin-off from chemical warfare research during World Wars I and II. Researchers found that mustard gas killed bone marrow and lymphoid tissue, so they injected it into mice with lymphomas and observed a remission. From those early beginnings chemotherapy was born. It is now dominated by creative combinations of drugs designed to kill the cancer cell. Over the years the method of delivery of the chemo drugs has improved. Instead of large doses given all at once, a fractionated drip infusion procedure evolved in the 1980s to control the powerful side effects these poisons have on the human body. [65] It is in the area of chemotherapy research that the search for the magic-bullet against cancer is focused. But what is the track record of this dangerous remedy? Dr. Albert Braverman, professor of oncology at the State University of New York, wrote in the *Lancet:*

Many medical oncologists recommend chemotherapy for virtually any tumor, with hopefulness undiscouraged by almost invariable failure. [66]

Dr. Ulrich Abel, Ph.D., of Heidelberg Tumor Center in Germany, reviewed the world literature on the use of chemotherapy alone as a cancer cure and found that it is helpful in only 3% of the patients with epithelial cancers, such as of the breast, lung, colon, and prostate. These forms of cancers kill 80% of cancer victims. Dr. Ulrich Abel then concluded:

... a sober and unprejudiced analysis of the literature has rarely revealed any therapeutic success by the regimens in question [the chemotherapy treatment of cancer]. [67]

The results of chemotherapy are often worse than the disease. Dr. Patrick Quillin quoted Dr. Johan Bjorksten as stating that chemotherapy can destroy the immune system beyond a point of no return, which increases the risk for early death from infections and other cancers. [68] Like its cousin, radiation therapy, chemotherapy causes cancer in the patients it is used against. In support of this opinion, Dr. Patrick Quillin cited the opinions of a number of researchers reported in the *New England Journal of Medicine.* These researchers found that the risk of developing leukemia from chemotherapy treatment of ovarian cancer outweighs the benefits of the therapy. [69] Dr. Patrick Quillin also noted that Tamoxifen, used in breast cancer patients, is carcinogenic. Recorded data shows that there is a 60% increase in cancer in the Tamoxifen-treated patients. [70] Tamoxifen works on the principle that there are receptors on cancer cells to which estrogen attaches, promoting their rapid growth. Tamoxifen attaches to these receptors on the cancer cells, blocking the activity of estrogen.

Chemotherapy suffers from similar defects that radiation therapy suffers from: healthy human cells are more easily damaged by the chemo drugs. Hence the net effect is to shrink the tumor by the reduction of non-cancerous cells, while leaving a residual mass of highly potent cancer cells. This potent mass of cancer cells is both resistant to further chemical poisoning and a factor in spreading the disease.

Similarly, blasting a typically malnourished cancer patient with
bolus (high doses once per week) injections of chemotherapy
alone may elicit an initial shrinkage of the tumor, but the few
tumor cells that survive this poison become resistant to therapy
and may even accelerate the course of the disease in the now
immune-suppressed patient. [71]

Chemo drugs are carcinogenic; that is they cause cancer. They are used
because physicians believe that they will kill off more cancer cells before
they kill the patient. But being carcinogenic they can initiate cancer growth
which shows up years later! The theory behind chemotherapy is that it
selectively attacks rapidly dividing cells. Apart from this, the chemo drugs
cannot distinguish between normal and cancerous cells. If the cancer cells
divide faster than normal cells, more cancer cells will be killed than normal
cells. This is true for some cancers. But if the cancer is slow growing, there
is no chance that the chemo drugs will work. In such cases more normal
non-cancerous cells will be killed than cancer cells. [72]

Other serious problems are associated with the use of chemotherapy.
Firstly, many human cells are rapidly dividing cells in their natural function. The rapidly dividing normal cells include cells of the hair, immune
system, and tongue. These cells are often the unfortunate victims of chemotherapy. Thus loss of hair, depressed immune function, and loss of taste
often plague the chemotherapy patient. [73] Secondly, the chemo drugs
also catch the blood cells in the act of dividing, thereby damaging them
and causing blood poisoning. Thirdly, the reproductive organs are also
affected. The result may be sterility. Fourthly, brain function, eyesight,
and hearing can also be impaired. This is only a partial listing of the side
effects of chemotherapy. Summing up the terrible side effects of chemotherapy, G. Edward Griffin observed:

Every conceivable body function is disrupted with such agony for
the patient that many of them elect to die of the cancer rather than
to continue treatment. [74]

Dr. John McDougall also noted that many women, if not most, being
treated for breast cancer by chemotherapy stop the course of treatment
prematurely because of the serious side effects of the drugs. He stated that
these side effects might include: hair loss, nausea, loss of nerve function,
anemia, diarrhea, cystitis, vomiting, and oral ulcers. [75] Because of the

depressed immune system he noted that viral infections are twice as common in women receiving chemotherapy for breast cancer. [76]

Chemo drugs are described as radiomimetic, because they mimic radiation therapy. However they are more deadly than radiation to the patient. While radiation affects the site of irradiation, these drugs travel to every cell, doing their baleful damage throughout the body. The immune system is weakened and the spreading of the cancer is often facilitated! Dr. John Richardson has emphasized this point:

> Both radiation therapy and attempts to "poison out" result in a profound hostal immunosuppression that greatly increases the susceptibility to metastasis. [77]

Ladies and gentlemen, let us now consider testimony concerning survival rates after chemotherapy. Does the evidence demonstrate the effectiveness of these drugs in terms of patient survival? Do the benefits outweigh the list of morbid and deadly side effects? Is life expectancy increased? Dr. John Trelford at the Department of Obstetrics and Gynecology at Ohio State University Hospital does not think so, at least as far as cervical cancers are concerned.

> At the present time, chemotherapy of gynecological tumors does not appear to have increased life expectancy except in sporadic cases. [78]

Dr. Saul A. Rosenberg, associate Professor of Medicine and Radiology at Stanford University School of Medicine, poignantly described the sad course of failure in administering chemo drugs to cancer patients in general.

> Worthwhile palliation is achieved in many patients. However, there will be the inevitable relapse of the malignant lymphoma, and, either because of drug resistance or drug intolerance, the disease will recur, requiring modifications of the chemotherapy program and eventually failure to control the disease process. [79]

Dr. Charles Moertal of the Mayo Clinic has admitted that only a small fraction of patients get a minor transient period of palliative relief. He stated that the failure rate of chemotherapy is as high as 85%.

Our most effective regimens are fraught with risks and side effects and practical problems; and after this price is paid by all the patients we have treated, only a small fraction are rewarded with a transient period of usually incomplete tumor regression ...

Our accepted and traditional curative efforts, therefore, yield a failure rate of 85% ... Some patients with gastrointestinal cancer can have a very long survival with no treatment whatsoever. [80]

This is a telling admission from the advocates of conventional cancer therapies: 85% failure rate is acceptable! For cancer that has metastasized, the hopelessness of chemotherapy is even more apparent. Here success is zero. Dr. Robert Sullivan of the Department of Cancer Research at the Lahey Clinic Foundation admitted that conventional medicine has no weapons against cancer that has already spread.

There has been an enormous undertaking of cancer research to develop anti-cancer drugs for use in the management of neoplastic [cancer] disease in man. However, progress has been slow, and no chemical agents capable of inducing a general curative effective in disseminated forms of cancer have yet been developed. [81]

Ladies and gentlemen, if this third method in the arsenal of orthodox methods of cancer cure is toxic, immunosuppressant, carcinogenic, and futile, why does the cancer establishment continue to promote it as a *proven* and *effective* cure for cancer? The answer is sobering. The cancer establishment, bowing to the wishes of a vast industrial oil and chemical industry, are boldly engaging in psychological conditioning to keep a misinformed public dependent upon their medical services. *The motive is profit.* The side effects are death and disability on a wanton scale. Even through chemotherapy is considered by many to be substantially void of value and positively harmful, it is prescribed as a remedy to an ignorant populace, to keep them from looking elsewhere for alternative cures that are not sanctioned by the establishment. The alternative cancer cures are effective and cheap because they are based on obeying the laws of nutrition and health. The cancer establishment is waging a deadly serious war against the natural laws of the Creator, and we are the victims of that war. The remedies that the Creator established for maintaining and achieving health are labeled as quackery even though they really work, while the so-called proven cures of modern medicine are deadly and substantial failures by their own admissions.

Although recognizing the ineffectiveness of chemotherapy, Dr. Victor Richard made an interesting admission in *The Wayward Cell, Cancer: Its Origins, Nature, and Treatment.* He wrote that even though a failure, chemotherapy is employed because it keeps the patient within the ambit of the cancer establishment. Although recognizing some of the shortcomings of chemotherapy, Dr. Victor Richard stated:

> Nevertheless chemotherapy serves an extremely valuable role in keeping patients oriented toward proper medical therapy, and prevents the feeling of being abandoned by the physician in patients with late and hopeless cancers. Judicious employment and screening of potentially useful drugs may also prevent the spread of cancer quackery. [82]

Should the goal of medicine be to retain patients within the orbit of conventional practice or to really help the cancer victim? You decide. His remark reveals the cold war against the nutritional approaches to cancer treatment.

The cancer establishment continues to assure us they are winning the war on cancer. How can this be when so many professionals have written on the failure of the so-called proven cancer remedies? The answer lies in the fact that they disseminate questionable statistical information to confuse the public. Many experts claim that they rig the statistics so that they can present a semblance of a claim of success in the war against cancer. The statistics are rigged in at least two ways. First, in controlled studies using their so-called proven methods versus untreated cases, they use a double standard, counting treated deaths differently from untreated deaths. The result is that the failures of their so-called proven remedies do not become apparent. Dr. Hardin Jones explained it this way, using for illustration a control study involving surgery and radiation:

> Evaluation of the clinical response of cancer to treatment by surgery and radiation, separately or in combination, leads to the following findings: The evidence for greater survival of treated groups in comparison with untreated is biased by the method of

defining the groups. All reported studies pick up cases at the time of origin of the disease and follow them to death or end of the study interval. If persons in the untreated or central group die at any time in the study interval, they are reported as deaths in the control group. *In the treated group, however, deaths which occur before completion of the treatment are rejected from the data, since these patients do not then meet the criteria established by the definition of the term "treated."* The longer it takes for completion of the treatment, in a multiple step therapy, for example, the worse the error ... With this effect stripped out, the common malignancies show a remarkably similar rate of demise, whether treated or untreated. [83] [Emphasis added.]

This use of a double standard in matters so vital to the public interest is unconscionable. The cancer establishment also rigs statistics by including some forms of cancer, such as skin cancer, in their studies of more malignant cancers that do not do well with their so-called proven remedies. Skin cancers respond well to treatment but often clear up without treatment. Seldom are they fatal; but since they affect large numbers of people, they alter the statistical tabulations drastically! [84] These questionable practices permit the American Cancer Society to state with a straight face, "There are on record a million and a half people cured of cancer through the efforts of the medical profession and the American Cancer Society with the help of the FDA." [85]

Dr. Hardin Jones contended that questionable grades of malignancies are also included in the tabulations to increase the number of cancer cures having normal life expectancies.

Beginning in 1940, through redefinition of terms, various questionable grades of malignancies were classed as cancer. After that date, the proportion of "cancer" cures having "normal" life expectancies increased rapidly, corresponding to the fraction of questionable diagnoses included. [86]

The American Cancer Society also confuses the public by claiming that patients are now surviving longer through orthodox therapies. This may be deceitful, for nutrition experts argue that people are not living longer after they *get* cancer; they are merely living longer after they are *diag-*

nosed with cancer due to earlier detection of the cancer. The length of life after diagnosis is longer, but the length of life after getting cancer is not increased.

Ladies and gentlemen of the jury, there is only one conclusion that can be drawn from the evidence. The so-called proven methods of treating cancer advocated by the cancer establishment are inefficacious. Dare we conclude that they constitute a malignant fraud upon an ignorant public? You be the judge. If you conclude that it is, then it is the worst form of medical malpractice ever devised by the mind of man. Expert testimony reveal that these so-called proven cures far too often deliver death, not life, compared to the simple but efficacious remedies provided by our Creator. Testimony in the next segment will show the successes achieved by nutritional and other means of cancer prevention and cure.

Section 3

IF WE CANNOT CHOOSE OUR REMEDIES, DO WE HAVE MEDICAL FREEDOM?

Ladies and gentlemen of the jury, after enduring the mutilations of radical breast surgery or the horrors of radiation burns and chemical poisoning, a great many cancer victims turn to alternative remedies. Studies show that up to 50% of all cancer patients will utilize some form of alternative remedy—even though they have to pay out of their own pockets. The medical monopoly of conventional medicine makes sure that insurance companies will not pay for anything but their so-called proven cures. [1] What is the cause of this mass exodus from conventional cancer medicine? Cancer victims learn from painful experience that the profit-making symptomatic cures prescribed by the Medical Deity frequently do not work. So, shattered in health and with spirits often crushed by the words *there is nothing more we can do for you*, they turn to those who not only offer hope, but who try to restore the entre organism of the cancer patient to health. Although the medical establishment labels these alternative remedies as unproven and quackery, their own alleged proven methods reveal the record of a dismal failure rate of 85 %. [2]

The semantic wordplay of *proven* and *unproven* reveal a double standard in judging healthcare options. For although those with monopolistic power classify their remedies as proven and blacklist everything else they disapprove of as unproven, the Federal Office of Technology Assessment states that only 10–20% of all procedures currently used in medical practice have been *proven* to be efficacious by controlled trial! [3] [4] In the case of cancer, the record is even bleaker for the alleged proven cures of the

cancer establishment. Recall the testimony of Dr. Charles Moertal of the
Mayo Clinic, who admitted:

> Our accepted and traditional curative efforts, [for cancer] therefore,
> yield a failure rate of 85%. [5]

Ladies and gentlemen, how could a failure rate of over 85% be classified
as *proven* cures? Even the National Cancer Institute only claims a 28%
survival rate for primary cancers. [6] In the case of long-term survival
after metastasis, the failure rate of conventional cancer medicine is close to
100%, for only one-tenth of 1% live five years after treatment. [7] By contrast nutritional experts claim that the success rate of vitamin B17 therapy
is 80%-85% for those who try this remedy before their health and immune
systems are shattered by radiation or chemo drugs. Additionally, vitamin
therapy can restore to health the ravaged and discarded victims of the
proven methods 15% of the time. [8] This data reveal the success of the
so-called unproven cures and failure of the so-called proven cures

Ladies and gentlemen of the jury, we will examine in considerable
detail the facts behind alternative nutritional remedies for cancer. Let us
look first at the trophoblast theory of cancer and the use of vitamin B17
to control the cancer. This is, of course, not a theory, but a fact. Cancer
cells *are* biologically trophoblast cells. The medical evidence demonstrates
that the immune system does not destroy these trophoblast or cancer cells
because they are surrounded by a negative electronic charge that ema-
nates from a thin protein coating surrounding the cancer cell. This protein
shield is called the pericellular sialomucin coat. [9] The normal defensive
mechanism of white blood cells consisting of lymphocytes, leukocytes,
and monocytes all have a similar negative charge. Since a negative charge
will repel another negatively charged particle, the trophoblast cancer cells
are protected from the body's immune defense. Their negative charges
repel the negatively charged white blood protector cells. This negatively
charged protein coating around the cancer cell also protects them from
antibodies. Dr. Ernst Krebs wrote:

> For three-quarters of a century classical immunology has, in effect
> been pounding its head against a stone wall in the vain quest for
> "cancer antigens," the production of cancer antibodies, etc., etc.,
> The cancer or trophoblast cell is non-antigenic because of the
> pericellular sialomucin coat ... [10]

How does the body protect itself from cancer if it recognizes trophoblast cells as normal tissue? Professor Beard gave us the answer to this puzzle in 1905. He discovered that among the ten or so pancreatic enzymes, two—trypsin and chymotrypsin—were important in the control and destruction of trophoblast cells. These two enzymes are produced in the pancreas and released in their inactive form, zymogens, into the intestines where they are converted into their active form. They are then absorbed through the bowel wall into the blood stream where they travel to the site of the trophoblast activity and digest the protein coating of these trophoblast cells. The immune system can then attack and destroy these unprotected trophoblast or runaway cancer cells. [11]

How wonderful are the mechanisms the Creator has designed to protect the body from self-destruction. If the scientific community would only cooperate with God's natural agents, they would find the answers to most of life's mysteries and bring disease under control. Many aspects of conventional medical remedies such as radiation and chemotherapy are good examples of how man's rebellious quest for autonomy from God, both intellectually and scientifically, leads him into the twilight paths of death.

G. Edward Griffin pointed out that as soon as Professor Beard published his findings, physicians everywhere began to experiment with pancreatic enzymes in the treatment of cancer and began to report favorable results. In 1906 Dr. Frederick Wiggins, in describing his success with cancer of the tongue, enthusiastically exclaimed:

> ... that further discussion of and clinical experience with Trypsin and Amylopsin within a reasonable time will demonstrate beyond question that we have at our disposal a sure and efficient remedy for the treatment of malignant disease. [12]

In 1950 Dr. Ernst Krebs, Jr., Ph.D. in biochemistry and past director of the John Beard Memorial Foundation, identified a nutritional factor that works with the body's natural metabolism to destroy cancer trophoblast cells. He isolated out a nutrient, later called vitamin B17, from the apricot kernel and named it Laetrile. The term Laetrile was coined by combining the first and last syllables from its two chemical characteristics: *Lae* (from laevorotatory because it was left-handed to polarized light), and *trile* (because chemically it was a Mandelonitrile). [13] Vitamin B17 is a non-toxic natural substance. It is a complex molecule containing two units of glucose sugar, one unit of benzaldehyde, and one unit of cyanide. Both benzaldehyde and cyanide are highly toxic in isolated form, and when working together synergistically, they are one hundred times more toxic. However, when nature combines these substances with glucose sugar into the complex vitamin molecule, these two toxic substances become harmless and non-poisonous. When acted on by the body's metabolism, these two substances work to destroy trophoblast cells while providing nutrients to healthy cells. How this works is another monument to the Creator's wisdom that he has locked into the tiny mysteries of life.

Vitamin B17 destroys antigens while providing nutrients to the body. To activate the benzaldehyde and cyanide within it, B17 requires an unlocking enzyme. The unlocking enzyme is beta-glucosidase, which is found everywhere in the body, but predominantly in the trophoblast cells. The result is that when the B17 vitamin comes in the vicinity of the trophoblast cancer cell, the beta-glucosidase enzyme unlocks the vitamin and releases the benzaldehyde and cyanide straight into the face of the cancer cell, killing it. If B17 is unlocked at other non-cancerous sites of the body, a protective enzyme called rhodanese converts the cyanide into by-products that are beneficial and necessary to the health of the cell.

Interestingly, the malignant cell not only has a greater concentration of the unlocking enzyme, but it is totally lacking in the protecting enzyme. Thus B17 becomes fatal to trophoblast cancer cells while providing nourishment to the rest of the body. [14] Mr. Griffin notes in passing that nature illustrates similar innovative uses of these toxic substances. The poisonous millipede found in Louisiana and Mississippi utilizes the chemicals benzaldehyde and cyanide as weapons in its arsenals for its protection. These substances are held in separate paired pouches in the body of the millipede; when attacked by predators, it releases them is such a way that they combine with deadly effect in the face of the aggressor. [15]

Another characteristic of the trophoblast and cancer cells demonstrates how benzaldehyde is deadly to cancer cells while supplying nutrients to healthy cells. Cancer cells are sugar feeders as earlier testimony has demonstrated. They live by utilizing energy from the process of fermentation. Dr. Otto Warburg demonstrated this fact in the work that earned him the Nobel Prize. Ordinary cells, on the other hand, depend on a complex oxygenation process for energy. Any benzaldehyde that diffuses away from the cancer cell is oxidized by the normal healthy cells into Benzoic acid, which has certain anti-rheumatic, antiseptic, and analgesic properties, hence the relief of pain felt by cancer patients who utilize Laetrile. [16]

Ladies and gentlemen of the jury, if the cancer establishment was interested in saving lives they would have jumped at this revolutionary breakthrough. But alas, that was not to be. Because Vitamin B17 is a naturally occurring substance that cannot be patented into a money-making drug, the cancer establishment and its pharmaceutical bosses rejected the harmless and nutritious B17 vitamin, embracing instead the deadly and more profitable chemo drugs—at the expense of the public's health, life, and pocket book. The use of Vitamin B17 has been suppressed. It has been blacklisted as merely another unproven cure despite its amazing effectiveness against cancer. In the fight against cancer, vitamin B 17 far outstrips anything conventional medicine has to offer. The cancer establishment and its big guns immediately went into action against this natural cancer cure as soon as it was discovered.

Dr. Ralph Weilerstein, former Public Health Medical Officer of California Food and Drug Administration, stated in 1972, nobody has come up with any reliable data that it [Laetrile] is of any value. [17] In August of that same year the FDA stated,

The Food and Drug Administration has seen no competent, scientific evidence that Laetrile is effective for the treatment of cancer. [18]

Closing their eyes to the available date, the American Cancer Society quickly lumped together Laetrile with other so-called unproven cancer cures.

After careful study of the literature and other information available to it, the American Cancer Society does not have evidence that treatment with Laetrile results in objective benefit in the treatment of cancer in human beings. [19]

In protest of these official statements against the effectiveness of vitamin B17, numerous prestigious and eminently qualified professionals have written extensively of the effectiveness of Laetrile in controlling cancer. G. Edward Griffin stated that the truth is, evidence for the effectiveness of vitamin B17 is everywhere. [20] The first of these experts to be cited is well known. In 1971 Dr. Dean Burk, then Director of the Cytochemistry

Section of the federal government's National Cancer Institute, made the
following remarks about the effectiveness of B17 in killing cancer cells:

Laetrile appears to work against many forms of cancer including
lung cancer. And it is absolutely non-toxic ...

In vitro tests with Ehrlich ascites carcinoma [a particular type of
cancer culture] revealed that, where cyanide alone killed one per
cent of the cells and benzaldehyde alone killed twenty percent,
a combination of the two was effective against all the cells.
Amygdalin [Laetrile} with glucosidase [the unlocking enzyme]
added also succeeded in killing 100 percent of the ascites tumor
cells, due to the freeing of the same two chemicals. [21]

Dr. Dean Burk was considered one of the foremost cancer specialists in
the world. He is not alone in promoting the effectiveness of vitamin B
17 against cancer. Ladies and gentlemen, you can sense we are in deep
trouble as a nation, when bean counters in the medical establishment fla-
grantly discredit world renowned medical geniuses, because their findings
threaten the profit margins of the cancer industry.

G. Edward Griffin noted that the use of Amygdalin (another name
for Laetrile), in the treatment of cancer is not new. Literally thousands
of people have had remission of their cancer by use of this vitamin. The
earliest know use of Amygdalin dates back to 1836 when a French woman
with extensive cancer began taking it; she was still surviving in 1845 when
the use of Amygdalin was written up in the *Paris Medical Gazette*. The
article also cited the use of Amygdalin by a young cancer patient in 1842.
[22]

The cancer establishment attempts to explain away the incidences of
cancer remission with Laetrile by saying either that the patient did not
have cancer in the first place or that it was a case of spontaneous remission.
It is funny how spontaneous remission only occurs to patients treated with
alternative remedies and not those treated by orthodox methods. It is true
that spontaneous remission can occur through the power of prayer or other
unknown mechanisms in a cancer patient, but it is very rare. With certain
cancers such as testicular chorionepithelioma, spontaneous remission is so
rare as to defy statistical analysis. [23] Hence testicular epithelioma is a
good test case to prove the effectiveness of Laetrile. Commenting on the

effectiveness of Laetrile on six of these cases, Dr. Ernst Krebs, Jr., stated sarcastically:

> And when we look at this scientifically, we know that spontaneous regression occurs in less than one in 150,000 cases of cancer. The statistical possibility of spontaneous regression accounting for the complete resolution of six successive cases of testicular chorionepithelioma is far greater than the improbability of the sun not rising tomorrow morning. [24]

Ladies and gentlemen of the jury, who do you think is right in this dispute? Surely something is wrong with this picture—world-renowned scientists opposing the claims of the cancer Cartel. Perhaps we should ask who stands to gain most if Laetrile is suppressed, the patient or the drug companies? The answer is obvious.

Let it be made clear that Laetrile or vitamin B17 therapy is not chemotherapy with vitamins rather than the use of drugs. Laetrile is not a drug; it is a food substance, a non-toxic vitamin. All chemo drugs are poisonous and work by destroying good cells as well as bad cells. Vitamin B17 is a natural nutrient that destroys bad cells while nourishing good cells. The use of chemo drugs is an incomplete symptomatic remedy; it does not reverse the causes that triggered the cancer in the first place, a poisoned and dysfunctional metabolism and immune system. B17 is a nutritional supplement that helps restore proper metabolic function in the healing system. Although there are other causes of cancer, one can, to a certain degree, accurately say that people with cancer have a vitamin B17 deficiency. Hence supplying the body with this vitamin not only assists it in fighting cancer, but in fighting other metabolic diseases. [25]

Laetrile, however, is not to be considered a nutritional magic-bullet. Its effectiveness is enhanced if it is taken along with a supporting nutritional program that consists of foods that do not consume the pancreatic enzymes Trypsin and Amylopsin. Such diets typically ban refined sugar (cancer cells are sugar feeders utilizing fermentation for their energy), poultry, and eggs and emphasize raw vegetables (a good source of live enzymes, vitamins, and minerals) and multiple vitamin supplements. [26] A living monument to the nutritional value of laetrile is the Hunzakuts who eat it in its natural form as found in the apricot and its seed. These people typically live well into their nineties and beyond.

Ladies and gentlemen, another alternative remedy that combines nutrition, enzymatic action, and detoxification was developed by Dr. Max Gerson, of whom Nobel Laureate Dr. Albert Schweitzer stated, "I see in Max Gerson one of the most eminent geniuses in the history of Medicine." One thing you will notice about these alternative cancer practitioners is that they are mostly numbered among world-class doctors and nutritionists who have achieved distinction and renown before being blacklisted and defamed by the cancer establishment. I speak of such men as Dr. Max Gerson, pioneer of the Gerson therapy for healing cancer and other degenerative diseases; Dr. Dean Burk, head of the Cytochemistry Section of the National Cancer Institute; Dr. Ernst Krebs, biochemist and the Louis Pasteur of the twentieth century; Dr. Ernesto Contreras, one of Mexico's most distinguished doctors; Dr. Linus Pauling, twice Nobel laureate; and Dr. Hans Nieper, the famous cancer specialist from Hanover, Germany.

Like other physicians who pursue nutritional cures for cancer, Dr. Max Gerson views cancer as a systemic disease, not a localized lesion. The local lesion or cancerous growth is a result of the more generalized disease. This makes a tremendous difference in one's approach to the treatment of this malignant disease. The systemic disease is caused by a gradual and general break down of metabolism through poisoning, which then manifests itself in a localized abnormal cellular growth of cancerous cells. Dr. Max Gerson stated that cancer is not a localized disease:

Cancer is not a single cellular problem; it is an accumulation of numerous damaging factors combined in deteriorating the whole metabolism, after the liver has been progressively impaired in its functions. Therefore one has to separate two basic components in cancer: a general one and a local one. The general component is mostly a very slow, progressing, imperceptible symptom caused by poisoning of the liver and simultaneously an impairment of the whole intestinal tract, later producing appearances of vitally important consequences all over the body. [27]

Dr. Max Gerson contended that it is the insistence by the majority of medical practitioners that cancer is a localized lesion, which has led to ineffective symptomatic methods of treatment. [28] This narrow view of cancer has dominated cancer research, leading to a lack of progress in the war on cancer. If the disease is not properly understood, the appropriate remedy cannot be fashioned. The inaccurate view of cancer as a regionalized problem is inculcated into the young minds of medical students and shapes their approach to research and practice.

> The scientifically accepted method is that these symptoms alone will be treated locally wherever they appear. That is what we physicians learn and how we are trained in university clinics. All research work adheres mostly to these local symptoms. This is, in my opinion, the reason why decisive progress in cancer treatment has been impeded, especially in the last 50 years, during which modern medicine made remarkable progress in many other fields. [29]

Ladies and gentlemen, the essential concept to grasp in dealing with cancer is to avoid focusing on the growth itself, which is merely the visible symptoms of a deep-seated problem. The extirpation of the cancer growth does not mean a cure of the disease. [30] The focus in cancer treatment should be on the damage that has been done to the whole metabolism, including loss of the body's defensive mechanism, its immunity, and healing power. Reversing this metabolic damage becomes the key to preventing and curing cancer. [31] Understanding the relationship between the generalized metabolic disease and the development of the local cancer lesion is also critical. Of course the mass of cancerous cells must also be destroyed; they contribute to a continuous poisoning of the body. The metabolic deficiencies contributing to and directing the growth of the cancer cells must be kept in focus. Both Dr. John Beard, past professor of embryology at the University of Edinburgh in Scotland, and Dr. Max Gerson believed that the local tumor mass consists of abnormal, immature, or damaged cells that fall back into a type of embryonic life. [32] These cancerous cells revert to a primitive metabolism, utilizing fermentation to sustain them, because they are no longer adequately supported by the activated (ionized) minerals of the potassium group. [33]

The general component of the systemic disease, which precedes the local lesion, comprises mainly the deterioration of the essential organs of the digestive tract and the liver. There the damage is done by a daily poisoning brought about by our modern civilization. The problem is basically one of improper nutrition, which started with the impairment of the soil when society shifted from organic to chemical fertilization. Dr. Max Gerson also asserted that the daily poisoning of our bodies begins with the depletion of the soil and continues with the refinement and over-processing of our food.

This [daily poisoning] starts with the soil which is denaturalized by artificial fertilizers and depletion, thus gradually reducing the top soil. In addition the soil is poisoned by DDT and other poisons. Furthermore, the food substances are damaged as they are refined, bottled, bleached, powered, frozen, smoked, salted, canned, and colored with artificial coloring. Carrots are sold in cellophane bags after having been treated for better preservation. Other foods contain damaging preservatives; finally, cattle and chickens are fed or injected with stilbestrol to accumulate more weight and be quickly ready for market. [34]

Other researchers have noted the link between improper nutrition and the degradation of the body's metabolism. In his book, *Cancer and Diet*, Dr. Frederick L. Hoffman reached the conclusion that cancer is not local in its origin; therefore treatment should not be limited to the local lesions. He argued that a deranged metabolism is the result of dietary and nutritional disorders, which then manifest themselves in various ways such as cancer and other degenerative diseases. [35] He also recognized that we must fight the war on cancer on the broadest possible fronts, beginning with those aspects of modern civilization that are contributing to the problem. Viewed in this broad light the narrow cut, burn, and poison remedies of the cancer establishment are readily seen to be hopelessly inadequate and in many respects, contributory to the problem by poisoning the human organism and diverting attention from correcting our nutritional inad-equacies. Dr. Gerson taught that because cancer is a disease of the entire metabolism, concentrated in the liver, patients must be taught what they have to do for the restoration of their vital organs. They must be educated in habits of proper nutrition so that they can stop poisoning themselves. [36]

In his treatment of the cancer victim, Dr. Gerson placed primary emphasis in restoring the functions of such vital organs as the liver and pancreas. The liver plays a vital role in proper metabolism and its derange-ment is a central aspect of cancer metabolism. Dr. Gerson observed that before cancer can develop, the liver must first be broken down by poisoning.

The experimental causation of cancer, first accomplished by Yamagiva and Itchikawa, through rubbing tar substance on the ears of rabbits for about nine months, is of importance insofar as they found that before the cancer started to appear, the liver was damaged and showed pathological changes, together with the kidneys, spleen and the lymphatic apparatus. The long period was required to poison the liver, before the damaged cells could perform the "mutation" into cancer. [37]

Not only does the poisoning of the body result in liver dysfunction, but it has also been demonstrated that the injection of certain toxins and poisons in the blood stream of rabbits resulted in the loss of electrical potentials, the loss of potassium minerals in the liver, and the invasion of sodium into liver parenchyma cells. The impairment of the liver and the loss of potassium from the cells and anodic organs from poisoning are critical factors in the development of cancer. [38] The poisoning of the liver interferes with the oxidizing enzymes and paves the way for the development of cancer. Dr. Gerson observed:

I think that the origin of the cancerous disease is more probable where the reactivation of the oxidizing enzymes, one of the first developed functions of the liver, is impaired. [39]

Dr. Gerson also pointed out that Dr. Kasper Blond, in his book The *Liver and Cancer*, was correct in concluding that:

95% of all cancers of the internal organs succumb not to the cancer but to the liver disorder. [40]

Consequently in treating cancer, Dr. Gerson emphasized that:

The metabolism and its concentration in the liver should be put in the foreground, not the cancer as a symptom. [41]

The nutritional rehabilitation of the liver is an achievable goal in cancer treatment. Dr. Gerson observed that the liver has a great capacity to regenerate itself. A partial destruction of the liver may be reversed so long as the deterioration is not too extensive and rapid. [42] Dr. Gerson also cited evidence from the work of several other authors who examined the function of the liver. In one case researchers followed fifty patients with various types of cancers of the gastro-intestinal tract. They found a pronounced hepatic dysfunction, but after removal of the tumors, the liver recovered to a certain degree. From these and other findings Dr. Gerson argued that the deterioration of the liver can be reversed. [43]

In the Gerson cancer therapy, the metabolic function of the liver as well as the body as a whole is restored by detoxifying the body of the poisons that have been produced by improper nutrition. As part of the detoxification process, Dr. Gerson placed his cancer patients on a diet that excluded salt, animal fat, and protein. In severe cases detoxification was accelerated by the use of coffee enemas. He observed that the process of detoxification begins to repair the body's healing mechanism, which a dysfunctioning metabolism had impaired. [44]

Dr. Max Gerson reasoned that since in a healthy body a healing apparatus is present and functioning, and since poisoning impairs this healing mechanism, it should be possible for this healing metabolism to be reactivated provided the body can be sufficiently detoxified during the treatment of degenerative diseases and cancer. [45] Detoxification is not only essential for the removal of years of accumulated poisons, it is an ongoing process that requires the constant removal of poisons released from the fatty tissues and cancerous mass as healing takes place. [46]

Dr. Gerson observed that patients who followed a dietary regime rich in potassium, void of salt, and low in protein and fat, responded much more favorably to his treatments. Therefore he began to experiment with reducing the protein content of the diet. He finally came to the conclusion that discontinuing all animal fat and proteins as much as possible reduced the damaging influence of animal proteins. [47] Dr. Gerson discovered that even small amounts of animal protein retarded the detoxification process and reduced the secretion of urine and sodium elimination. [48] He found that the end products of protein metabolism, urea nitrogen, and uric acid from the cell metabolism, are eliminated in greater amounts the smaller the amounts of animal proteins present. [49] Dr. Gerson further noted that animal proteins in the diet of those suffering from degenerative diseases over stimulated the visceral nervous system and resulted in frequent spasms in the diaphragm, the intestinal tract, and even in the heart vessels. [50]

From these experiments with his patients, Dr. Max Gerson concluded that detoxification was only one part of the healing process, though an important part. He contended that the mineral balance of the body has to be restored so as to assist in the restoration of proper metabolism. The proper types and nutritive ratios of minerals help activate the enzymes and hormones essential to the functioning of a healthy body.

Simultaneously, the metabolism has to be balanced at least to a certain degree. The sick organs are unable to do so themselves for a long period, especially in advanced cases. The body needs essentially the important minerals ... the oxidizing enzymes and coenzymes, and the hormones. All of them must be activated in the body and must be re-activated there, otherwise they are lost. Equally important is the restoration of the pH (mineral in the cells) so that the enzymes can function again step by step. [51]

Dr. Max Gerson wrote that the diet of the cancer patient has to be saltless because restoring the mineral balance is vital. He believes that all acute and chronic degenerative disease, including cancer, begins by an infiltration of sodium (Na) chloride and water into the cells of the anodic (positive) organs, replacing potassium and other positive ions. [52] All the essential metabolic processes of the organism, such as hormonal function, vitamin activity, and enzymatic function, are based on and dependant on the potassium/sodium relationship. Potassium (K) plays an indispensable and unique role in tissue protein synthesis and potassium ions are indispensable in certain enzymatic reactions. [53] To understand why Dr. Gerson believed the potassium and sodium groups of ions play a fundamental role in human growth, and conversely in the development of disease when the Na/K ration is reversed, I will quote extensively from him.

It is my opinion that K and Na also play an important part in the cancer problem. These two minerals are the leaders of the two electrically opposite groups. They are in close connection with the development and maintenance of the human body as well as with the origin and progress of the disease ...

The human organism is, in embryonic life and early infancy, a sodium-animal, due to the relative preponderance of Na throughout the entire organism, but in adult life, a potassium-animal. The potassium predominance must be maintained throughout life. To a certain degree it gives the basis for important developments in both directions—normal and abnormal ...

The unfertilized human egg cell is full of K-group or intracellular minerals (K, P, Mg, Mn, Cu, Fe, Au), electro-positive and has the corresponding enzymes, vitamins and protein-compounds. The sperm contains the Na-group minerals and is electro-negative (Na, Cl, H_2O, I, Br. Al and the ionized part of Ca), together with the other group of enzymes and vitamins ...

The fertilized egg becomes, through a process of discharging some compositions and absorbing a great deal of Na from the surrounding lymph fluid, distinctly negatively charged; an "Na-animal" is created and remains one throughout the entire pregnancy and up to six months after birth (Frank Golland) ...

The months of pregnancy and six months of extra-uterine life ... (are only a "transitional stage" of a living being, which continues to pass over into normal life with an excess of K-group minerals in vital organs, until disease or old age makes it lose some of the K-minerals, together with the corresponding enzyme-functions, etc ...

Each cell carries in itself some potentialities of a normal living cell under normal internal and external environmental conditions, or else they fall back to their original embryonic stage. R.R. Spencer and other investigators, with keen foresight, compare cancer cells not to cells of old age but, rather, to embryonic ones ... [54]

The purpose of the saltless diet is to eliminate excess sodium and increase the proportion of potassium, thus helping to restore proper metabolic activity. Dr. Max Gerson also observed that the reduction of sodium salt also assisted in the removal of toxins and poisons from the body.

The main task of the saltless diet is to eliminate the retained Na, Cl, H_2O, together with toxins and poisons from the tissues all over the body. [55]

When patients were placed in a detoxification regime and a saltless diet, Dr. Gerson observed that they eliminated copious amounts of sodium, chlorine, and water. [56] He therefore argued that the higher sodium chloride content in the urine of cancer patient during the first weeks of the saltless treatment proves that sodium chloride and water are retained in cancer patients. [57] The replacement of sodium with the potassium group minerals in the cells and organs forces the cancer cells to revert to a normal oxidative metabolism, but since they are programmed to ferment only, they die. [58] Other researchers have observed the role of salt in promoting cancer growth. [59] Yet other researchers feel strongly that excessive amounts of salt *is* the root cause of cancer. [60]

In his nutritional therapy Dr. Gerson included supplements such as vitamin B12 to help the body make the correct use of amino acids. In treating cancer it is essential to restore the conditions under which foodstuffs can be properly metabolized by the body. Dr. Gerson mentions other nutritional modalities that, when combined with a saltless diet, help restore the mineral balance. Thus when the body's healing mechanism is restored, by whatever means, the body has the ability to destroy cancer.

I have seen two cancers of the breast disappear with the use of Fenugreek seeds tea in large amounts, combined with a saltless vegetarian diet. Two others were cured after the patients drank green leaf tea juice only for six to eight months... . This helps to transform the relations of the minerals of the body and to bring them into the organs where they belong ... The effect of the diet is that the potassium group is enriched in the essential organs and the abnormal sodium content in these organs reduced to a minimum and eliminated into the extra-cellular fluids, where they belong. [61]

Dr. Max Gerson cautions that merely because nutritional treatment is unspecific and even unexplainable, to reject any dietary regime because of insufficient physiological proof is unwise. [62] By its very nature, the detoxification therapy that Dr. Gerson advocated helps not only cancer

patients but other degenerative diseases such as diabetes. He cited the
work of Dr. Ernest Leupold in support of this.

The combination of liver therapy and diet was necessary in serious
cases of osteoarthritis, asthma, angina pectoris and malignancies.
The combination of a saltless diet, poor in fat and proteins, with
the liver therapy, regularly lowers the blood sugar considerably, so
that the diet increased the effect of the liver enzymes, increased
the effect of insulin, and decreased the adrenalin effect to a great
extent. According to Ernst Leupold, the lowering of the blood
sugar level is of great significance in cancer patients. [63]

As a whole the liver therapy can be looked upon as a kind of hormone-
enzyme therapy, but in a very mild dosage and in a natural manner. It was
found helpful in returning glycogen, K-group minerals, and vitamins to
the liver and other tissues; as well as in preparing the conditions for the
re-functioning of the oxidizing enzymes. [64]

In the closing decades of his life (Dr. Max Gerson died in 1959), Dr.
Max Gerson treated a great number of patients, mostly difficult or terminal cases, with relatively favorable results with his vegetarian diet and
detoxification regime. [65] Of course it is a known fact that vegetarians
also get cancer occasionally. For this reason many have questioned the
efficacy of the Gerson therapy in helping cancer patients, because it relies
heavily on a vegetarian approach. Dr. Gerson anticipated this question
and pointed out some vegetarians get cancer not because of their vegetarian diet, but from their ignorance of other aspects of nutrition which even
vegetarians must implement or suffer the consequences. He provided four
reasons for cancer in vegetarians:

1. Even vegetarians may not know what conditions are necessary
to maintain the normal metabolism.

2. Our modern agricultural methods decreased potassium
and iodine in our nutrition, precisely the minerals essential for
prevention of cancer.

3. Some people with weak organs are not sufficiently protected by
diet alone.

4. The therapy comprises much more than a vegetarian diet and is successful in healing vegetarians of cancer. [66]

Of course, being a vegetarian is of no value to a person if that person consumes refined, un-nutritious foods. Dr. Nancy Appleton has ably demonstrated the link between refined sugar and cancer in her bestselling book, *Lick the Sugar Habit*. Many vegetarians unwisely consume tons of refined sugar while rejecting animal products. But refined foods may be even more toxic and cancer causing than animal products for they deplete the body of its nutrients.

Cancer is a disease of our industrialized civilization. Its cure must embrace a wide variety of modalities, but above all we must focus on restoring the health of our soil. With proper soil nutrition, we can then restore the health of our bodies through proper nutrition and healthy choices. In this respect Dr. Gerson observed that our civilization faces a life and death choice.

The coming years will make it more imperative that organically grown fruit and vegetables will be, and must be, used for protection against degenerative diseases, the prevention of cancer, and more so in the treatment of cancer.

According to present government statistics, one out of every six persons in our population will die of cancer. It will not be long before the entire population will have to decide whether we will all die of cancer or whether we will have enough wisdom, courage, and will power to change fundamentally all our living and nutritional conditions. [67]

Since Dr. Max Gerson wrote this gripping warning, the proportion of cancer deaths in our country has worsened. What will it take for us to take action and save our civilization? It is because of the urgency of the situation that you, the jury, have been empanelled to hear this case. Will you have the courage to return a verdict of indictment upon those institutions that are denying us the choice of remedies and the vital information we need to save our sons and daughters from the dread scourge of cancer pandemic in our land?

Ladies and gentlemen, another so-called unproven remedy that is showing great potential for curing certain types of cancer is the use of natural shark cartilage. The theory behind this modality is not new, but its implementation in human clinical trials is new because of road blocks erected by the FDA, National Cancer Institute, and the medical establishment. The story of the use of shark cartilage is another example of the triumph of industrial profit over nutritional medicine and of inertia and prejudice over progress. The major pioneer in the use of shark cartilage to fight cancer was Dr. I. William Lane, Ph.D. In his influential book, co-authored with Linda Comac, *Sharks Don't Get Cancer*, Dr. William Lane wrote:

> Orthodox medicine's reaction to the use of shark cartilage sometimes brings to mind scientists of yesterday—men like Galileo, Pasteur, and Lester, who were scorned, ostracized, or excommunicated when their investigations broke with the accepted wisdom of the times. [68]

Why is the medical and cancer establishments so opposed to the use of shark cartilage? Is it toxic? No. Is it ineffective? No. The preliminary trials demonstrate its efficacy. Is it too costly? No. The secret of their opposition lies in the fact that, like Laetrile, it is a cheap, natural product that cannot be patented into a drug, and therefore is not profit-making to the pharmaceutical companies and the medical bureaucracy that depend on the high cost of medicine for their existence. With over two trillion dollars being spent annually on conventional symptom-oriented medicine, Dr. Lane asked us to imagine the pressure groups of pharmaceutical companies, doctors, hospitals, clinics, therapists, and auxiliary services that may get involved when a relatively low-cost item aimed at preventing some of mankind's major diseases is presented to the market place. Lane contended that *medicine has become big business, and cancer is the most profitable of all medical businesses.* These powerful businesses pressure governmental agencies to pass regulations to preserve their financial monopoly and exclude all other low-cost, natural modalities. Governmental forces thus become arrayed against the patient's health and interests. In the case of cancer treatment, Dr. Lane stated:

> A loss of income—directly or through pressure from the pharmaceutical industry—may be one of the reasons that government agencies resist conducting or funding research into

natural products such as shark cartilage. Each year, the National Cancer Institute spends more than $1 billion on research in its own facilities and on outside research at universities and other centers—more than $1 billion from our taxes. But this organization has consistently refused to fund research into or to investigate natural products except in token amounts. [69]

In an earlier portion of our testimony, we learnt that Hippocrates defined medicine as the use of good food coupled with moderation and temperate living. This form of medicine focuses on keeping the human organism healthy and disease free. Ladies and gentlemen of the jury, we have come a long way from this concept of medicine. The concept of medicine has changed because we focus on killing the germ and not keeping the human organism healthy. By redefining medicine to include, for the most part, only pharmaceutical drugs and excluding natural products, herbs, and nutrients, the FDA has discouraged medical institutions from conducting research on beneficial natural products. If a natural product shows any medically beneficial potential, the medical cartel proceeds to financially exploit it. They try to discover the active ingredient in the product. When this is achieved, they chemically isolate the active ingredient and introduce it into the market place as a wonder drug. Then they lobby the government agencies to outlaw use of the natural product, thus suppressing all competition. The whole process can cost over $231 million and twenty years in getting FDA approval. This not only drives up the cost of healthcare, it also directly contributes to the suffering and death of untold millions of Americans (half a million die from cancer alone annually) by making the natural products unavailable for medical use. Meanwhile, a financial burden is placed on society while the scientists search for the chemical counter part of the natural product through a prolonged process of purification, isolation, and synthesis. [70]

The process of isolating a so-called active ingredient from a natural herb or substance can pose grave dangers to the health of the patient. Whereas the natural product, such as shark cartilage, may be beneficial and non-toxic, the chemicalization of its active ingredient opens the door to toxicity, side effects, and high cost for consumers. The chemical drug may also be less efficacious than the natural product. Often there is not just *one* active ingredient, but a host of compounds acting synergistically, and it is this combined influence that makes the natural product so effective. In the case of shark cartilage, the active ingredients appear to include two or more angiogenesis-inhibiting proteins. These active ingredients are in an environment that includes anti-inflammatory complex carbohydrates such as mucopolysaccharides. Dr. Lane soberly asks if the isolated protein or proteins would be as effective? How long will it take to find out, decades or more? How many people are we prepared to allow to die while we suppress a non-chemical whole product that could be saving lives?

Ladies and gentlemen of the jury, the way in which shark cartilage works is simple; its discovery constitutes a fascinating tale of medical detective work. The evidence is compelling. To understand how it works, we must examine a typical tumor. We know that cancer is a runaway growth of a cell, which, if unchecked, eventually suffocates vital organs, depriving them of oxygen, nutrients, and other life resources. These malignant cells may proliferate and spread via the blood stream or lymphatic system to other parts of the body, forming colonies of proliferating cells. We call this process metastasis. For certain cancers—such as breast, cervical, prostate, bladder, central nervous system, and pancreatic cancers—growth beyond a certain size is dependent upon the cancer establishing its own vascular network to facilitate blood supply and thereby bring nutrients to the cancer cells. This process is called neovascularization. Neovascularization is a normal biological process that accompanies the growth of most tissues in the body. The process is also called angiogenesis, from the Greek, *angio*, meaning blood, and *genesis*, meaning creation or formation. The term was coined in 1935 to describe the formation of new blood vessels in the placenta during pregnancy. [71] By logical inference, if the blood supply of a cancerous tumor can be cut off or destroyed, the tumor should die of malnutrition, a process called necrosis. It stands to reason too that if one could prevent a mass of cancerous cells from developing a blood network, the cancer can be nipped in the bud.

In the 1890s a medical researcher by the name of Dr. William Coley, while working at Memorial Hospital in New York, found that he could cause tumors to hemorrhage, turn necrotic, and die by injecting the cancer patient with a vaccine made from dead bacteria. The substance or factor that caused the death (necrosis) of cancer cells was called the tumor necrosis factor or TNF. After Dr. Coley's work, the search was on in earnest to identify this tumor necrosis factor. [72] After studying the blood supply of tumors in the 1960s, Dr. Judah Folkman of Children's Hospital and Harvard Medical School concluded that without tiny blood vessels to nourish them, tumors cannot grow. In 1971 he published his famous hypothesis in *The New England Journal of Medicine* and stated, among other things, that:

> Tumors cannot grow without a network of blood vessels to nourish them and to remove waste products. Inhibiting the development of blood vessels could be a potential cancer therapy. [73]

Without a blood network to supply the larger tumors with nourishment and to remove toxic wastes, the tumor will die. [74] It is that simple. The question now became one of knowing where to look for and how to identify the factor that would limit or destroy the blood supply to tumors. By logical deduction researchers began to look for an angiogenesis inhibitor in cartilage, for the simple reason that cartilage does not have a blood vessel network. Cartilage is essentially avascular. The researchers correctly reasoned that there may be some biological factor in cartilage that inhibits the formation of blood vessels in cartilage tissue. Their thinking was correct. In 1973 researchers at the Rush-Presbyterian St. Luke's Medical Center in Chicago implanted small amounts of cartilage into the fetal membrane of a chick embryo and found that blood vessels in the embryo did not invade the cartilage although they invaded other tissues implanted. [75]

A break-through occurred soon after this finding. Dr. Robert Langer, Sc. D., and Dr. Anne Lee, Ph.D., reported in the journal *Science* that when cartilage from calves is injected into rabbits and mice, inhibition of the vascularization of solid tumors occurs. [76] Because the cartilage found in mammals was infused with fat, it was difficult to obtain a reliable quality and quantity of cartilage for experimentation. The fats, if not completely removed, would cause the cartilage extract to become rancid. [77]

Drs. Langer and Lee therefore turned—like other researchers, such as Dr. Carl Luer, Ph.D., a biochemist at Mote Marine Laboratory in Sarasota, Florida—to the shark to obtain their cartilage. Sharks have no bones, only cartilage where bones should be. They therefore have an abundant supply of cartilage. Dr. Luer recognized that sharks rarely if ever get cancer, even when exposed to massive amounts of carcinogenic chemicals. And he probably reasoned that this may be due to the plentiful supply of cartilage, which contain substances with angiogenesis inhibiting influences. Testing protein extracts from cartilage, he discovered that there are six or seven proteins that have the ability to inhibit blood vessel growth. Dr. Luer found that shark cartilage have only 20% of liver enzymes (compared to calves) that activate pre-carcinogens such as Aflatoxin B1. Thus he reasoned that sharks may be 20% less likely to develop cancer than calves. Meanwhile Drs. Langer and Lee discovered that 0.5 grams of shark cartilage provided as much inhibitors as 500 grams of calf cartilage. In other words, gram for gram, shark cartilage is 1,000 times as powerful as calf cartilage in inhibiting new vessel growth. [78] Although Drs. Langer and Lee had proved the efficacy of shark cartilage in inhibiting tumor growth, no one paid much attention to this groundbreaking news. Incredibly, its potential for the treatment of cancer in human beings was disregarded.

In 1972 Dr. John Prudent, MD., Med. Sc. D., a Harvard-trained surgeon, began a study utilizing bovine cartilage to treat cancer patients. He selected thirty-one patients with a variety of cancers considered hopeless cases in reference to treatment with the standard surgery, radiation, and chemotherapy. The cartilage extract was administered first by injection and then orally. He reported no toxicity or interference with kidney or liver function. He reported tumor regression without the debilitating effects of chemotherapy, radiation, or surgery. In all, 35% of his patients had a complete response (tumor disappearance), 26% had a complete response with relapse, 19% had a partial response of tumor regression, and only 6% showed no benefit from the therapy. Dr. John Prudent wrote in the *Journal of Biological Response Modifiers:*

> When confronted by entities such as pancreatic cancer, squamous or adenocarcinoma of the lung, glioblastoma mulitforme, and other situations where present therapeutic impotence is clear, the use of Catrix [powered calf cartilage] therapy as the primary agent should be considered. One persuasive argument for using it in this way is that, in happy contrast to chemotherapy, it burns no immunological or hematological bridges. [79]

Again, there was little or no follow-up to Dr. Prudden's clinical study. Contemporaneously, Dr. Brian G.M. Durie of the Department of Internal Medicine at the University of Arizona Health Sciences Center was doing his own clinical studies. He found that when bovine cartilage was applied to tumor cells in a test tube, all of the tumor cells were killed. Following this up, he applied bovine cartilage to human cancer cells and found good responses against ovarian, pancreatic, colon, testicular, and sarcoma cancers. This should have been very exciting and important news in the case of ovarian cancer; for one-half of all ovarian cancer is considered inoperable. [80] Again, there was silence from the medical and cancer societies. There was little or no follow up to these findings by the medical community. It would appear that maintaining the *treatment of cancer* is more profitable to the medical community than finding a cure. It is incredulous how the research of the best and brightest of medical scientists are so completely shunted aside by mental peons in the pharmaceutical/industrial complex, who place profit over health.

In 1988 Dr. Patricia D'Amore tried to generate interest in anti-angiogenesis approaches to curing cancer. Her work centered on the vital area of metastasis of cancers, a condition that drastically reduces the success rate of the standard treatment approaches of cut, burn, and poison.

The only event that stands between maintenance of metastatic cells in a dormant state and their establishment into a secondary tumor is the development of a vasculature [system of blood vessels] Thus, therapies aimed at interfering with vascularization represent viable strategies for antimetastasis ... [81]

Simply stated, vascularization is as essential for primary cancer sites as it is for the establishment and subsequent growth of metastatic colonies of cancer cells. If shark cartilage can prevent cancer growth and its spread, why not use it? Why wait indefinitely for chemists to isolate and synthesize so-called active ingredients while scores of cancer victims die needlessly? Ladies and gentlemen of the jury, is this not medical malpractice in its most virulent form? You be the judge. You must speak for the dead cancer victim who can no longer protest, and for the uninformed public who do not know that they should protest.

Breast cancers begin to metastasize when quite small and are undetectable by any known method. This is what makes breast cancer such a destructive disease. Shark cartilage can prevent breast cancer from metastasizing and shrink the original tumor. [82] In 1990 Dr. Robert Langer and his associates published a paper in *Science* in which they claimed to have isolated a macro-protein from cartilage that had anti-angiogenesis

properties. Later that year the Japanese identified two other macro-pro-
teins that inhibited vascularization. [83]

And so the search for the magic-bullet in shark cartilage would have
continued decade after decade in the back drop of accumulating and esca-
lating cancer deaths year by year had not a courageous chemist with doc-
torates in biochemistry and nutrition from Rutgers University entered the
fray. In the 1970s Dr. William Lane was working as a consultant to the
Shah of Iran when the Shah asked him to develop a fishery in the Persian
Gulf. He suggested to the Shah that he fish for and market sharks, which
were very populous in the Gulf. It was at this time that William Lane
began an intense study of sharks. In 1981 he met Dr. John Prudent and
learned of his experiments with bovine cartilage in cancer treatment. Dr.
William Lane then determined to utilize the cartilage from his shark business for cancer research. Later in 1981 he met with Dr. Robert Langer
who had made headlines with his use of extracts from shark cartilage in
cancer research. Dr. Langer agreed that the use of whole shark cartilage
might provide even better results because all the active ingredients in the
cartilage would be working synergistically.

By 1985 Dr. Lane had devised a method of pulverizing the cartilage
under nitrogen and freeze drying it so that the active proteins would not
be degraded by oxygen. That same year Lane sent some of this specially
processed whole-shark cartilage to Dr. Prudden and asked him to compare
it with the bovine cartilage he was using. Dr. Prudden sent it to Dr. Durie
at the University of Arizona who did the comparative tests. Dr. Durie
reported that the shark cartilage was providing better results that the
bovine cartilage he had been using. [84] Dr. Lane took Dr. Durie's data
to Europe, which was more open to the use of natural products in cancer
research than the United States. He was introduced to Dr. Henri Tagnon,
head of the prestigious Institut Jules Bordet in Brussels. Dr. Bordet was
so impressed with the data that, after reviewing exiting literature on the
subject of anti-angiogenesis inhibitors, he had his team of top researchers
do the preliminary toxicology tests. When these tests came back favorable,
he immediately commenced to do the necessary animal and then human
studies. First rats were fed large quantities of the processed shark cartilage.
They showed no signs of toxicity. Next Dr. Ghanem Atassi fed test animals which had leukemia cell implants with oral doses of shark cartilage.
Depending on the doses received, the test animals lived 34% longer than
cancerous animals not fed the cartilage. [85]

Encouraged by these positive results, Dr. Atassi tested the shark cartilage against metastasized cancers. Rats with an induced melanoma metastasis were fed 1,200 milligrams of cartilage per 1 kilogram of body weight
for twenty-eight days. The tumors in the control group doubled in size in
twenty-one days. The tumors in the rats fed the cartilage reduced in size
by 17% in twenty-one days. The Bordet researchers were ecstatic, because
the results were better that those obtained by even the most aggressive chemotherapy procedures. [86] This experiment showed that tumor masses
release angiogenesis substances after two weeks of growth, at which time
the tumors, now richly supplied by blood vessels, grew rapidly.

A repeat of the experiment with a slight modifier achieved a 40%
reduction of tumor mass, while the untreated animals had their tumors
increase by two and a half times in the same period. This latter experiment
established that if the blood network can be kept from forming, cancer
growth can be prevented—confirming that shark cartilage can be used as
a *preventative* in cancer treatment as well as a *cure* for cancer, especially
when combined with a nutrition program. [87] Despite these impressive
results, Dr. Lane was still not able to get the American medical establishment to get excited about the use of shark cartilage in cancer research.
Because the medical establishment has substantially curtained medical
freedom in America, Dr. Lane turned to countries south of the border
that have greater medical freedom than America.

In the late 1980s Dr. Lane supplied Dr. Carlos Luis Alpizar of Costa
Rica with shark cartilage for use with a patient with inoperable abdominal
cancer that was as large as a grapefruit. Dr. Alpizar administered 12 grams
per day in three equal portions before meals. Within a month the tumor
stopped growing; after six months the tumor had reduced to the size of a
walnut. The patient recovered and was able to return to work and a normal
life. [88]

Seeking a greater outlet for cancer research using human subjects,
Dr. Lane flew to Mexico in 1991 and was able to obtain the cooperation
of the directors of the Ernesto Contreras Hospital in Tijuana, Mexico.
Dr. Ernesto Contreras, Sr. has an untarnished reputation in Mexico as a
first-class physician. He and his sons, Dr. Ernesto Contreras, Jr. and Dr.
Francisco Contreras, are the physician-directors of the Ernesto Contreras
Hospital. They agreed to use Dr. Lane's purified shark cartilage in large
doses in eight late-stage cancer patients whose conditions were all considered terminal. They were each given 30 grams of the cartilage in a water

suspension. For female patients, one-half was given as an enema and the other half via the vagina cavity later in the day. The men were given two retention enemas daily. This method ensured maximum absorption by the body of the cartilage product. After two months, seven of the eight patients showed a reduction of tumor size from of between 30 and 100%.

These case histories are available for review in Dr. Lane's book, *Sharks Don't Get Cancer*. Just a few examples of the efficacy of whole shark cartilage will be cited here. A forty-eight-year-old woman with Stage 2 inoperable uterine cervix cancer, which had spread to the bladder, that had not responded to radiation therapy showed an 80% reduction of the tumor after seven weeks of treatment with shark cartilage. After eleven weeks the tumor had completely disappeared. Dr. Lane explained that shark cartilage can cause the necrosis of tumors because it interferes with the routine breakdown and repair process that goes on in the blood vessel network within a tumor mass. [89]

In May 1992 Dr. Roscoe L. Van Zandt—a gynecologist in Arlington, Texas, who is forced to do his cancer research and treatment in Mexico, at the Hoxsey Clinic in Tijuana—released his clinical studies of eight women with advanced breast tumors. They had all received 30 to 60 grams daily of shark cartilage orally. In all eight patients the tumors significantly reduced in size. Surgical examination of the tumors revealed that they had turned from pink to grey, a sign of necrosis or death of the tumor. One important finding was that two of the tumors, which had been attached to the chest wall of the two respective patients, had reduced in size and had become free floating, allowing for surgical removal—something that rarely, if ever, happens once the tumors anchor themselves in the bone. [90]

Some more spectacular outcomes were obtained by Dr. Ella Ferguson in Panama in 1991. He treated a forty-three-year-old male suffering from terminal lung cancer, which had spread to the bone and into the brain. After three months of taking capsules of shark cartilage, the patient stopped feeling pain in his chest and hips. Thereafter the dosage was increased from 30 grams daily to 60 grams. Within seventy-two hours the pain in his brain subsided and his double vision cleared up, indicating that the brain tumor had shrunk. [91] In another case a patient with advanced liver cancer experienced complete remission after eight weeks when treated with 60 grams of shark cartilage given in 15-gram retention enemas. [92] Bear in mind that the medical monopoly in America maintains that once cancer has metastasized, treatment is virtually hopeless.

Dr. Lane's work with shark cartilage was given great exposure in 1992 and 1993 through a 60 *Minutes* expose of the use of shark cartilage in Cuba. The Cuban Government arranged for twenty-seven terminally ill, stages 3 and 4 patients with a variety of cancers to receive treatment using 60 grams daily of shark cartilage daily. Later on, the dosage was changed to 1 gram of shark cartilage per every 2 pounds of body weight. This meant that a 180-pound man would receive 90 grams daily and a 110-pound woman 55 grams daily. In early January 1993 the eighteen patients who had remained in the study were evaluated. Despite a diet poor in minerals and vitamins, almost 40% of the patients experienced significant improvement in their conditions. Tumors shrank, pain decreased, and where present, symptoms such as rheumatoid arthritis, osteoarthritis, and psoriasis disappeared. [93]

Ladies and gentlemen, you would think that with all of their grandiose talk about waging war on cancer, the National Cancer Institute, the American Cancer Society, and the medical establishment would rejoice at these spectacular breakthroughs in the treatment of cancer. After all, in standard drug approaches, any drug that achieves a modest 3 to 4% response is considered a breakthrough. Shark cartilage was achieving considerably greater success, 100% cures in many instances. Don't hold your breath for this one. Predictably, there was no response from the medical establishment on the use of shark cartilage to destroy cancers. Shark cartilage is not synthesized by chemists or prescribed by physicians. There is just not enough money to be made by the use of this natural product. With steel-cold financial calculation, the pharmaceutical oriented researchers placed all of their focus on trying to isolate the active protein ingredients in the shark cartilage, which they then hoped to synthesize and sell as a drug at tremendous profit.

The FDA has aided and abetted this mercenary practice by refusing to give approval for the use of the pure shark cartilage product because it is a natural product. [94] Dr. Lane found that it was impossible to get the National Institutes of Health and the National Cancer Institute involved in the shark cartilage research. Apparently their position is that if it could not be used in drug form, they were not interested. [95] This is another example of how sinful man, in rebellion against his Creator, turns from the simple, natural remedies the Creator has abundantly supplied for the healing of disease to man-made substitutes. Good, wholesome food supplied by our Creator is the best of preventative medicines. It is, along with the herbs and natural products of nature, the best remedy for disease—acting together, they supply nutrients to restore the human frame, thus allowing the body to heal itself.

The FDA's identification of medicine with drugs has warped the concept of medicine and confounded people's ideas as to the source of good health. The force of government acting through the FDA is thus enlisted on the side of lucrative efforts of resolving disease and against the inexpensive natural remedies of the Creator. Is it not true that there is a way that seems right onto a man, but the path thereof leads to death? Proverbs 14: 12.

In 1993 Dr. Richard Passwater, author of *Cancer Prevention and Nutritional Therapies*, acknowledged that shark cartilage may prove to be the most promising weapon against cancer tumors, achieving cure rates as high as 90%. He said that shark cartilage would achieve this by preventing tumors from developing and maintaining their blood supplies. [96] Yet no one was listening, at least not in the medical establishment. Is it not high time that the American people wake up to the politics being played with their health and very lives?

Ladies and gentlemen of the jury, Dr. Richard Passwater is a top nutritionist and scientist who has been at the forefront of nutritional approaches to cancer prevention since the 1960s. When he first published *Cancer and Its Nutritional Therapies* in 1978, the idea that diet affected the course of cancer was considered medical heresy. He has lived long enough to see many leading scientists admit the causal relationship between diet and cancer. Most scientists now concede that diet may be the cause of up 80% of all cancers. [97] Even the National Cancer Institute now concedes that diet may be the leading cause of cancer. Dr. William DeWys of the NCI estimated that diet causes 35% of all cancers, tobacco causes about 30%, viruses about 5%, occupation about 4%, alcohol about 3%, excess sunshine about 3%, environmental pollution about 2%, medicine and medical procedures about 1%, and food additives 1%. [98]

Dr. Richard Passwater welcomes this endorsement of his life's work but states that these establishment doctors are still not looking at the whole picture. While they are focusing on the roles of saturated fat and fiberless diets as a cause of many cancers, he states that they are overlooking the part played by *micronutrients* such as vitamins and minerals that can protect us from cancers caused by smoking and chemicals. Smoking and diet, Passwater maintained, are the cause of the majority of cancers. [99]

Passwater contended that one can achieve a 90% reduction in cancer risk and incidence by using micronutrients and reducing one's exposure to cancer-initiating agents. [100] Dr. Passwater also had stern criticism for the cancer establishment, particularly the National Cancer Institute, which he felt has misused and misdirected the enormous governmental funds made available through the National Cancer Act of 1971. This was the same Act that inaugurated the so-called war on Cancer. The NCI budget went from $180 million in 1971 to $400 million in 1972, and then escalated to $2 billion annually in 1993. He contended that the vast majority of this additional money was channeled into the old lines of research, primarily chemotherapeutic, instead of into other innovative approaches. He regretted this, especially in light of the paucity of good results from the standard approaches of surgery, radiation, and chemotherapy. [101]

Dr. Passwater has not been the only voice criticizing the cancer establishment and calling for new approaches. He cited Dr. Ralph Moss, former public affairs director at Memorial Sloan-Kettering Cancer Center in New York.

> Our country is waging a billion-dollar war on cancer, and we seem to be losing ... Conventional surgery, radiation and chemotherapy treatments are often more devastating to the patient than the disease itself ... the cancer field continues to be marked by political power grabs and economic selfishness. With billions of dollars in research and treatment money ... there is fierce competition ... Cancer patients seem to be the losers ... while orthodoxy appears to have all the cards—money, power, prestigious credentials, influence in the major media—the continuing failure of orthodox medicine to deal satisfactorily with the major forms of cancer guarantees the growth of non-conventional approaches. [102]

Dr. Passwater firmly believes that nutritional therapies can be a valuable adjunct to conventional treatments. It is not always an either/or situation. He asserted that at the very least, nutritional supplements can strengthen the immune system, which is the body's last line of defense for overcoming existing cancer. [103] Holding that the best defense is a good offense, he contended that nutritional therapies can do more than merely strengthen the immune system. He argued that preventing cancer is more important than waiting until you get cancer and then trying to eliminate it.

He believes that adequate *micronutrients* can prevent cancer in several important ways: they can help activate the liver so that it can more effectively destroy invading chemicals that cause cancer; and they can fortify the body's second line of defense—the membranes that are the skin of every cell, which will keep cancer agents from entering the cells. If the carcinogens do penetrate the cells, antioxidant micronutrients can prevent harmful reactions from occurring by destroying the free radicals that actually do the damage. Micronutrients can also repair free radical damage and strengthen the immune system.

Ladies and gentlemen of the jury, let us now examine the ways in which supplementing with micronutrients can prevent and cure cancer. Combating free radicals is a good point in which to introduce the beneficial action of micronutrients. It is now well known that free radicals can cause up to sixty human diseases, including cancer. [104] Keep in mind that the harm done by free radicals depends on their number, where they are formed, and the biological system involved. [105] Although the body in its normal metabolic processes produce some free radicals, it is also known that carcinogens readily produce free radicals, adding to the load of free radicals in the body and increasing the cancer risk. Nutritional experts state that it is one of the tasks of antioxidant nutrients such as vitamin A, vitamin C, vitamin E, coenzyme Q-10, beta-carotene, and the trace mineral selenium as well as various enzymes to protect the body from free radical activity. In so doing they protect us not only from cancer but from other degenerative diseases, such as heart disease. [106]

Free radicals can exist in the form of molecules, atoms, or chemical fragments called ions. What is common among these chemicals is that they have lost or gained one or more electrons and have a net electrical charge instead of being neutral, thus making their behavior radical. Free radicals that have lost an electron try to regain one by taking an electron from another molecule. This is how they do their damage. In taking an electron from another molecule, that molecule becomes a free radical in turn, and so on and on in a destructive chain reaction. [107] When a molecule becomes a free radical, it loses its normal function while in that state. For example, when a metal ion gains an electron, it is called a *reduced* metal free radical. When the reduced metal passes on this extra electron to an oxygen atom, the oxygen is transformed into a free radical called superoxide. This superoxide can be converted into hydroperoxide, which is fairly stable. But if the superoxide acquires yet another electron from a reduced metal, it becomes a hydroxyl free radical, which is very reactive. [108]

Hydroxyl radicals and other free radicals can damage cellular fats, proteins, and DNA, impairing their function. Enzymes can repair much of the damage to proteins, but when the enzymes themselves are damaged by free radicals, the body's ability to repair metabolic damage is impaired. Thus an excess of free radicals can be very destructive to the body's repair and defense mechanism and so compromise the immune system. [109]

It is important to keep in mind that while the beneficial action of antioxidant nutrients are being discussed separately for the sake of simplicity and clarity, in the human body they do not work alone; rather they function synergistically, that is, as a team, assisting each other directly or indirectly. Ladies and gentlemen, while supplementing with vitamin and mineral micronutrients play valuable roles in preventing and reversing chronic degenerative diseases, it must be made very clear that micronutrients prepared from live fruits and vegetables and preserved in their food matrix is superior to commercially prepared micronutrients because they are more easily assimilated by the body. Dr. Colin Campbell is emphatic in *The China Study* that the best source of micronutrients is natural fruits and vegetables. Micronutrients prepared by such companies as Mannatech and Dr. Richard Schulze's Superfood Plus protocol are preferred above the chemically prepared brands. Besides being more absorbable, they are found in the context of natural phytochemicals, fibers, and enzymes with which they act synergistically. The physiology and metabolism of the body is extremely complex, so be wary of silver-bullet remedies, even in the area of micronutrients. The following evidence will show that micronutrients work best to reverse chronic degenerative diseases in the context of a broader nutritional and lifestyle reform. Let us consider how supplementing with vitamin A and carotenoids can protect us from cancer. Both vitamin A and beta-carotene can protect us from cancer, but they do so in different ways. Generally speaking, vitamin A is found only in animal products; its precursor, beta carotene, is found in plant foods such as fruits, leafy green vegetables, and yellow or orange vegetables. The vegetarian can take comfort in the fact that the body has an enzyme that can cleave a beta-carotene molecule in half, producing two molecules of vitamin A. Vitamin A was associated with cancer protection shortly after its discovery in 1913 by McCollum and Davis. In 1922 Dr. S. Mori published studies describing cancer-like changes with vitamin A deficiency. [110] In 1925

Drs. S. B. Wolbach and P.R. Howe described similar cancer-like changes in tissue following vitamin A deprivation. [111]

Over the next few decades other studies demonstrated that vitamin A plays a vital role in the maintenance of normal tissue and actually helps controls cellular growth. Hence a vitamin A deficiency can lead to metaplastic changes. These studies also showed that vitamin A helps determine cell differentiation. Since cancer is unregulated cellular growth, vitamin A helps prevent cancer by regulating cell growth and development. [112] Since over half of all human cancers starts in the specialized cells making up epithelial tissue, one can readily see the link between vitamin A deficiency and cancer of the lining of organs, the mammary glands, the respiratory tract, the digestive tract, the urinary tract, the reproductive tract, and skin, all of which are lined with epithelial tissue. These specialized epithelial cells depend upon vitamin A for their normal development. Dr. Michael Sporn of the National Cancer Institute stated in 1977 that:

Vitamin A is a hormone-like controller of cell differentiation... . If you are vitamin A deficient, there is no question that you may be more susceptible to development of cancer ... Probably one of your best investments that you can make in your food budget is to spend a few cents a day and take a multivitamin capsule. [113]

Vitamin A and carotenoids are also antioxidants, providing yet another way in which these micronutrients can protect us against the action of free radicals. In 1975 Dr. E. Bjelke did a study of 8,278 men in Norway and found that carotenoids provided protection against lung cancer. [114] Vitamin A and carotenoids protect us against cancer by enhancing normal cell communication while preventing mutated cells from communicating and growing. Additionally, carotenoids help synthesize specialized proteins called *connexin* or gap-junction proteins, which facilitate intercellular communication. [115]

Now that we understand something about the protective function of vitamin A and beta-carotene, let us look at some of the clinical studies proving their efficacy against cancer. Dr. T. Hirayama did a study of 25,000 Japanese in 1979 with beta-carotene. He demonstrated that beta-carotene does prevent cancer of the lung, stomach, colon, prostate, and cervix. [116]

While doing research on cholesterol and heart disease in 1981 some

internationally famous researchers observed vitamin A's potential for protecting us from cancer. In that year Dr. Jeremiah Stamler of Northwestern
University School of Medicine and colleagues at three other institutions
published a joint paper showing the results of following 1,954 middle-
aged men for nineteen years. The study compared the incidence of cancer
on four different groups that had different amounts of vitamin A and
beta-carotene in their diets. The amount of vitamin A and beta-carotene
consumed was divided into four levels. It was found that the men who
consumed the smallest amount of these two nutrients had seven times
the incidence of lung cancer compared to the group who consumed the
greatest amount of vitamin A and beta-carotene. What was even more
significant was the finding that smokers who consumed only the amount
of vitamin A and beta-carotene in the first and lowest quartile had 8.1
times the incidence of cancer than those who consumed the highest level
of these nutrients. In other words, when vitamin A and beta-carotene are
taken at certain levels, even smokers can obtain protection from lung cancer. [117]

In 1982 a Committee on Diet, Nutrition, and Cancer selected by the
National Research Council, which is a part of the National Academy of
Sciences, published a report demonstrating the link between beta carotene
and reduced cancer risk. The Committee stated: "Epidemiological evidence is sufficient to suggest that foods rich in carotene or vitamin A are
associated with a reduced risk of cancer." [118]

Dr. Passwater stated that these and other findings have moved scientists to put pressure upon the FDA and other cancer institutions to
examine the evidence with a view of re-examining their positions on anti-
cancer nutrients. At the same time he advised the public to take steps to
protect themselves with these supplements and not wait for the voice of
officialdom to approve the use of these beneficial antioxidants. The most
important step to take, he stated, is to eat natural, unprocessed foods high
in these nutrients. One should also supplement one's diet with 5,000 to
10,000 IU of vitamin A and 15 to 25 milligrams of beta-carotene daily
to reduce one's risk of cancer. [119] Dr. Passwater felt that conventional
medical cancer therapies can benefit from the concurrent use of natural
nutritional remedies consisting of generous amounts of fruits and vegetables and their juices rich in vitamin A and beta-carotene; however other
nutritional doctors would discourage the use of radiation and chemotherapy as an adjunct to nutritional remedies because theses modalities impair

the immune system, the very defense mechanism that helps one destroy cancer. [120] Many experts recommend juicing fruits and vegetables (separately, of course) as an excellent way of concentrating and using these micronutrients.

Prominent among those doctors who utilize primarily nutritional modalities is Dr. Lorraine Day, former chief of orthopedic medicine at San Francisco General Hospital, who cured herself of breast cancer by nutritional remedies alone. [121] Other cancer patients following her natural foods diet have achieved reversal of their breast cancers and leukemia. Dr. Lorraine Day advised us to limit the amount of processed food we eat. She called processed foods *dead* foods because almost all the micronutrients have been removed in the processing. To get sufficient micronutrients she urged us to eat natural foods, eating them raw as much as possible.

Dr. Day also recommended juicing fruits and vegetables (separately) so as to get concentrated amounts of these micronutrients. She also advocated the use of Barley Green, a powered form of the barley leaf extract. The leaf is harvested at twelve weeks, juiced, and then reduced to a powder. Dr. Day's regime is comprehensive. It includes utilizing all of God's tools for the maintenance and restoration of health. Her nutritional modalities are supplemented with exercise, rest, sunlight, water, fresh air, and trust in God; a regime also advocated by Weimar Institute in northern California.

Ladies and gentlemen of the jury, let us look at testimony regarding the use of vitamin C in cancer prevention and cure. The testimony will demonstrate that large doses of vitamin C can prevent cancer. When two-times-winner of the Nobel Laureate, Dr. Linus Pauling proved to the world that vitamin C in large doses can prevent cancer, the cancer establishment ridiculed him. But Dr. Pauling had the last say when the National Cancer Institute's Cancer Prevention and Control Division convened a symposium in the summer of 1990 consisting of the world's top scientists to discuss vitamin C's efficacy against cancer. They had before them evidence from over one hundred epidemiological studies demonstrating the benefits of vitamin C in preventing cancer. One of the explicit findings of this conference was that:

> Evidence continues to accumulate that vitamin C has numerous biologic effects, including some that may relate to the prevention of cancer. [122]

This was a clear endorsement of the work of Dr. Linus Pauling and a rejection of the position of conventional medicine. Yet, despite the vast and overwhelming evidence of the efficacy of vitamin C in the prevention and control of cancer, and despite its endorsement by world renowned scientists, the FDA still refused to officially endorse this nutrient's role in fighting cancer. In protest of official intransigence, Dr. Gladys Block left the National Cancer Institute for work with the University of California at Berkeley, and in 1992, she appealed to other top scientists to petition the FDA to recognize the health role of vitamin C in cancer prevention.

I have reviewed the epidemiologic literature, about 140 studies, on the relationship between antioxidant micronutrients or their food sources and cancer risk. The data are overwhelmingly consistent. With possibly fewer than five exceptions, every single study is in the protective direction, and something like 110 to 120 studies found statistically significant reduced risk with high intake. [123]

Her appeals fell on deaf ears. One may well ask, who is the FDA working for. Is the function of the FDA to protect our heath or to maintain industrial and medical monopolies that are at best injuring us? The power of the FDA has to be curtailed. Its adulterous relationship with big business—particularly the pharmaceutical industry, the medical associations, and the fast food industry—has to be ended.

The evidence is very clear that vitamin C protects us against cancer through a number of biologic mechanisms. It serves as an antioxidant that traps and defuses free radicals, thus protecting body tissue from being damaged by these free radicals. When vitamin C reduces an oxidized free radical mineral, this mineral is now available as a coenzyme to the enzymes in the body. Since enzymes control body chemistry, the net result of vitamin C's antioxidant activity is to restore proper metabolic activity to the body by ensuring that enzymes are paired with their mineral coenzymes. Dr. Harish Padh at the University of Chicago noted this twofold function of vitamin C.

The available data suggest that perhaps the most significant role of ascorbate [vitamin C] is as a reductant that, along with other reducing agents, minimizes damages by oxidative processes. This role includes keeping iron and copper ions in some enzymes in their required reduced form and neutralizing harmful oxidants and free radicals. [124]

Vitamin C also directly enhances the immune system in a variety of ways. It has been discovered that vitamin C can concentrate in neutrophils and lymphocytes, thus supercharging them against viruses and bacteria. In their protective role white blood cells can engulf bacteria, but is has been discovered that without large amounts of vitamin C, they cannot break down the bacteria. [125] Despite the claims of the FDA, this ability of vitamin C to concentrate in white blood cells vindicates the practice of taking mega doses of vitamin C supplements as advocated by Dr. Pauling and others. Vitamin C also enhances immune function in working synergistically with vitamin E. It is now known that vitamin C repairs vitamin E after it is destroyed in the act of fighting free radicals. [126]

Ladies and gentlemen of the jury, physicians practicing nutritional medicine will testify to you that vitamin C is not only useful in *preventing* cancer, it can help *cure* cancer. In 1971 Dr. Linus Pauling—working with Dr. Ewan Cameron at the Vale of Leven Hospital, Loch Lomondside, Scotland—demonstrated the beneficial action of vitamin C in treating cancer patients. They treated 100 terminally ill cancer patients with 10 grams of vitamin C daily and compared the results with 1,000 cancer patients not treated with vitamin C. When they published their findings in 1978, the patients treated with vitamin C had lived four times longer than those not treated. By 1978, thirteen of the vitamin C treated patients were still alive; twelve were cancer free while all 1,000 non-treated patients were dead. [127] *The evidence is clear: vitamin C in large doses can cure some cases of cancer.* Other experts would argue that combined with other nutritional modalities, vitamin C would do even better in reversing cancer in all types of cancer patients.

Dr. Pauling's 1978 report showed that colon cancer patients treated with vitamin C lived seven times longer than non-treated patients; breast cancer patients treated with vitamin C lived six times longer than non-treated patients; and kidney cancer patients treated with vitamin C lived five times longer than non-treated patients. [128] Dr. Pauling wrote two books that can be helpful to cancer patients and those interested in a more healthy life: *Cancer and Vitamin C* and *How to Live Longer and Feel Better.* Since his pioneering work with vitamin C, new methods of production have produced even more potent forms of vitamin C. The vitamin C metabolite L-threonic acid, sold under the trade name Ester C, is reputed to be more absorbable than other commercial forms of vitamin C.

Between 1988 and 1989 Dr. Pauling and Dr. Abram Hoffer of Victoria, British Columbia, treated terminally ill cancer patients who were not expected to live more than five to six months with large doses of vitamin C. Most of those treated were alive in 1992 when Dr. Richard Passwater reported on this study. The average vitamin C patient had at that time lived fifteen times longer than the non-treated patient. [129] Passwater observed that the cancer establishment did not only scoff at Dr. Pauling's work, they tried to destroy it by conducting rigged studies. One such study by the Mayo clinic treated cancer victims with large doses of vitamin C for ten weeks. They then reported the death of all the treated patients. What they failed to say is that the cancer patients did not die while receiving the vitamin C. They only died after the vitamin C was stopped! Apparently fraudulent medical research and reporting is acceptable when it protects the financial bottom line of the cancer industry. In Dr. Pauling's protocol, the patients are to remain on vitamin C for the rest of their lives; unless of course they radically change their harmful life styles and eating patterns. Clearly vitamin C in large doses can be useful in controlling cancer. But it is not to be used alone; combined with other nutritional modalities, vitamin C would reverse cancer in more cancer patients.

What is clearly demonstrated by the results of Dr. Pauling's work and the response of the cancer establishment to his work, is that orthodox medicine does not have a genuine interest in finding a cure for cancer. They are interested only in the economic benefits flowing from the high cost of conventional cancer therapy. But the lives of millions of cancer patients are the pawns in their high-stake economic gambit.

The evidence also shows that vitamin E plays a vital role in controlling cancer. Researchers have found that, although vitamin E by itself is a powerful antioxidant, in the treatment of cancer it must act synergistically with other nutrients, such as vitamin C and the trace mineral selenium. Dr. Paula Horvath and Dr. Clement Ip reported:

Vitamin E, although ineffective by itself, was able to potentiate the ability of selenium to inhibit the development of mammary tumors. [130]

These two researchers found that although selenium alone was able to reduce tumor development, it worked much more efficiently in the presence of vitamin E. [131] A large scale study in Finland involving 21,172 men showed a statistically significant relationship between vitamin E levels and cancer. [132] Nevertheless, the overwhelming data revealed the futility of testing the antioxidant nutrients one by one, as is often done by the cancer establishment. If the cancer institutions were to use antioxidants *synergistically* during their treatment of cancerous tumors, their results might very well match the results obtained by nutritional doctors.

In light of the fact that micronutrients act synergistically, Dr. Passwater emphatically remarked:

Looking at vitamin E by itself, or any antioxidant by itself, is a waste of time. [133]

But this is what conventional medicine does in their rigged studies aimed at discrediting the use of micronutrients! If the true effect of antioxidants on cancer is to be determined, they must be tested in their synergistic combinations. Even when working in combinations, certain antioxidants inhibit cancer only at specific stages in the development of the tumor, and this must be taken into account. For example, Dr. Passwater observed that vitamin E facilitates the anti-carcinogenic action of selenium only during the *promotion* or *proliferation* phases of cancer development. [134]

In 1984 a British team of researchers led by Dr. N. J. Wald discovered that vitamin E and beta-carotene levels tended to be lower in breast cancer patients. [135] Unfortunately, they did not study these nutrients in combination, thus they missed the chance of discovering the potent synergistic effect of the two nutrients against cancer. In 1985 the synergistic effect of vitamin E and selenium against cancer was studied by Dr. Jukka Salonen at the University of Kuopio in Finland. Dr. Jukka had been following 12,155 Finns for several years in the famous North Karelia Project. Four years after blood samples were drawn from these participants in the study, fifty-one died of cancer. These fifty-one were then matched by age, sex, and smoking habits with surviving members of the group, and their blood samples were compared. Both vitamin E and selenium levels in the blood were studied. For persons with low selenium levels who also had low vitamin E levels, the risk of cancer was 11.4 to 1 compared with those with high selenium and vitamin E levels. Reviewing the data from this study, Dr. Passwater noted that there was a reduction in cancer risk of 91% with the intake of just these two antioxidants. [136]

Besides its role as an antioxidant, vitamin E has been found to act in a number of other ways to prevent cancer. For example it can react with some cancer-causing chemicals to deactivate them. It can also inhibit nitrate and nitrites from being converted into carcinogens. [137] Vitamin E plays a key role in enhancing immune function, thus improving the anti-cancer defenses of the body. Vitamin E also assists in white blood cell intercommunication, and it helps maintain lymphocyte membrane fluidity, which is vital for immune response. [138] Dr. Passwater criticized the inadequate RDA of 15 IU for vitamin E consumption. He recommended 100 to 1,000 IU of vitamin E daily to prevent cancer. [139]

As has been shown, chemotherapy is a chemical poisoning of the body in the hope that the cancer is killed before the patient. But vitamin E can help control the effects of such drug poisoning. Passwater observed that vitamin E in large doses of 1600 IU has been found to prevent chemotherapy patients from losing much of their hair. [140] Dr. Patrick Quillin is a nutritionist who has used nutritional modalities as an adjunct to conventional cancer remedies. He has had great success in this approach. Recognizing that cancer is a metabolic disease and hence the remedy must be a nutritional one, Dr. Patrick Quillin wrote in *Beating Cancer with Nutrition:*

> Cancer is an abnormal growth, not just a regionalized lump or bump. Chemo, radiation and surgery will reduce tumor burden, but they will do nothing to change the underlying conditions that allowed this abnormal growth to change the underlying conditions that allowed this abnormal growth to thrive. In a nutshell, this book is designed to change the conditions in the body that favor tumor growth and return the cancer victor to a healthier status. [141]

In November of 1992, Dr. Patrick Quillin organized the first scientific conference on nutrition for the cancer patient. There were twenty-six speakers and 3,000 scientists and clinicians from around the world in attendance. He reported that the evidence presented is substantial. The data pointed to an inexpensive and low-risk method for extending the quality and quantity of life of cancer patients. [142] In his insightful book Dr. Patrick Quillin devoted a chapter to reviewing the more prominent alternative approaches to cancer treatment. Recognizing that there is promise with many of these nutritional approaches, he called for further research and study along these lines. He stated, however, that there is one major impediment to advancement along alternative treatment lines: *Government bureaucracies in alliance with the cancer establishment.* He exposed some of the same cast of characters, whom other experts have identified as unfairly controlling the direction of medicine in America today.

There is one problem with this long menu of alternative therapies for cancer: the gatekeepers of the Food and Drug Administration, the insurance industry, the American Medical Association and the American Cancer Society have been quick to "throw out the baby with the bath-water." That is, some of these approaches warrant further study, yet they have all been lumped together under the tainted reputation of "fringe" and either discouraged or outlawed. We need to separate the chaff from the grain in these therapies and expose them to some much needed research scrutiny. [143]

Ladies and gentlemen of the jury, if there is one thing better than curing cancer, it is preventing cancer. All of the nutritional regimes discussed in this chapter will of course help stave off the dreaded disease. The nutritional approach is not a single-bullet remedy. No one advocates utilization of herbs or vitamins in a vain attempt to reverse the effects of an improper diet and lifestyle. Nutritional regimes include eating a wholesome diet, excluding animal products, refined foods and sugar, besides the use of supplements, preferably in their food matrix. Dr. James Duke, in his exhaustive and well-researched book *The Green Pharmacy*, made this point well:

> When it comes to preventing cancer, the key seems to be eating as wide a variety of fruits and vegetables as possible. In a sense, then, if you want to lower your risk of cancer, you can create a whole diet—excluding or minimizing meats and dairy products—that consists of healing herbs. So singling out individual plants would be giving you a false picture of how to use herbs to prevent cancer ... the research is very clear. As fat and meat consumption increases, cancer rates rise. But as fruit and vegetable consumption increases, thereby lowering fat in the diet and increasing the amount of fiber and helpful phytochemicals, cancer rates fall. [144]

Dr. James Duke provided us with a Cancer Prevention Herbal Salad that consists of the following ingredients: garlic, onions, red peppers, tomatoes, red clover flowers, chopped cooked beets, fresh calendula flowers, celery, fresh chicory flowers, chives, cucumbers, cumin, peanuts, poke salad, purslane, and sage. [145] For a salad dressing he used flaxseed oil, evening primrose oil, garlic, rosemary, a dash of lemon juice, and that Latin American favorite, hot peppers. [146] Some of the anti-cancer phytochemicals found in this salad include the sulfides in garlic, the capsaicin in red peppers, the limonene in citrus fruits, and the lycopene in tomatoes. [147]

Dr. Mike Colgan, the world-famous sports nutritionist, also advocated prevention. He felt that the war *against cancer will be won not by the symptomatic remedies of the cancer establishment but by preventing the disease through educating the people on proper nutrition.* Noting that 90% of cancers are preventable, he wrote in *Prevent Cancer Now* that the cancer establishment must reverse its course and emphasize prevention.

> The answer to all major cancers lies not in surgery, drugs or radiation therapy. These procedures, though essential for treatment, have such a high failure rate, that we have to find another way.

> The answer lies in prevention. Yet even now, in 1990, less than 1% of cancer dollars is spent on prevention. Over 99% is spent on treatment, much of it ineffective, all of it wholly expensive ...

> Prevention happens slowly, by education, by the dissemination of information that you can use yourself. Prevention happens when you realize that no physician, hospital, or government agency can protect you against cancer. You have to learn to protect yourself. Self protection is what this book is about. [148]

Dr. Colgan emphasized that cancer is a metabolic disease and therefore the key to cancer prevention must be found by following a nutritious diet that builds up the body's immune defense mechanism. He stated that healthy bodies do not get cancer, only sick ones do.

> Cancer is predominantly a degenerative disease. Most cancers grow silently inside you for decades, before being discovered. They do not occur at all in healthy bodies.

> Before you can develop cancer, your body has to lose or damage many of its defense mechanisms. In the healthy person, these mechanisms destroy cancer cells every day. Esteemed British scientist and physician, Sir Peter Medawar, was fond of saying in lectures, that the average person gets cancer a million times in his

life. The healthy body destroys every one of these budding cancers long before they become established. [146]

Dr. Mike Colgan pointed out that certain unwholesome foods should be stricken from our diets if we are to avoid cancer. [147] In particular he singled out refined foods such as white bread and pastas made from white flour. Because white flour has been stripped of much of its micronutrients, its metabolism increases the chemical imbalance of the body and hence degrades the body's nutritious status and defense mechanisms. He explained that the metabolism of carbohydrates requires the following vitamin and minerals working together: thiamin, riboflavin, niacin, pantothenic acid, pyridoxine, phosphorus, and magnesium. [148] If even *one* of these ingredients is not present in adequate amounts our bodies cannot digest the carbohydrate. [149] These ingredients are largely removed by processing and only three are replaced in enriched bread. Obviously not enough of the essential micronutrients are replaced to permit us to digest the white flour. To digest the refined carbohydrate the body has to rob itself of these essential micronutrients—a process that degrades the body chemistry and so upsets the metabolism that degenerative diseases are the result.

> Virtually all of the eight essential nutrients are lost in the processing of white flour. Only three, thiamin, niacin and riboflavin, are added back in so-called enriched flour. So, in order to use enriched flour breads and baked goods, the body has to rob itself, depriving nerves and muscles of pantothenic acid, depleting bones and heart of phosphorus and magnesium. In this way, high use of processed foods creates degenerative processes in the body that indirectly prepare it for cancer. [150]

Dr. Colgan cited a study in which a group of rats were fed regular commercial white bread. All the rats were dead within sixty days. [151] He stated that if tough creatures such as rats cannot subsist on white bread, how can humans conceive that they can? Clearly we do not any longer eat for nutrition but for deceptively injurious pleasure. Dr. Colgan recommended that we buy whole grains, stone ground, and certified organic bread. [152]

In addition to eating wholesome foods with plenty of fresh fruits and vegetables, Dr. Colgan advocated that we supplement with vitamins and minerals, especially the antioxidants which prevent cancer. He included the antioxidant Coenzyme Q 10 in his list of supplements. [153] His primary reason for promoting the use of supplements was that our soils have been depleted of essential micronutrients and our foods are over processed. [154] He stated that lettuce loses half of its vitamins if kept a mere three days in the refrigerator. Asparagus, broccoli, and green beans lose half of their vitamin C in cold storage, and cooking vegetables can destroy up to 25% of their vitamin C and 70% of their thiamin. [155] The canning of foods can deplete their nutrients even more than storage or cooking. He cited Dr. Henry Schroeder, who demonstrated that canning carrots removes 70% of their cobalt and canning tomatoes removes 80% of their zinc. And canning green vegetables destroys half of their B vitamins. [156] Dr. Colgan also recommended supplementing with essential fatty acids such as omega 3, which has been shown to be a cancer inhibitor. [157]

Along with a nutritious diet, Dr. Mike Colgan advocated that we get plenty of the right form of exercise in order to prevent cancer. He feels that weight training combined with an appropriate aerobic sport will help us build up lean muscle and slow down the aging process than can predispose us to cancer. [158] In summary Dr. Mike Colgan's anti-cancer lifestyle included quitting smoking and the consumption of alcohol; maintaining a low body fat; eating a low-fat diet with high levels of fiber, vegetables, and fruits; taking a complete vitamin/mineral supplement with a high level of antioxidants; getting enough essential fatty acids such as omega 3 oils; drinking pure water; and exercising regularly. [159]

Building the immune system can help protect us against skin cancer, according to Dr. Neal Barnard in his inspirational book, *Eat Right, Live Longer.* [160] He stated that the immune system can be built up so as to protect us against skin cancer by increasing the antioxidant foods in our diet, by reducing the oils in our diet, and by avoiding ultra-violet light. [161] Immune changes made by ultra-violet light affect the whole body. This is shown by the fact that melanomas crop up in parts of the skin *not* exposed to the ultra-violet light. [162] Nutrients such as beta-carotene can help build the skin's immune strength. [163]

Dr. Barnard observed that the effect of reducing fats in the diet is dramatic. Studies show that cutting the fat intake in half dramatically reduced the risk of pre-cancerous skin changes. [164] The fat and oils in our diet end up in the cell membranes, and the proportion of mono-unsaturated, poly unsaturated, and saturated fats in our cells mirror the proportion in our diets. [165] People who eat more monounsaturated fats have less skin cancer; and those who eat more polyunsaturated fats have more skin cancer. [166]

Dr. Barnard's skin-protecting diet resembles most diets designed to prevent or reverse degenerative diseases in general.

Have plenty of vegetables each day. Include orange and yellow varieties like sweet potatoes and carrots, as well as dark green vegetables.

Include whole grains and legumes such as beans, peas and lentils, which provide vitamin E and selenium.

Avoid animal products.

Keep oils to a minimum. [167]

Ladies and gentlemen, one of the more recent and promising broad-based nutritional approaches to treating cancer is that advocated by Dr. Harvey Bigelsen, who was forced out of the United States and is now consultant for the Instituto De Medicina Biologica in Tijuana, Mexico. [168] Building on the work of Drs. Bechamp, Enderlein, Rife, Livingston-Wheeler, and Naessens, Dr. Bigelsen believed that diseases, including chronic degenerative disease like cancer, are caused by a breakdown of the internal environment of the organism. [169] This concept involves a radical departure from the conventional rationalistic teaching held by Galen, Descartes, Pasteur and Allopathic medicine today—that diseases are externally caused and can be identified by a specific antigen or germ, which can be in turn identified and destroyed by pharmaceutical weapons. [170] Rather, Dr. Bigelsen agreed with Dr. Bechamp that *the germ does not cause the disease, but the disease the germ.* Dr. Bechamp identified certain living protein entities he called the fundamental biological units of life that can become pathogens when exposed to a toxic, unhealthy environment.

If [Claude] Bernard provided the concept that it was the internal terrain that was important, Bechamp provided the mechanism that determines health or disease, and he showed how the system works. The fundamental question being argued was really Does the germ cause the disease, or does the disease cause the germ?

Bechamp showed that the latter is generally the case, and he showed how.

He identified fundamental biological units, which he called *microzymes*, which are the building blocks of microbes as well as other cells and which are today considered the precursors of DNA. *When the body becomes toxic, the microzymes survive by changing into pathogenic microbes.* Pasteur's concept that infectious disease can be caused only by external microbes was wrong. [171] [Emphasis added.]

The war on cancer is failing because it is based on some erroneous assumptions, assumptions such as Pasteur's that disease stems from external germs. This has led to a narrow focus on the symptom of cancer, the tumor, and the discovery of ways of killing it. Dr. Bigelsen argued that to successfully combat cancer we must make a 180-degree shift in our thinking about disease. He stated that we must adopt the approach of Dr. Naessens and others who held that cancer as well as other diseases are in fact caused by the internal bodily response to a toxic lifestyle and environment.

If the environment is out of balance, if it is toxic, deficient, or damaged, (e.g., due to radiation), and if that imbalance or toxicity continues for an extended period of time, then the microzymes will change into pathogenic forms and disease will be the result. Many chronic diseases, from chronic fatigue syndrome to candida albicans to mononucleosis to arthritis to cancer and AIDS, can result. Remove the stressors, restore the internal environment and the immune system to health, and the body will itself heal the disease. [172]

The ability of the microzymes, those fundamental biological units of living things, to change into pathogenic forms and back again into healthy forms is called pleomorphism. Dr. Bigelsen stated that *blood acidity* is a primary cause of pathogenic microorganism production in the pleomorphic cycle. [173] Dr. Bigelsen's cancer treatment therefore utilized a number of modalities to restore the internal environment to health. These modalities build the immune system, which then destroys the cancer. Dr. Bigelsen provided his patients with a list of foods to avoid. These included most processed foods, sugars, animal proteins, and fats, especially red meats, pork, and factory chickens that might contain pathological bacteria. Also on the prohibited list was meat contaminated with hormones and antibiotics and preservatives. He advocated instead a diet that freely embraces fresh, natural foods, such as fruits, vegetables, and grains free from preservatives, herbicides, and additives. [174]

Recognizing that our emotions can bring on diseases, Dr. Bigelsen emphasized the importance of stress reduction and exercise, encouraging health-giving emotions such as love and laughter. Norman Cousins showed us that laughter is a live-giving tonic. [175] Dr. Bigelsen also followed Drs. Linus Pauling and Livingston-Wheeler in supplying his patients with natural dietary supplements, which included dietary enzymes, vitamin C, and multiple vitamins and minerals. [176] In order to cleanse the body of toxic material and rid it of pathogenic microorganisms, Dr. Bigelsen endorsed Dr. Enderlein's practice of utilizing biological remedies, such as plant medicines and fungal extracts, that are capable of changing the disease-producing microorganisms back into harmless forms.

The Enderlein remedies join with and break down the harmful microbes, and also work with the body's immune system to eliminate any toxins dumped into the blood during the healing process. The remedies contain a "tame" version of the disease-producing microbe that reduces it to a harmless form. [177]

Dr. Bigelsen is not the only modern physician who has turned from the conventional cut, burn, and poison remedies of the cancer establishment to various types of immunosupportive therapies. The list of doctors crossing over to nutritional therapies is growing. The bottom line is that they are discovering that while degenerative diseases like cancer are serious, they can be cured. [178] By understanding the true causes of disease and the role of the immune system in both preventing and curing disease, we can have hope. We can have hope because change is in the wind all along the darkened medical horizon. Dr. Larry Dossey, chairman of one of the panels of the National Institute of Health's Office of Alternative Medicine, stated that one-third of the medical schools in American are now offering courses on alternative medicine. [179] But the warning of physicians like Dr. Richard Passwater is not to wait for the medical establishment to direct your health; rather, take back your God-given medical freedom and educate yourself about the cycle of life and health he has imprinted into nature.

Ladies and gentlemen, the role of nutrition in the prevention and reversal of cancer has been brought into sharp focus by the seminal work of Dr. Colin Campbell in his China Study. We have already considered some of his findings. But it will be beneficial to briefly review his work. The *Saturday Evening Post* called his China Study a landmark study that should shake up medical and nutrition researchers everywhere. [180] What was this earth-shaking discovery about the causes and prevention of cancer and other chronic degenerative diseases? Simply this, doctor Dr. Campbell had discovered what Hippocrates had known 2,500 years ago.

Our most powerful weapon against cancer [and other degenerative diseases] is the food we eat every day. [181]

Dr. Colin Campbell discovered that eating more than 10% animal protein promotes the onset and growth of cancer in all three phases—*initiation, promotion,* and *proliferation.* [182], [183], [184] Astonishingly, he discovered that we can turn cancer off and on by the amount of protein we consume! If cancer promotion commences at 20% protein intake, the growth stops when the protein is reduced to 5%. If we then increased the protein intake, the cancerous cells began to grow once more. [185] This was a revolutionary finding in cancer research.

Ladies and gentlemen of the jury, it should be very clear to you by now that we need not be hapless victims of this dreaded modern-day scourge we call cancer. Nor need we surrender our freedom and lives to the medical establishment, which would ruin our health and rob us of our lives by their drug nostrums. We can control our destinies. By our dietary habits and our lifestyles, we can determine whether a genetically damaged cell starts to grow within us in a cancerous fashion, remain dormant, or is destroyed and removed by the body's internal defense mechanisms.

Note this well—cancer cells will not grow and multiply within our bodies unless the right conditions are met. [186] Dr. Campbell stated that this is one of the most profound findings about cancer. Discussing the need for the right conditions to occur before cancer cells begin to multiple, Dr. Campbell wrote:

This is one of the most profound features of promotion. Promotion is reversible, depending on whether the early cancer growth is given the right conditions in which to grow. This is where certain dietary factors become so important. These dietary factors, called promoters, feed cancer growth. Other dietary factors, called anti-promoters, slow cancer growth. [187]

Moreover, a significant discovery by Dr. Campbell was that not all proteins have the same effect on the body. He discovered what Drs. Gerson, McDougall, and Whitaker and others were telling us for years; plant-based proteins and animal-based proteins are totally different in their affect on cancer initiation and promotion. Rats fed 20% plant-based proteins did not reveal any cancer initiation or formation *despite* exposure to carcinogens! [188]

Dr. Campbell's China Study confirmed his cancer research using rats. He found that as blood cholesterol in rural China rose in certain counties, as a result of eating animal-based proteins, the incident of Western diseases such as cancer and heart disease increased. [189], [190] In the West the average cholesterol is around 170 to 290mg/dl, and we consider 150mg/dl as normal. But in China the average cholesterol level is as low as 94 mg/dl!

As blood cholesterol levels decreased from 170 mg/dl to 90 mg/dl. cancers of the liver, rectum, colon, male lung, female lung, breast, childhood leukemia, adult leukemia, childhood brain, adult brain, stomach and esophagus (throat) decreased. [191]

Dr. Campbell also found that the high-fiber diets of rural Chinese were linked to lower blood cholesterol and lower rates of cancers of the rectum and colon. [192] The study also showed that high vitamin C intake in the form of fresh fruits was linked to lower levels of cancers of the esophageal, breast, stomach, liver, leukemia, colon, and lung. [193] It was not only excess animal-based protein that was linked to cancer, animal fat was also implicated. Dr. Campbell found that reducing dietary fat from 24% to 6% was linked to lower breast cancer rates. [194]

Finally, ladies and gentlemen of the jury, because breast cancer is so devastating to our mothers, wives and daughters and sisters, we will end our testimony on how to cure cancer nutritionally by reviewing the work of Dr. Johanna Budwig, a German biochemist trained in pharmaceutical science, physics, botany and biology. In 1951 she discovered that the blood of cancer patients was deficient in certain important and essential ingredients such as phosphatides and lipoproteins, while the blood of healthy individuals always contained sufficient quantities of these essential nutrients. What was revolutionary about her finding is that when cancer patients were fed specially prepared foods designed to introduce these essential ingredients into their blood, their cancer tumors receded and disappeared. [195] After ten years of clinical trials, she developed a natural formula that heals and prevents not only cancer but prevents arteriosclerosis, strokes, cardiac infraction, and other immune disorders. Her dietary regime has been used extensively all over Europe since those early days with impressive results, succeeding where conventional medicine has failed. [196] Dr. Joanna Budwig has authored several books on nutritional medicine, including *Cancer—A Fat Problem*, *The Death of the Tumor*, and *True Health Against Arteriosclerosis, Heart Infarction, and Cancer*.

Budwig found that when flax or linseed oil is mixed with foods containing protein compounds of sulphuric content, the synergistic effect of these foods provided the body with the essential phosphatides and lipoproteins that it needed to ward off diseases such as cancer. Her formula consists of mixing in a blender 1 cup of organic low-fat cottage cheese plus 2–5 Tbsp. of flaxseed oil with enough water to blend it into a soft food. Other foods rich in these sulphuric proteins can be substituted for cottage cheese, such as certain nuts, onion, leek vegetables, and garlic. [197]

Her testimony is essentially consistent with other nutritional doctors. She advocated a broad dietary reform. Absolutely forbidden is refined sugar, all animal fats, all salad oils (including mayonnaise), all meat (because of the presence of chemicals and hormones), butter, margarine, and preserved meats (the preservatives block metabolism of the flax oil). She recommends a healthy plant-based diet and freshly juiced vegetables such as carrots, celery, apples, and red beet. She stated that warm peppermint, rose hip, or grape teas, all sweetened with honey, are beneficial to the patient. [198]

Diabetes

America's Third Leading Cause of Death.

Section 1:

FAT AND A CLUSTER OF VILLAINS

Over 2,000 years ago, physicians noticed that some people produced urine that attracted ants. Tasting the urine confirmed that it was indeed sweet to the taste. They named the condition *diabetes mellitus*, or *fountain of honey* from the Greek word for *fountain* and the Latin *mellitus* for *honey*. [1] People with high blood sugar also had high urine sugar levels and thus became fountains of honey in the process of urination. Tasting urine for sweetness became a diagnostic tool for diabetes in many ancient cultures. [2]

Ladies and gentlemen of the jury, diabetes is one of the major killers of Americans. In 1987 it was determined that diabetes was the *third* leading cause of death by disease; the *second* leading cause of peripheral nerve disease; and the *leading* cause of blindness, non-traumatic amputation, and renal failure in adults. [3] An estimated 10 million Americans are diabetic. Diabetes greatly enhances the risk of developing heart disease, stroke, kidney disease, and loss of nerve function. [4] Many people are diabetic, but they do not know it. Another 20 million Americans have impaired glucose tolerance, a condition that could lead to full-blown diabetes. [5]

In 1987 Americans spent $15 billion dollars on this disease. [6] If you are suffering from the classical symptoms of frequent and excessive urination as well as excessive appetite and thirst, and you are an overweight adult or an underweight child, you may have diabetes without knowing it. [7] [8] The major contributing factor for the development of diabetes is obesity, so much so that a new term has been coined to describe this condition—Diabesity. [9] You may have anticipated my next statement. Yes, ladies and gentlemen, as in the case of other chronic degenerative

diseases, managing diabetes is a lucrative source of profits for the pharmaceutical and medical industries, which treat the symptoms of this disease
and not its cause.

The major symptom of the diabetic is that their blood sugar level is
too high. Normal blood sugar level for the average person is in the range
of 70 to 105 mg/dl. When your blood sugar level is 140 mg/dl, you know
you have the disease. [10] Sugar or glucose is one of the primary fuels of
the body. It is taken from the digestive system and conveyed by the blood
to the cells of all tissues where it can be stored and used for energy production. The hormone insulin, which is produced in the pancreas, is generally
responsible for getting the cells to take in sugar, thereby regulating the
amount of blood sugar. I say generally, because there are two exceptions
to the insulin-glucose relationship: brain cells can absorb glucose directly
from the blood, and during physical exercise the cells have the ability to
absorb glucose directly from the blood. This is why exercise is so very
important to the diabetic in controlling glucose levels in the blood. [11]

Normally then, for all the cells of the body except the brain, insulin
is vitally important in moving glucose out of the blood and into the body
cells. The insulin binds to the glucose and takes it into the cell. [12] You
can think of insulin as the key that unlocks the door of the cell to allow
the sugar or glucose to enter the cell. As the transfer of glucose from the
blood to the cell takes place, the blood sugar level falls proportionately.
High blood sugar levels signal that there is a problem with the transfer of
glucose from the blood to the cells.

The diabetic condition is not, strictly speaking, a disease; rather it is a
metabolic disorder. [13] Metabolism is a term that seeks to describe the
chemical and physiological processes by which our bodies assimilates and
utilizes food. In the case of diabetes, the body has begun to malfunction
in the way it assimilates and utilizes glucose, the primary fuel of the body.
This is a serious condition, and if not reversed or checked, it can lead to
serious medical complications and eventually death.

Ladies and gentlemen, let us take our investigation of this metabolic
disorder another step further. It is important to understand that high
blood sugar is not the real problem; it is merely a symptom of the problem. Therefore treating the symptom will not cure the disease. In order
to understand diabetes and thus arrive at a cure, we must penetrate to the
origin of the metabolic problem producing the symptom. We need to ask
why the blood sugar level is running too high. This inquiry will move us

farther in the direction of discovering the causes of the problem. When we determine the cause, we will be in a position to determine the best course of treatment. Reducing the blood sugar by external means is merely suppressing the symptom while giving the patient a false sense of well being.

The search for causes can be complex. There are immediate causes, and there are more remote underlying causes. To attempt to *cure* a problem, we need to get as close as possible to the more *remote* and *final* causes. The immediate cause of high blood sugar resolves around the hormone insulin. The failure of the body to transfer glucose or sugar from the blood to the cells means one of two things. Either the pancreas is not producing enough insulin; or if it is, the insulin is not doing its job. Two separate problems are at work here, and they give rise to two different types of diabetic disorders, commonly referred to as Type I and Type II or Juvenile onset and adult onset diabetes. Type I diabetes is characterized by a lack of insulin in the body. So the immediate cause of high blood sugar in Type I diabetes is the lack of insulin in the blood stream. But why is there a lack of insulin in the Type I diabetic? Asking this question moves us toward a deeper underlying cause.

The absence of insulin in the body is brought about by the failure of the pancreas to produce sufficient insulin. We must ask yet another question to get nearer to the original cause; why does the pancreas produce too little insulin? This is how the problem occurs. The beta-cells of the pancreas are responsible for manufacturing insulin. In Type I diabetic individuals, the white blood cells develop antibodies that destroy the beta-cells of the pancreas. This type of diabetes is actually an immune disorder. What causes the white blood cells to start attacking its host? White blood cells can develop these destructive antibodies in response to chemicals, viruses, free radical activity, or food allergies. [14] At this stage of the analysis we are dealing with some fundamental causes. Eliminating these causes can avoid or cure the disease or problem. Remedies at this level are more meaningful than superficial remedies which just deal with the symptom—high blood sugar.

Let us examine one of these fundamental causes—food allergy, and the corresponding remedy. An article in the *New England Journal of Medicine* on the relationship of cow's milk and juvenile diabetes throws some light on this destructive process. The article related how doctors at the Hospital for Sick Children in Toronto discovered that children who drank cow's milk had a higher than normal level of an antibody that attacked a protein in cow's milk. The bodies of juvenile diabetics target this milk protein for elimination. So far so good, the body's immune system is doing its job. A problem arises because a component of this milk protein is almost identical to a protein on the surface of the insulin-producing cells of the Islets of Langerhans in the pancreas. The doctors in Toronto discovered that when the child's antibodies attack the milk protein, the look-alike pancreatic protein is also destroyed along with the milk protein. The result is a reduction of the number of insulin producing cells in the pancreas and a corresponding fall in the production of insulin. Not surprisingly the child develops Type I diabetes. [15]

Because the pancreas of Type I diabetic individuals does not produce enough insulin, Type I individuals need external insulin. This condition is called Insulin Dependent Diabetes Mellitus. [16] Only 10% of diabetics fall into this Type I category. It usually develops in children and adolescents. Hence, Type I diabetes was formerly called juvenile diabetes. [17] These individuals have to take insulin by injection because insulin cannot be absorbed orally. Type I diabetics must have their insulin supplied externally all their lives. In section three of this chapter, we will discover that whereas a nutritional diet cannot reverse the destroyed parts of the pancreas, it can greatly enhance the quality and length of life of the Type I diabetic. Together with exercise, weight control and stress management, a proper diet can help preserve the faculties of vision, hearing, balance, coordination and tactile sensitivity of Type I diabetics. [18] Dr. Andrew Weil also believes that Type I diabetics can reduce their requirement of insulin by diet, stress reduction, and other lifestyle modifications. [19]

Ladies and gentlemen of the jury, our main focus in this trial will be on Type II diabetes. Over 90% of the diabetic population in America is Type II diabetics. [20] Type II diabetics fall into two classes: Type II lean and Type II obese individuals. In Type II lean, there is an under production of insulin by the pancreas for various reasons. These individuals also need externally supplied insulin. But let us focus on the Type II obese diabetic, which is the most prevalent type of diabetes.

With Type II obese diabetes, the pancreas produces enough insulin, but for various reasons the tissues have become insensitive to insulin. In these individuals insulin has lost its ability to act as the key to open the cell door to glucose, thus the cells fail to take in glucose and the blood sugar level remains high. *The result is a simultaneous rise in blood sugar and insulin levels in the blood.* It is this dual elevation that is responsible for many of the long-term consequences of diabetes. [21] Type II diabetes is called Non-Insulin Dependent Diabetes Mellitus because lack of insulin is not a problem.

Let us consider the causes of adult onset diabetes (we are speaking of Type II obese diabetics). Remember—unless we know the causes we cannot intelligently treat the condition. Again, we are not interested in suppressing the symptoms of diabetes. Symptom management leaves the underlying causes operating to the detriment of the patient. What causes adult onset diabetes? We could ask this question in another way. Why does the body become insensitive to insulin? There are several known factors that produce insulin insensitivity. A review of the leading authorities in natural medicine reveals that there are several factors that play a primary role in the development of insulin insensitivity:

1. A high fat diet.

2. High refined sugar intake.

3. Overweight or obesity.

4. A high protein diet.

5. A low carbohydrate diet.

6. A low fiber diet.

7. Inactivity or lack of exercise.

Ladies and gentlemen, we are now dealing with the fundamental causes of adult onset diabetes. Solutions at this level can be meaningful in avoiding and even reversing the diabetic condition. So let us consider some of these causes of insulin insensitivity in depth.

A high fat diet. In 1927 Dr. W.D. Samsum of Santa Barbara, California demonstrated that a high fat diet can produce the diabetic condition. He took a group of twenty-three healthy medical students and divided them into four groups. Group 1 was given a high fat diet. Group 2 was put on a high protein lean meat diet; Group 3 on a high carbohydrate diet. Group 4 was simply starved for the duration of the experiment. Those on the high fat diet developed a diabetic condition as indicated by the glucose toler-

JAMES HENDERSON

ance test. The high carbohydrate diet group did not develop a diabetic condition. [22]

Dr. S. Sweeney performed a similar test in 1927 and found that medical students put on a high fat diet of olive oil, butter, and mayonnaise made with egg yolks and 20% cream, developed blood sugar levels high enough to classify them as diabetics. [23] This was earth-shaking news in 1927; at that time the standard dietary treatment for diabetics was a high fat diet and a restricted carbohydrate diet. The reasoning behind the low carbohydrate diet was that since carbohydrates are converted into sugar in the digestive system, and diabetics had a problem with too much blood sugar, then restricting carbohydrates and increasing the consumption of fat would cure the condition. They were deadly wrong. They were attempting to treat the symptom, not the real cause. Dr. Julian Whitaker stated that the culprit was not complex carbohydrates but fat. [24] Conventional medical wisdom was actually compounding the problem. *Incredibly, the cause of the problem, saturated fat, was advocated as the remedy!* This is a classic example of how faulty science can confuse our thinking, leading us to advocate the problem as the remedy.

How does a high fat diet create the diabetic condition? The evidence is overwhelming that excess fat and oils in the diet interferes with insulin activity. [25] Thus although the pancreas may be producing enough insulin, the insulin is not doing its job in facilitating the transfer of blood glucose through the cell membrane and into the cells, because the fat in the blood inhibits it. According to Dr. John McDougall, high triglycerides levels also decrease insulin sensitivity. [26] A study by the University of Sydney, Australia, published in the March 11, 2008, *American Journal of Clinical Nutrition,* linked the consumption of white bread and white sugar to elevated triglyceride levels in the blood (and thus to insulin insensitivity). Triglycerides are the chemical form in which most fats exist in foods and in the body, thus it is not surprising to learn that in 1930, Dr. I. M. Rabinowitch demonstrated that a high meat and fat diet transformed potential diabetics into full-blown diabetics. [27]

A high refined sugar intake. Ladies and gentlemen of the jury, the link between highly refined sugar intake and diabetes is almost as strong as the link between a high fat diet and diabetes. [28] Sugar causes a calcium/phosphorus imbalance which renders the body incapable of breaking down proteins into amino acids which are the essential building blocks of hormones. Without adequate amino acids to construct hormones, the insulin supply begins to diminish. The resulting insulin deficiency can cause hyperglycemia and diabetes. [29]

Research has shown that eating excessive refined sugar can cause an increase of urinary excretion of chromium. Without chromium many other minerals do not function properly, and the result is an impairment of metabolism. Many diabetics have shown to be deficient in chromium. [30] The increase of diabetes in America has paralleled the consumption of sugar in this country. The evidence shows that during World War II, when sugar consumption dropped, the incidence of diabetes dropped proportionally. [31] The consumption of refined sugar disrupts the mechanism that controls blood glucose. High sugar intake correlates with high blood glucose and high insulin blood levels, thus signifying that the insulin has been rendered insensitive and is not effective in removing glucose from the blood. [32]

Overweight or obesity. There is ample evidence that excess weight contributes to the development of diabetes. This factor is associated with the high fat diet. Too much tissue fat prevents the cells of the body from responding to insulin. [33] The major contributing factor for the development of diabetes is obesity, hence the new term coined to describe this condition: Diabesity. [34]

Ladies and gentlemen, despite denials by the protein industry, *a high protein diet* is also a significant factor in the development of diabetes. As long ago as 1927, Dr. W. D. Samsum, in Santa Barbara, California, demonstrated that a high protein diet can produce the diabetic condition. As we stated earlier, he rounded up twenty-three healthy male medical students and divided them into four groups. Group 1 was put on a high fat diet. Group 2 was fed a high protein diet of lean meat and egg whites. Group 3 had a high carbohydrate diet; and group 4 was placed on a starvation diet, no food for two days. We are interested here in the results he had with Group 2, the high protein group. He found that the high protein group had developed the diabetic condition as demonstrated by the glucose tolerance test. [35]

It is significant to notice that the high protein diet that Dr. Samsum put his volunteers on was an *animal-protein diet*, not a *plant-based* protein diet. This makes a lot of difference. While we need to keep our protein intake from *any* source within certain limits, it is more important to reduce or eliminate animal protein from our diets. Why is excessive animal protein dangerous and how does this relate to diabetes? Dr. Dean

Ornish stated that animal protein has been found to increase the level of cholesterol in the blood. [36] The high cholesterol inhibits the action of insulin. Experiments were tried in which all the fat and cholesterol were removed from the animal protein; animal protein was still found to produce increased levels of cholesterol in the blood.

The evidence shows that animal protein inhibits the excretion of cholesterol from the blood by slowing the conversion of cholesterol into bile acids, thus allowing blood levels of cholesterol to rise. On the other hand, plant-based proteins bind to cholesterol in the intestines, thus slowing its absorption into the blood. Some tentative studies in Canada and Italy show that plant protein may actually reduce blood cholesterol levels. [37]

This information on the dangers of a high animal-protein intake may come as a shock to some. Growing up we were bombarded with the propaganda that protein from milk and meat were absolutely essential to grow strong and healthy bones. *The more protein the better* was the fad. Scientific studies now demonstrate that this was absolutely wrong and positively harmful. Most of the degenerative diseases in America, including diabetes, can be traced to a meat-based diet; and it is not just the saturated animal fat, but also the animal protein that is responsible for this epidemic of chronic degenerative diseases. [38]

Dr. Julian Whitaker has testified that one of the most dangerous opinions being sold today is that protein is an *energy* food. Protein is *not* an energy food; it has other vital functions, such as enzyme production and for maintenance of other body proteins in the muscles, bones and other tissue. [39] Protein is not burnt as energy by the body unless under starvation conditions. The body burns primarily carbohydrates and some fat for energy. [40] When you eat excess protein, the body has to break it down and eliminate it through the kidneys. The typical American diet can provided us with as much as 300 to 400% excess protein. This excess protein puts an overload on the liver and kidneys. This can stress the body and accelerate aging and disease. The kidneys are particularly vulnerable to destruction by high protein intake. This is really bad news for the diabetic, because the diabetic condition is itself the number one cause of kidney failure. [41]

We can measure this kidney failure by observing how inefficient the kidney becomes in removing the broken-down products of protein from the blood. When protein is broken down by the liver, the level of blood urea nitrogen (BUN) and creatinine rises. Creatinine is the by-product of the metabolism of creatine, a nitrogenous substance commonly found in blood, urine and muscle tissue. The most sensitive test for kidney failure is the creatinine clearance test. The amount of creatinine excreted by the urine is measured over a 24-hour period. When the level of creatinine in the urine goes up, the kidney has been damaged. [42] Dr. Julian Whitaker noted that one of the glaring oversights of many medical doctors is to not put diabetic patients on a low protein diet at the first signs of kidney failure: elevated creatinine levels. The doctor typically advises a diabetic that he or she has elevated creatinine levels and one day they may have to be put on a dialysis machine. But they do not advise them to decrease their protein intake until after their kidneys fail and they are hooked up to a dialysis machine. [43] This should be considered medical malpractice, and it is high time it is stopped. I note that Dr. Whitaker made this observation in 1987, and hopefully this mercenary practice is changing.

How much protein is adequate for the average American? Many authorities, including the World Health Organization, feel that half a gram of protein per kilogram of body weight per day is adequate. [44] Although he felt a diet of 10% protein is far more than we need, Dr. Colin Campbell will not contest this recommended daily allowance (RDA). [45]

A low complex carbohydrate diet. It is refined carbohydrates, and not naturally occurring complex carbohydrates, which contribute to the development of diabetes Refined carbohydrates, especially white rice, white bread and refined white sugar have all their fiber, minerals, enzymes and vitamins stripped from them, and therein lays the problem. These essential nutrients are indispensable to a proper metabolic functioning of the body. The complex carbohydrates of whole foods produce an opposite effect on the body than does fat. Complex carbohydrates have been shown to *increase* the power of insulin. Hence Dr. John McDougall concludes that inadequate intake of complex carbohydrates in our diet contributes to the development of diabetes. [46]

Ladies and gentlemen, let us for a moment consider the harm done by *a low fiber diet.* A lack of natural fiber in the diet contributes to the development of diabetes. There are several mechanisms at work here. There are two kinds of fiber, soluble and insoluble. Soluble fiber slows the absorption of sugar in the blood stream. By controlling the release of sugar into the blood stream, fiber assists insulin in regulating the level of blood sugar in the body. Soluble fiber also binds to cholesterol and removes it from the body, thus lowering the cholesterol level and increasing the body's sensi-

JAMES HENDERSON

tivity of insulin. [47] Insoluble fibers provide roughage that helps stool formation and elimination. Insoluble fibers thus work in tandem with soluble fibers; the former is eliminated in the stool along with the cholesterol bound to it. Adequate elimination also helps with weight reduction and the control of the amount of fat in the body.

Inactivity or lack of exercise. Inactivity is a serious factor in the development of diabetes. Lack of exercise is thought to destroy insulin sensitivity. We will consider the value of exercising for treating the diabetic condition at some length later. It is considered to be one of the most important factors in reversing diabetes.

Ladies and gentlemen, Drs. Agatha & Calvin Thrash explored the problem of insulin dysfunction from a slightly different perspective. They have asserted that there is insulin receptors in every cell of the body that permit the insulin to enter the cell bound to a glucose molecule. If the number of insulin receptors in the cell is reduced, then the insulin cannot enter the cell. They list several factors that reduce the insulin receptors in the cells of the body. [48]

1.   Overeating.

2.   Use of Alcohol.

3.   Overuse of sugar.

4.   Overweight.

5.   Habitually eating too great a variety of food at one meal.

6.   Overuse of very concentrated foods.

7.   Eating between Meals.

8.   Late night meals.

9.   Use of meat, milk, eggs and cheese.

Alcohol damages the exocrine and endocrine functions of the pancreas. The Islets of Langerhans, which produce insulin in the pancreas, become smaller, and vital cells are destroyed by alcohol, thus reducing the supply of insulin. This increases the risk of developing diabetes. [49] Alcohol also upsets the insulin/glucagon balance, producing the well-known morning-after hangover, which is really a result of low blood sugar. Glucagon is an important hormone produced in the pancreas by alpha cells and is responsible for increasing the blood sugar to optimum levels, whereas insulin, which is also an important hormone produced in the pancreas by the beta cells, is responsible for reducing blood sugar to low manageable levels. A severe hypoglycemic reaction can make an alcoholic mean and abusive. [50]

There are other factors which contribute to diabetes. Caffeine is thought to damage the insulin producing cells of the pancreas. The exact methodology of the damage is not fully understood. [51] After eating a meal the blood sugar levels of diabetics are increased considerably when coffee is ingested. The level of free fatty acids also rises in the blood stream after drinking coffee. [52]

Spoiled fruit should be avoided. The protein from rotten and spoiled food produces a substance called nitrosamine that is known to contribute to the development of diabetes. Foods that show the least spoilage should be discarded. [53]

Drugs such as the corticosteroids group can also promote the development of diabetes. Implicated are Cortisone, Prednisone and Ilosone. The long-term use of birth control pills can also cause diabetes. [54] The Diuretics, Diamox, Lasix, Aldactone, Dyazide, Diuril and Hydrodiuril contribute to high blood sugar because of their dehydrating effect. [55]

Chronic dehydration can be an independent cause of diabetes, and it can compound the harmful effects of the other known causes of diabetes. Without proper water intake the body cannot adequately utilize the nutrients ingested. Dr. F. Batmanghelidj, in his inspiring book *Your Body's Many Cries for Water*, explained how chronic dehydration can lead to the development of diabetes by interfering with the metabolic function of the body. Dehydration promotes insulin-dependent adult diabetes in at least two ways: by interfering with the function of the pancreas and by decreasing tryptophan levels in the body. Dr. Batmanghelidj stated that the pancreas plays at least two vital roles. It produces insulin to facilitate the movement of potassium, sugar, amino acids and water into the cells. [56] Secondly it is engaged in the production of copious quantities of bicarbonate containing water solutions to neutralize the acids coming from the stomach. When there is chronic dehydration of the body, the pancreas partially shuts down its insulin production. It does this to conserve water loss to the cells, in order to carry on the vital role of digestion through the production of aqueous bicarbonate. Insulin insufficiency is thus a symptom of dehydration. Dr. Batmanghelidj stated:

> This phenomenon of insulin inhibition with dehydration shows that the primary function of the pancreatic gland is directed at the provision of water for food digestion. Insulin inhibition is an adaptation process of the gland to the dehydration of the body. [57]

Inasmuch as dehydration is a primary cause of diabetes, the remedy should be to rehydrate the body, not treat the symptom, in this case, insufficient insulin. Dr. Batmanghelidj also stated that dehydration causes a depletion of tryptophan in the brain. [58] Water shortage is accompanied by the release of histamine and an increase of the rate of tryptophan breakdown in the body. With a decrease in tryptophan there is a proportionate decrease in the efficiency of all functions in the body, including pancreatic function, thus ultimately resulting in diabetes. [59]

Ladies and gentlemen of the jury, the evidence is very clear that diabetes is one manifestation of a more general metabolic dysfunction of the body. It does not occur by itself but is usually accompanied by a variety of other degenerative diseases in various stages of intensity. When nutritional and lifestyle abuses create insulin insensitivity, then high blood pressure, coronary artery disease, as well as diabetes can develop. Insulin insensitivity can be an initiating factor in all these diseases. [60] Consider how the mechanism works. When dietary and other factors cause insulin insensitivity, the pancreas produces more insulin to make up for the ineffective insulin. The result is an excess of insulin in the blood stream. Several harmful consequences follow. The excess insulin increases the conversion of ingested sugar into fat, promoting obesity. Insulin also stimulates a liver enzyme, HMG-CoA reductase, which causes the liver to make more cholesterol, thus increasing the risk of heart disease.

Excess insulin may also enhance the growth of the smooth muscle cells found in the lining of the artery. The excessive growth of the smooth muscle cells may in turn clog up the arteries. Dr. Dean Ornish reported that people with high insulin blood levels have higher rates of heart attacks. [61] Over a period of time the excess insulin results in insulin insensitivity which in turn causes the pancreas to produce more insulin, leading to greater insulin insensitivity and so on in a vicious cycle. [62] High triglycerides levels, high blood pressure and high blood sugar and low HDL cholesterol follow in the wake of excessive insulin. [63]

Insulin also plays a vital role in the production of VLDL by the liver. VLDL stands for *very low-density lipoprotein*, a blood fat. The VLDL then decomposes in the blood stream into IDL (intermediate density lipoprotein) which is one of the fats know to produce considerable damage to the lining of the arteries. [64]

Excess insulin also helps to produce high blood pressure. Insulin activates the sympathetic nervous system to trigger the release of the hormone norepinephrine in the blood which normally operates to raise the blood pressure under stress. [65] Excess insulin can result in high blood pressure through different pathways. Insulin stimulates the proliferation of smooth muscle cells in the arteries and encourages connective tissue growth. The inner diameter of the blood vessels is consequently reduced and high blood pressure and heart disease is the result. [66]

High insulin levels can upset the chemical balance of minerals in the cells, which is yet another pathway to high blood pressure. Insulin adversely alters the sodium pumps in the cell membranes which increase the flow of sodium into the cells. The cells can go into a cramp, a condition called vasospastic activity. This condition can cause high blood pressure. Excess insulin also results in too much calcium flowing into the cells, which in turn, can result in vasospasm and high blood pressure. [67] Breast cancer in women and pancreatic cancer are known to result from excess insulin in the blood. [68]

The complications of diabetes can be very serious. Illness, trauma or emotional stress can cause a diabetic to go into a condition called ketoacidosis. Ketones are the byproduct of fat metabolism and they acidify the blood, hence the name ketoacidosis. This is how it works. Stress promotes the release of hormones into the blood stream that lower the insulin levels. The result is an increase of blood sugar, but the lack of insulin makes this sugar unusable by the body cells. The body then tries to burn fat as a substitute for sugar. The byproduct of fat is ketones which begin to accumulate in the blood, acidifying it, and producing the very serious condition of ketoacidosis. [69]

Ketoacidosis can promote excess urination—a defensive mechanism the body employs to wash out excess sugar from the body. An unquenchable thirst may develop as well as chronic dehydration. Yeast vaginitis, bladder, skin, eye and mouth infections can develop. [70] The excessive fat breakdown produces ketones and acetones which bring on nausea and loss of appetite. The acetones produce that fruity breath of the diabetic. The symptoms may progress to drowsiness then coma. If not relieved in time, ketoacidosis can lead to diabetic coma and sometimes death. [71] While ketoacidosis is usually a complication of Type I diabetes, Type II diabetics can also experience ketoacidosis during severe illness. [72]

Treating the diabetic person can become medically complicated. The diabetic can have simultaneous problems in the blood vessels, circulation and the nervous system. The small capillaries and arterioles in the eyes can become damaged and cause hemorrhages in the retina and other parts of the eyes, leading to impaired vision or blindness. The optic nerve can degenerate and cataracts can occur at an early age. [73]

Ladies and gentlemen, in our analysis of the cause of diabetes, we may preliminarily conclude that treating one symptom of diabetes, high blood sugar, is not a wise or adequate remedy. The evidence will show that pumping excessive insulin into the body to offset insulin insensitivity eventually results in a cluster of secondary diseases. Because diabetes is a general metabolic dysfunction and is associated with many companion degenerative diseases and related illnesses, it is of the utmost important to address the problem at the root of the disorder—faulty nutrition and other harmful lifestyle choices. The limited benefits and long term harmful consequences of drug therapy as a treatment for diabetes is discussed in section two.

THE DRUG THERAPY RACKET

Ladies and gentlemen of the jury, now that we have some understanding of the causes and medical complications of adult onset diabetes Type II, we can now proceed to discover the best approach to treatment. As you may have anticipated, there have been two general approaches:

1. Treating the symptoms; or
2. Eliminating the causes.

The first has generally been the approach of modern medicine. To be fair, modern medicine did try to address the dietary causes—when in the 1930s it recommended a high fat diet. But, ignorant of the true causes of diabetes, this approach proved disastrous. Although it is now well known that a high fat diet is the major contributing factor in developing diabetes—a fact that should give us the clue to its successful treatment—conventional medicine has placed an undue emphasis on pharmaceutical approaches that have provided bitter-sweet results for the diabetic and rich profits for the drug industry.

The use of modern anti-diabetic drugs—such as tolbutamide, tolazamide, chlorpropamide, acetohexamide and sulfonylureas—have produced short-term benefits but long-term detriment. Basically these drugs attempt to do two things:

1. Enhance the body's sensitivity to insulin; or
2. Stimulate the pancreas to produce more insulin.

This approach appears to be beneficial until you look at the results. First, the effectiveness of these drugs is usually short term in normal dosages. In 40% of cases blood sugar levels cannot be controlled beyond three months. [1]

Second, with some of these drugs, such as tolbutamide, studies show that the death rate due to heart attack or stroke increases by 250% for users of these drugs, compared to those that use dietary measures. Tolbutamide

(Orinase) increases the level of the enzyme adenylate cyclase in the heart muscle fibers. This enzyme increases the oxygen demand of the heart, thus causing it to overwork. This can induce irregular heart rhythms.[2] With all of these drugs the side effects can be terrible: hypoglycemia, allergic skin reactions, headaches, fatigue, indigestion, nausea, vomiting, and liver damage which can facilitate the development of cancer.

In 1998 Dr. Neil Nedley, wrote in *Proof Positive: How to Reliably Combat Disease and Achieve Optional Health through Nutrition and Lifestyle* that the sulfonylureas class of drugs, which include DiaBeta, Micronase, Glucotrol, Glynase, Amaryl and Diabinese can cause increased cardio-vascular mortality. This warning is also found in the Physician's Desk Reference.[3] Dr. Nedley also noted that the new class of drugs used in the treatment of diabetes, such as Precose, Glucophage and Rezulin have not been on the market long enough to accurately assess their side effects. [4] His preference, based on published research, is therefore to treat his diabetic patients by dietary means. [5], [6] Third, the use of drugs to control diabetes faces the same problem with drug therapies in general. The danger of multiple drug interactions is a major problem with the *disease management* approach of modern medicine. [7]

Ladies and gentlemen of the jury, let us consider testimony regarding the use of insulin to control blood sugar levels. Since this hormone is applied externally, it is part of the drug approach to diabetic treatment. Insulin treatment has of course been beneficial for Type I and Type II lean individuals who are insulin dependent. Normal insulin production is thirty-one units per day. Since Type I diabetics produce only 4 units of insulin per day and Type II lean diabetics produce only 14 units of insulin per day, insulin therapy has proven to be a blessing. [8]

However, insulin treatment of Type II obese individuals does not deliver a clear benefit. You see, Type II obese individuals produce about 114 units of insulin per day! [9] That is 400% over normal. Clearly insulin *insufficiency* is not the problem. So why pump more insulin into Type II obese diabetics? To do so is equivalent to mega dosing the individual with insulin. Dr. Julian Whitaker stated that as of 1986, most non-insulin dependent or Type II diabetics were treated by oral drugs or injected insulin. While this treatment may reduce the blood sugar to some extent, the excess insulin also produces undesirable side effects. Since the problem with Type II individuals is not with the quantity of insulin in their blood but the ineffectiveness of the insulin, the remedy should focus on increasing insulin sensitivity in these individuals. [10]

Ladies and gentlemen, you may remember that when discussing the causes of diabetes, we paused to notice some of the medical complications of excessive insulin in the blood. Let us now consider some additional drawbacks of insulin therapy. One of the most common problems of insulin therapy, especially in thin diabetics, is episodes of hypoglycemia, a condition of dangerously low blood sugar levels due to too large a dose of insulin. [11] Dr. Whitaker noted that several studies have been done to document the frequency of hypoglycemia in diabetics. Over 90% of diabetics on insulin claim to have these episodes. Hypoglycemic episodes account for 3 to 7% of deaths in insulin-treated diabetics. [12] A greater percentage of Type II diabetics suffer brain damage in some degree. Since glucose is the only fuel source of the brain, low blood sugar can destroy brain cells permanently. [13]

The hypoglycemic episode can set up a vicious cycle known as the Somogyi effect, named after Dr. Michael Somogyi who made significant contributions to the science of diabetic medicine between 1930 and the mid 1960s. [14] He noted that the body reacts to the abnormal low blood sugar by stimulating the production of hormones that reduce insulin levels. Cortisol and Epinephrine from the adrenal gland, growth hormone from the pituitary gland and glucagon from the pancreas are released into the blood stream and they elevate the blood glucose levels. [15] Epinephrine acts on the liver and muscle cells while glucagon acts on the liver. Epinephrine is responsible for the cold clammy feeling and racing heart of the hypoglycemic episode. [16] The body next goes into a reverse condition—too high levels of blood sugar. To survive, the body reverses itself again, releasing insulin antagonists to lower the blood sugar. [17]

Another serious problem of treating the Type II diabetic with insulin is the grave complications that can arise from excessive insulin in the body. One of the major health risks of diabetics is progressive damage to the retina that often leads to total blindness. Aggressive treatment with insulin in Type II individuals may actually increase the rate of eye damage especially where tight control of blood sugar levels is achieved too rapidly. [18] It is believed that the increased retinal damage is associated with the production of excessive amounts of the hormone called *Insulin-Like Growth Factor* 1, by the pituitary gland. [19] Several large-scale studies suggest that achieving *tight control* of blood sugar levels by use of insulin *increases* the incidence of retinopathy.

In one study reported in the 1984 issue of the *New England Journal of Medicine*, the researchers divided seventy diabetics with mild eye damage randomly into two groups. One group was treated aggressively with the insulin pump and the other group by insulin injections in the conventional manner. After one year, those treated by the insulin pump had greater control of blood sugar levels but worsening of their eye problems, compared to the other group. But after two years the insulin injection group caught up with the pump group in degree of eye damage. [20]

Another drawback of aggressive insulin use in controlling blood sugar is the danger of blunting the body's defense mechanism for combating hypoglycemia. Patients may get use to the swings of low blood sugar and so not act soon enough to combat the drop in blood sugar. The result could be a dangerously low level of blood sugar that could produce insulin shock and coma before the patient has time to eat something to raise the blood sugar. [21]

The evidence is clear that the use of drugs or insulin to treat Type II individuals is a classic case of the symptom management of disease. High blood sugar is the symptom of a deeper metabolic problem that can lead to some very serious medical complications, including heart disease, blindness and death. Treating the symptom of high blood sugar does nothing to stop the relentless progress of these life impairing diseases that the diabetic is prone to. Ladies and gentlemen, there is convincing evidence that the symptom management of diabetes standing alone is or should be medical malpractice. It is therefore shameless profiteering through the pharmaceutical drug racket.

Consider some more evidence of the harm done by the symptom management of diabetes. To the surprise of many, some alarming findings came out of an eleven-year study by The University Group Diabetic Program (UGDP) funded by the National Institutes of Health. Patients were selected between 1961 and 1965 for a nine-year study. The goal of the study was twofold:

a. To determine if oral medications reduced the incidence of medical complications in Type II diabetics.

b. To determine if controlling blood sugar by use of insulin in Type

II individuals reduced the medical complications of diabetics as everyone assumed it did.

The study divided 619 Type II diabetics into three groups.

* Group 1 was given variable amounts of insulin to maintain blood sugar levels as normal as possible.

* Group 2 was placed on a fixed amount of insulin regardless of their day-to-day blood sugar levels.

* Group 3 was placed on a placebo and had only dietary restrictions.

All the patients were followed for nine years and 75% were followed for eleven years. Over the nine-year period the group on variable amounts of insulin showed a significant reduction of the blood sugar levels. However, despite the marked difference in blood sugar levels, there was no significant difference between the three groups in either the death rate or the medical complication rate. [22] By 1974 there were fifty-four deaths among the placebo group, forty-eight among the fixed insulin group, and forty-nine among the variable insulin group. [23] This was not a statistically significant difference. You can interpret this study to mean that the pharmaceutical companies were benefitting, but not the patients. The study also demonstrated that there was no difference in the nonfatal complications of diabetes in any of the three groups. The following is a comparison of the complications rates for eye, kidney and blood vessel damage as cited by Dr. Julian Whitaker. [24]:

Medical Condition	Placebo %	Insulin-fixed %	Insulin-variable %
Eye Complications:			
Reduction in visual acuity	11.2	11.7	11.4
Acute damage to the retina	9.2	10.6	11.6
Kidney Function:			
Presence of protein in the urine	4.2	2.1	5.8
Serum creatinine 1.5 mg/dl	16.2	8.3	9.1
Blood Vessel Complications			
Calcification in the leg arteries:	29.6	28.8	28.4
Claudication painful walking	17.6	19.4	16.0
Amputations:	1.5	0.5	1.6

Except for the slight elevation in creatinine levels in the placebo group, indicative of kidney damage, the researchers found insulin conferred no significant benefit to the diabetics in reducing medical complications when compared to the placebo group. These expert medical researchers concluded:

Thus over the time period studied with an average follow-up of 12 years, insulin used in a fixed dosage or used in a variable dosage to normalize glucose levels was no better than diet alone in prolonging life or in preventing the vascular complications considered in this report in the adult-onset, non-ketosis-prone diabetic.

The UGDP findings provide no evidence that insulin or any other drug lowering blood glucose levels will alter the course of vascular complications in the type of diabetes that is most common, adult-onset diabetes. [25]

Considering the additional danger that excessive insulin poses and the serious side effects of the diabetic drugs, the researchers recommended that weight reduction and dietary means of controlling blood sugar be given greater emphasis in the treatment of adult-onset diabetes.

> Weight reduction has been shown to be feasible and effective in lowering blood glucose, thus dietary management deserves greater emphasis in this type of diabetes than it has received to date, as others have suggested. In any case, the UGDP results suggest that the use of any other additional therapeutic agent must be justified on grounds other than the prevention ... [26]

Reviewing this study in his 1998 classic, *Proof Positive,* Dr. Neil Nedley concluded that the use of insulin and oral agents in these individuals carries the potential to do more harm than good. [27] Despite these scientific findings, it is difficult for many physicians to abandon their commonly held beliefs on the benefit of drug and insulin therapy for the Type II diabetic. It is not difficult to see why drug companies would ignore these findings: it cuts into their bottom line—profits.

Ladies and gentlemen, we have seen again and again that the use of pharmaceuticals and insulin therapy to control blood sugar focuses on the *symptom* of the diabetic—high blood sugar—and not the *metabolic causes.* The symptom management of disease has become big business and it drives our healthcare system and also drives up the cost to the taxpayer. These approaches purposely do nothing about the causes of the diabetic condition, which are all lifestyle causes. If the real causes are treated, the profit pipeline will dry up. The health of our nation is held ransom to a powerful oil, drug, chemical and financial cartel. It is high time America woke up to this shameless exploitation. Unless the diabetic is simultaneously taught how to avoid the causes of diabetes, the symptom management approach, standing alone, will continue to do a great disservice to the patient.

Physicians are also prone to utilize pharmaceutical approaches to treat the medical complications that are common to diabetics, such as high blood pressure and heart disease. But the evidence shows that the use of drugs to combat the medical complications of diabetics can worsen the diabetic condition. Doctors commonly use beta-blockers such as Inderal, Corgard, Lopressor and Tenormin, to combat high blood pressure. These drugs block the body's response to epinephrine (adrenaline) and thus lower the blood pressure and the heart rate. [28]

However, beta-blockers can worsen the diabetic condition by *suppressing* insulin production by the pancreas. [29] Additionally, by blocking the production of epinephrine, the beta-blockers interfere with the body's ability to respond to hypoglycemia. [30] When hypoglycemia occurs, the body's defensive mechanism swings into action to raise the blood sugar level. It does so by stimulating the production of epinephrine which raises the blood sugar levels. Beta-blockers interfere with this mechanism. [31] Dr. Whitaker insisted that every effort should be used to control high blood pressure by diet and exercise, to avoid exposing the diabetic to these additional risks. [32]

Physicians also often prescribe diuretics to the diabetic to control high blood pressure. However it has been shown that diuretics such as Thiazide may cause a worsening of the diabetic condition by promoting the loss of potassium through the urine. Low potassium levels impair the ability of the pancreas to produce insulin. [33] Diuretics can even *cause diabetes* in otherwise normal people. [34] Thiazides also cause magnesium loss, which can increase the risk of eye disease in diabetics. [35] To make matters worse, Thiazide diuretics have been implicated in elevations of cholesterol and triglycerides levels, increasing the risk of cardiovascular disorders in diabetics. [36]

Ladies and gentlemen, the tightly held secret is that there *are* alternatives to the use of drug therapy to control diabetes. Dietary approaches to controlling diabetes are not new or untried procedures. In 1930 Dr. I. M. Rabinowitch successfully treated his diabetic patients with a high complex carbohydrate and low fat diet. In many patients the diabetic condition was reversed. [37] Also in 1930, Dr. E. P. Joslin, the founder of the famous Joslin Diabetic Center in Boston, suggested that the high fat and cholesterol diet of diabetics was contributing to their accelerated coronary artery disease. [38] In 1948 Dr. Walter Kemper of Duke University demonstrated that a diet of rice and fruit was effective in lowering high blood pressure. [39] Dr. Lynne Paige Walker outlined in *The Alternative Pharmacy* many alternative and natural remedies for controlling diabetes. [40] When diet is used in the place of drugs the patient experiences none of the health risks or side effects of drugs. Their quality of life is enhanced as they take charge of their destiny.

If dietary approaches to controlling diabetes have been successfully used for over half a century, why do not more physicians and health authorities advocate it? Many physicians that seek to reverse diseases using natural remedies assert that the problem is that there is no money in *curing* degenerative diseases. However *managing* the symptoms of degenerative disease is big business. Dr. John McDougall believes that drugs and medical procedures generate business for drug companies and physicians; therefore there is no incentive to advocate the more cost effective natural remedies. [41] Many people are getting rich on our misery. It is imperative that we do all in our power to stop this financial and health hemorrhage.

In our next session we will look in depth at evidence which indicates that dietary approaches not only control, but actually reverse, the diabetic condition.

Section 3

PREVENTING & CURING DIABETES: THE NUTRITIONAL APPROACH

Ladies and gentlemen of the jury, in the last session you heard testimony that drug therapy was not only ineffective in controlling diabetes, but it was accompanied by dangerous side effects that undermined the health of the diabetic. Let us now look at some real solutions to the diabetic condition. Nutritional approaches to the treatment of diabetes fall into four broad interlacing categories:

a. Dietary;

b. Herbal; and

c. Supplementation with vitamins and minerals.

d. Exercise.

The dietary approach is primary, but should be accompanied by the use of certain herbs and supplements, as well as other lifestyle changes such as becoming more active. Dietary approaches are cheaper, more effective and more pleasant than most of the pharmaceutical alternatives. [1]

Drs. Agatha and Calvin Thrash stated that Type II diabetes can be completely controlled in most cases by the control of the appetite, weight reduction and adequate exercise. [2] Dr. Dean Ornish reports that people who follow his recommended diet in his program for reversing heart disease also become more insulin sensitive and thus gain some control of their diabetic condition. [3]

The dietary approach addresses the fundamental cause of Type II diabetes: Excess animal fat and protein, and refined sugar in the diet. The link between highly refined sugar and diabetes is almost as strong as the link between high fat and diabetes. [4] Let us go back to Dr. W.D. Samsum's research work in 1927 to review the role of fat in causing diabetes. Dr. W.D. Samsum of Santa Barbara California convincingly demonstrated that a high fat diet can produce the diabetic condition. He took a group of twenty-three healthy medical students and divided them into four groups:

* Group 1 was given a high fat diet.

* Group 2 was put on a high protein lean meat diet; and

* Group 3 was on a high carbohydrate diet.

* While the group 4 volunteers were simply starved for the duration of the experiment.

Those on the high fat diet developed a diabetic condition as indicated by the glucose tolerance test. What is even more interesting is that when he put the high fat group on the high complex carbohydrate diet, their diabetic condition was reversed! [5]

In 1979 Dr. James Anderson outlined the dietary treatment for diabetes in an article in the *American Journal of Clinical Nutrition*. He stated that the best diet for the control of diabetes was a high complex carbohydrate, high fiber diet, which emphasized cereal grains, legumes, and root vegetables while restricting sugar and fat intake. He contended that this diet results in the following benefits:

1. Increased sensitivity of the body tissues to insulin.

2. Reduced blood sugar levels.

3. Reduced body weight.

4. Reduced levels of bad LDL cholesterol and increased levels of good HDL cholesterol.

Although the American Diabetes Association (ADA) no longer promotes the extremely detrimental high fat diet for the diabetic, it has not yet (as of

234   JAMES HENDERSON

this writing) endorsed the high complex carbohydrate, high fiber (HCF) diet as the primary means of treating diabetes, even in the face of compelling evidence. Some years ago a number of Type I diabetics were put on the high complex carbohydrate, high fiber and low fat diet. Their insulin needs decreased. When placed back on the ADA diet, their insulin needs increased. [6] The best diet conventional medicine advocates consists of:

50% to 60% of calories from carbohydrates.

20% to 38% of calories from fat.

12% to 20% from proteins.

Dr. John McDougall would argue that this diet still has much too little complex carbohydrates and fiber, and consequently too much fat. [7] Because of the vital role played by fiber in controlling blood sugar levels, Dr. Julian Whitaker emphasized that the diet should be rich in fiber. He considered the fiber of the legume family to be of chief importance. High fiber intake also has the added benefit of reducing many of the complications of diabetes. It helps reduce weight. It helps increase good HDL cholesterol and it reduces bad LDL cholesterol.

Dr. Whitaker recommended that the diabetic get their calories from the following sources:

1. 55 to 60% from complex carbohydrate: 50% of which should come from grain products; 48% from fruits and vegetables; and 2% from skim milk.

2. 20% from protein: 50% of which should come from fruits and vegetables; 36% from grain products; and 14% from skim milk and lean meat.

3. 20 to 25% from fat: 60% of which should come from grain products; 20% from fruits and vegetables; and 12% from skim milk and lean meat. [8]

He also recommended 100 grams of fiber daily. [9] For hospitalized diabetics Dr. James Anderson recommended the dietary formula:

Complex carbohydrates: . . . . 70 % - 75 %

Fat:. . . . . 5 % - 10 %
Protein:. . . . . 15 % - 20 %

Although any of these dietary approaches will provide great benefit to the diabetic, the evidence will show that the best dietary approach is based on Dr. John McDougall's research and recommendations for dietary control of diabetes for it is more consistent with the findings of Dr. Colin Campbell as reported in his China Study. Dr. Campbell reported a study in which twenty-five Type II diabetics were put on a high-fiber, low fat and high complex carbohydrate diet.

Of the twenty-five Type 2 patients, twenty-four were able to discontinue their insulin medications! Let me say that again, all but one person were able to discontinue their insulin medication in a matter of weeks! [10]

Dr. McDougall's program most readily achieves the goal of *reversing* the metabolic dysfunction that gives rise to diabetes. This natural foods diet also has the added benefit of reversing a host of companion degenerative diseases. Dr. McDougall recommended the following therapeutic diet to reverse diabetes:

80 % to 90 % carbohydrates, mostly complex.

5 % to 10 % fat

5 % to 12 % protein.

Dr. John McDougall also recommended that we consume no cholesterol. Since cholesterol is only found in animal products, his Diabetic Reversal diet is a vegetarian diet. [11] His clinical experiences demonstrated that 75% of diabetics who go on this diet can stop their insulin and almost all can stop oral medication completely. [12] This diet consists of a high percentage of *complex* carbohydrates which have the power to increase insulin sensitivity. [13] However carbohydrates in any form is much better for the diabetic than excess fat. [14]

Dr. John McDougall also recommended that the diet also consist of as much natural fibers as possible. [15] Fiber slows the absorption of the sugars from complex and simple carbohydrates. And dietary fiber brings about the gradual release of sugar into the blood stream. Thus dietary fiber is the key regulator of sugar from the digestive system into the blood stream. The role of fiber is considered as vital as the role of insulin which regulates the absorption of sugar into the cells from the blood stream. [16]

Ladies and gentlemen of the jury, it is vital to grasp the fact that insulin, complex carbohydrates and fiber work hand in hand to regulate the blood sugar level. Fiber regulates the absorption of sugar into the bloodstream; and complex carbohydrates increase the power of insulin to transport sugar into the body cells where it can be stored or used as energy. It has been shown that simply adding foods containing fiber to a high fat meal can reduce the blood levels of sugar. [17] The importance of fiber in the diet underscores the great disservice that the refined foods industry does to the American consumer. Stripping all of the fiber, vitamins, minerals, and enzymes from natural foods and serving it to the consumer is equivalent to sentencing them to a life of slow death by chronic degenerative diseases. The type of fiber which is most helpful to diabetics is that found *naturally* in foods. Dr. John McDougall noted that merely adding extra bran fiber to one's meal often does little more than provide gas and bowel pains. [18]

Fibers taken naturally are of two kinds: soluble and insoluble. They have different functions. Soluble fibers, found plentifully in oats, wheat, and fruits, have a greater effect in lowering blood sugar and cholesterol levels than insoluble fibers. [19] Insoluble fibers have a different, though complementary, function. They bind to cholesterol and eliminate it from the body. [20] Insoluble fibers also assist in stool formation, acting like a broom to promote proper elimination. [21] Thus both soluble and insoluble fibers work hand in glove to prevent or reverse diabetes. The first regulates blood sugar levels, and the second reduces the dietary fat and cholesterol which are inhibitors of the function of insulin.

This natural diet first provided to mankind in the Garden of Eden, was high in complex carbohydrates and fiber. This type of diet helps one to achieve one's ideal weight and size, preventing the onset of degenerative diseases. We cannot improve on God, Dr. Lorraine Day often emphasized, and she is absolutely right. In the case of obese diabetics, simply bringing weight down to optimum levels can cure them of the diabetic condition. [22]

Nutritional experts advise that upon commencing a high complex carbohydrate diet to reverse diabetes, one should always consult with a physician if one is on insulin or oral medication, because this diet immediately increases the body's sensitivity to insulin. With increased insulin sensitivity, taking extra insulin externally or by oral medication can result in an insulin overload. Dr. McDougall recommends the following procedure:

1. Cut your insulin by 50% the day you start the carbohydrate/fiber based diet.

2. Test urine sugar levels four times per day, daily, before meals and at bedtime. The urine test becomes your guides for adjusting insulin dosages.

3. If all the urine sugar tests are negative for two days then cut your insulin intake by another 5 to 10 units.

4. Test daily as above. If the tests are negative for two days cut insulin by another 5 to 10 units. Repeat this procedure until you eliminate your insulin needs.

5. If the urine tests are strongly positive for two days after lowering insulin, then adjust upward by 5 to 10 units until the tests are negative once again, before proceeding.

6. Carry simple sugar or candy if hypoglycemic reactions occur.

Dr. John McDougall stated that most people are able to get off insulin by this method within one to six weeks. [23] For diabetics on oral medication, the procedure is rather straight forward. Simply stop all oral medication the day you start the diet. [24]

Type I diabetics can rarely eliminate their insulin requirements, but with this diet, coupled with exercise, they can *reduce* their dosages of insulin and improve their health. [25] Reporting on a study of Type 1 diabetics who were put on a high fiber and low fat diet, Dr. Campbell observed,

Type 1 diabetics cannot produce insulin. It is difficult to imagine any dietary change that might aid their predicament. *But after three weeks, the Type 1 diabetic patients were able to lower their insulin medications by an average of 40%! Their blood sugar profiles improved dramatically. Just as importantly, their cholesterol levels dropped by* 30%! Remember, one of the dangers of being diabetic is the secondary out-comes, heart disease and stroke. Lowering risk factors for those secondary outcomes by improving the cholesterol profile is almost as important as treating high blood sugar. [26] [Emphasis added.]

Ladies and gentlemen, the evidence is also very convincing that exercise is a key factor in the treatment of diabetes. Dr. Andrew Weil contended that it is the most important factor. He stated that thirty minutes of daily aerobic exercise may prevent the onset of diabetes in those at risk and may cause complete disappearance of symptoms in those who have it. [27] Dr. Neil Nedley agreed that exercise should be the first element in a regime of comprehensive diabetic lifestyle management for, simply put, exercise helps sugar to leave the blood stream and flow into the muscles where it is consumed as energy. [28] Under the stress of exercise, the muscle cells have the ability to extract sugar directly from the blood—they do not need insulin to do this. Thus lack of exercise can result in not enough sugar being removed from the blood of a diabetic. [29] Both Drs. Weil and Whitaker concur that exercise may entirely eliminate the need for insulin therapy or the use of oral drugs in some diabetics. [30]

How does exercise have this positive effect? The mechanism is still unclear. Some researchers feel that as the level of calcium increases in exercising muscle cells; the calcium then unlocks certain receptors in the cells, allowing the cell to take in sugar. Others feel that the lactic acid and carbon monoxide that is produced by the exercising cells play this role in unlocking the cell receptors, permitting glucose to enter the cell. [31]

The effect of exercise on blood sugar levels raises a red flag for Type I diabetes. If they are tightly controlling their blood sugar with too much insulin, exercise can cause a severe drop in blood sugar because blood sugar is being removed by two methods, by the insulin in the blood and by the exercise. The result is that there is too much insulin in the blood and this can cause a severe drop in blood sugar levels, a condition called hypogly-cemia. The Type I diabetic should always lower their insulin intake before commencing exercise. When commencing an exercise program, a physician's advice is important.

Dr. Julian Whitaker advises Type I diabetics to carry some source of glucose with them while exercising in case hypoglycemia sets in. [32] Type I individuals should not start exercising if their blood sugar levels are too high; exercise may have the effect of increasing blood sugar, thus creating a dangerous condition called ketoacidosis. [33]

The timing of the exercise is also important. Exercising after eating tends to lower blood sugar because sugar is absorbed directly into the cells during exercise without the help of insulin. Dr. Whitaker noted that exercise after breakfast in the morning has the added benefit of making exercise after lunch and dinner even more effective in lower blood sugar levels. [34] Morning exercise sets the metabolic thermostat at a high rate thus helping in the burning of calories.

Exercise also reduces other medical complications of the diabetic. Research by Dr. Peter Forsham at the University of California, San Francisco School of Medicine, has shown that exercise can reduce platelet stickiness and hence increase the fluid capacity of the blood. This, in effect, reduces clotting in the small blood vessels of the eye and kidney, thus protecting the Type I diabetic from eye damage and kidney dysfunction. [35]

Stress can affect the course of diabetes dramatically. Stress management is of great importance to the diabetic. [36] Exercise can be of great help for all types of diabetics in reducing stress. Jogging, bicycling, swimming and other aerobic activities can be great mood elevators. Such activities release beta-endorphins that improve the mood and relieve depression. [37] Exercise also helps manage or reverse any cardiovascular problems the diabetic may have. It elevates the good HDL cholesterol while reducing triglycerides fats in the blood. It can also strengthen the heart muscle. [38] Other forms of stress management, such as trusting in God and meditation on the wonders of his Creation, are of great value to the diabetic.

The use of herbs can be of significant benefit to the diabetic. The Ayurvedic medical tradition of India has used the herb Gymnema sylvestre for the control of diabetes. In the West we call it Gurmar. The chief action of this herb is to regenerate the insulin producing beta cells of the pancreas. [39] [40] This herb has helped Type I diabetics reduce their insulin needs while reducing their blood sugar levels. Some Type II individuals have been able to stop their oral medications completely by use of this herb. [41]

Ladies and gentlemen of the jury, let us for a moment consider testimony regarding use of herbs to treat diabetes. The evidence demonstrates that garlic and onions can be beneficial to the diabetic. The oils in the garlic help reduce cholesterol and triglyceride levels, and they enhance the function of the immune system which is vitally important to the diabetic. A clove of garlic juiced into an unsweetened mixture of freshly juiced tomatoes and celery makes a healthful cocktail that cuts the odor of garlic. [42] The oils in the onion provide the substance Quercetin which has been shown to help with eye problems that are often associated with diabetic retinopathy. [43] Dr. Lynne Paige Walker in *The Alternative Pharmacy* reported on a number of herbs that have beneficial effects for the diabetic: The herb *milk thistle* containing the anti-oxidant *silymarin* was show by Italian researchers to significantly drop and stabilize glucose levels without hypoglycemic episodes. [44] The Chinese use the herb c*hrysanthemum* in the treatment of diabetes. Its extract *Stevia Rebaudiana* is a sweetener which reduces plasma-glucose levels in normal adults without affecting blood-sugar metabolism. [45] The Indians have used *Gymnema Sylvestre* for centuries for supporting the pancreas and regulating blood-sugar levels. [46]

Various types of beans help regulate blood sugar. Beans are high in fiber which reduces the rise of blood sugar after meals, and because of the slow absorption of these complex carbohydrates, acceptable blood sugar levels are maintained for hours. [47] Peanuts also seem to keep blood sugar levels at acceptable low levels. [48] Other herbs that lower blood sugar include *Bitter Gourd;* eaten raw or juiced, it helps lower blood sugar according to Dr. Melvyn Werbach assistant clinical professor of psychiatry at the University of California, Los Angeles School of Medicine. Dr. Michael Murray, author of *Botanical Influences on Illness* also recommended b*itter gourd* for the diabetic. [49] The herb *Fenugreek* contains the soluble fiber mucilage that helps regulate sugar levels. [50]

Green Tea, *Camellia Sinensis,* contributes to cardiovascular health by reducing platelet formation and hence the development of blockages in the coronary arteries. [51] Green tea is also known to lower the blood sugar. Animal experiments show that animals that maintain lower blood sugar live longer. [52] In the island of Trinidad people have used a weed called *jackass bitters* (Neurolaena lobata) to regulate blood sugar levels for hundreds of years. Some adult onset diabetics have been able to stop their insulin use altogether with this herb. [53]

Ladies and gentlemen of the jury, we must one again consider testimony regarding micronutrient supplementation. While the use of vitamin and mineral supplements has been frowned on by conventional medicine, the evidence demonstrates that they play a role in releaving the diabetic condition. Some nutritionists argue that in light of the depletion of our soils and the loss of these nutrients in processed foods, supplementation of one's diet with vitamin and mineral supplements is essential. Again, the use of micronutrients in their food matrix is preferred above commercially prepared brands from chemicals. Micronutrients found in live foods are absolutely essential for the health of the body and its proper metabolism. Dr. Julian Whitaker stated that research shows that diabetics are usually deficient in the following nutrients: Vitamins C, E and B6 and the minerals, chromium and magnesium. Therefore he recommended that supplementation with these nutrients is beneficial. [54]

Dr. James A. Duke also recommended manganese, phosphorus, zinc and omega-3 and omega-6 fatty acids to one's list of supplements. [55] The evidence shows that a vitamin C deficiency in diabetics results in some common problems such as poor wound healing, depression of immune function, high cholesterol levels, and degradation of the capillary walls, a condition that can lead to bleeding. [56] Vitamin C is absolutely essential to the health of many organs and tissues of the body. Its concentration in the blood is usually 0.5 milligrams per deciliter. [57] But the liver, spleen and lens of the eye require 20 times this concentration of vitamin C. The adrenal and pituitary gland require 100 times the concentration of vitamin C that as is found in the blood. [58] Dr. Whitaker recommended 1,000 to 2,000 mg; and as much as 5,000 mg in some cases. Since excess vitamin C can cause gas and diarrhea, it must be used to bowel tolerance. [59]

Vitamin C is also important to the diabetic because of their proclivity for wound infection and poor healing of tissue. Vitamin C plays a very important role in many immune mechanisms. [60] It appears in high concentrations in white blood cells such as the lymphocytes. The body repairs wounds with a protein substance called collagen. Collagen is critical for cartilage, tendons and other connective tissues. Vitamin C plays a vital role in the manufacture of collagen. [61]

Vitamin E improves the action of insulin, making it more efficient. Studies show that doses in the level of 400 to 600 IU reduce insulin requirements. [62] The active form of vitamin E is alpha-tocopherol. Tocopherol means to bear offspring. *Tokos* in Greek is *offspring* and *phero* means *to bear.* The vitamin got its name from studies in 1922 when the vitamin was discovered. Researchers found that rats deprived of vitamin E were unable to reproduce. When vitamin E was returned to their diet they bore offspring. Hence the term tocopherol—to bear offspring. [63]

Vitamin E also functions as an antioxidant in protecting cell membranes from damage. Without vitamin E the cells of the body, particularly the nerve cells, would be vulnerable to damage. [64] Vitamin E protects the lining of the arteries from damage from cholesterol in the blood. Dr. Whitaker contended that low levels of vitamin E in the body are a better predictor of impending heart attacks, than high levels of cholesterol or high blood pressure. [65] Studies in Europe show that high cholesterol levels predicted heart attacks 29% of the time and high blood pressure 25% of the time, while low levels of vitamin E predicted heart attacks 70% of the time. [66] Selenium acts in synergy with vitamin E, therefore Dr. Whitaker recommended that they be taken together. About 240 to 400 mg per day of selenium is recommended. [67]

Vitamin B6 is also commonly deficient in diabetics. [68] The neuropathy produced by B6 deficiency is indistinguishable from diabetic neuropathy, a nerve dysfunction that often leads to pins and needles, or numbness and loss of feeling in the hands and feet. [69] [70] The danger of experiencing neuropathy in the extremities is that diabetics may hurt themselves and not know it, thus creating the risk of infection.

Research has found that the mineral chromium helps insulin open the cell doors to glucose. In 1854 researchers became aware that brewer's yeast improved the diabetic condition. Later it was discovered that the active ingredient in brewer's yeast was chromium and several amino acids. These nutrients have been labeled Glucose Tolerance Factor (GTF). [71] GTF chromium enhances insulin sensitivity. Dr. Whitaker recommended 400 micrograms daily. [72] Dr. Lynne Paige Walker cautioned diabetics with enlarged prostates to avoid free chromium, but reported that in other cases, chromium lowered heart disease risks by lowering insulin resistance, blood cholesterol and blood pressure. [73] Not all experts disagree on the various nutritive roles claimed for chromium, yet all agree that chromium plays an important role in blood sugar metabolism, which is very important to the diabetic. [74]

The mineral Magnesium is also commonly low in diabetics, especially those suffering from retinopathy. Magnesium supplementation is therefore recommended. Dr. Whitaker recommended 100 milligrams per day; [75] however he cautioned that magnesium should be balanced with calcium by a 2 to 1 ration. [76] The diabetic condition itself contributes to low magnesium levels in diabetics. Elevated blood sugars stimulate excessive urination which can wash out magnesium and other essential minerals from the body. [77] Additionally many diabetics take hypertensive medication or diuretics. Use of diuretics can lead to excessive mineral loss, including the loss of magnesium. [78]

Magnesium is very important to cell function. Magnesium and potassium are the most important minerals *within* the cells of the body. [79] Combined with chloride, they become mineral salts that conduct electricity when dissolved in water. Along with other electrolytes, magnesium helps maintain many important body functions. It helps regulate water balance and distribution throughout the body. It regulates the acid-base balance in muscle and nerve function. [80] Magnesium and potassium are involved in many other cellular functions such as energy production, protein formation and cellular replication. [81]

Magnesium Aspartate plays a role in the conversion of glucose, fatty acids and amino acids into chemical energy (A process called ATP). [82] Magnesium is essential to the metabolism of carbohydrates, and it therefore plays a key role in the efficient action of insulin. [83] These functions are vital to the health of the muscle and nerve cells.

Magnesium helps the heart muscle to contract. Low levels of magnesium have been found in individuals who die from sudden heart attacks. [84] Magnesium deficiency can produce coronary artery spasm which further reduces the flow of blood and oxygen to the heart. Magnesium deficiencies are also associated with high blood pressure. [85] Magnesium is also essential to kidney and adrenal function. Magnesium helps prevent the formation of kidney stones by increasing the solubility of calcium in the urine. [86] One can readily see how a host of chronic degenerative diseases can result from magnesium deficiency. White bread and refined sugar, which leach magnesium from the system, can contribute to the development of many degenerative diseases linked to magnesium deficiency. Dr. Julian Whitaker recommended a daily intake of 1,000 milligrams of elemental magnesium. [87]

Potassium is also beneficial to the diabetic. Potassium plays an important role in nerve function which is often impaired in the diabetic. [88] However, for people with kidney dysfunction, excess potassium can be harmful. [89]

Most Americans take in more sodium than potassium, so the ratio of potassium to sodium is reversed. This can result in cancer, heart disease, and high blood pressure. [90] Dr. Whitaker believes the ideal ratio of potassium to sodium should be 5:1; [91] while, we have seen from earlier testimony, that Dr. Max Gerson thought the ration should be 4:1 ratio. To bring the potassium to sodium ration into line one should reduce excess sodium salt intake and eat plenty of legumes, bananas, and citrus fruits. The ratio of potassium to sodium in fruits is 50:1. [92]

Ladies and gentlemen, the evidence demonstrates that the proper intake of water is also very important, perhaps more so than proper micronutrient supplementation, for without proper hydration, nutrients cannot be utilized by the body. Dr. Batmanghelidj stated that chronic dehydration is a disease producer. [93] He demonstrated that dehydration of the body causes the pancreas to shut down its insulin production in order to carry on the more vital production of aiding the digestion through the production of bicarbonate which helps neutralize excessive acids. [94] Because Type II diabetes can be caused by inadequate water intake, its treatment should include the daily hydration of the body. At the same time they should be aware that the use of diuretics could contribute to dehydration.

Many physicians feel that you can get all the essential minerals and vitamins from your food and therefore supplementation is not generally necessary. The facts are against this posture. It is well known that our soils are depleted of important minerals and only NPK (Nitrogen, Phosphorous and Potassium) are replaced by chemical fertilizing. What is not in the soil cannot get to us via the normal food chain. Hence the value of micronutrient supplementation. It is also known that cold storage and refinement of foods deplete them of essential nutrients. In the case of the diabetic, supplementation is even more important because of the excessive urination and the action of diuretics which wash out minerals from the body. Dr. Whitaker and other experts treating degenerative diseases have made a convincing case for supplementation. [95] The nutritional evidence is clear that the diabetic should use supplements or eat richly of organically grown foods. To do otherwise is reckless and can be detriment to their health and life.

Ladies and gentlemen of the jury, the most important thing to remember in the treatment of diabetes is that it is a metabolic disorder caused by incorrect habits of eating and drinking. Excess animal fats and proteins and refined, denatured foods—especially refined sugar—creates the metabolic disorder that results in diabetes. This means that the proper treatment of diabetes must involve correcting our eating and drinking habits.

We have to decide whether we shall eat for life or for death; for health and strength or for disease. Of course the use of herbs, along with vitamin and mineral supplementation is no *substitute* for proper nutrition. Supplements must not become nutritional *silver-bullets*. A proper nutritional program with plenty of exercise and trust in our Creator is the foundation of good health. Supplementation is only an adjunct to proper eating and lifestyle choices.

Heart Disease
America's #1 Killer

Section 1:

THE DEADLY TRIO: EXCESS FAT, CHOLESTEROL, AND PROTEIN

Ladies and gentlemen of the jury, in his ground-breaking book *Reversing Heart Disease*, Dr. Dean Ornish attempted to dramatize the astonishing reality that over one and a half million Americans have heart attacks every year. He stated that it is equivalent to 125,000 heart attacks every month; 4,100 every day; 173 every hour; and approximately 3 people have heart attacks every second of the day in the United States. [1] The figures are so mind numbing that we fail to comprehend them. In 1990 forty million Americans suffered from some degree of cardiovascular disease. [2] Millions more today have the disease but do not even know it. About one third of these will first learn that they have heart disease after their first heart attack. [3] Not a very pleasant way to find out!

We loudly lament the deaths caused by firearms, car accidents and air disasters; but did you know that more Americans die from heart disease than from all other causes of death put together? Dr. Julian Whitaker stated in 1985 that this was about half of all the deaths annually. [4] In 1999 the situation was no better. In a *Special Medical Alert* he stated:

> Heart disease is our nation's #1 killer. Half of all Americans who die this year will die from it. [5]

That is frightening, folks. Statistics on the precursors to heart disease are just as staggering. An article in the 1990 issue of the *Journal of the American Medical Association* estimated that one half of all adult Americans have cholesterol levels that require some degree of treatment. That is about eighty million adults! [6] Almost sixty million Americans have high blood pressure which can lead to heart disease.

Heart disease is not a disease of the elderly. Young people in the prime of life are being struck down by this silent killer. Neither wealth nor fame can shield you from this disease. At the age of forty-eight, David Janssen, the star of the TV series *The Fugitive*, was struck down by a massive heart attack although he had no prior history of the disease. Another well-known personality is Peter Sellers who died at age fifty-four of heart disease. [7] Ladies and gentlemen while heart disease is America's number one health concern, there are cultures in which heart disease is so rare it is virtually unknown. Clearly something is wrong with our culture.

What is becoming increasingly clear is that we are not *victims* in this national tragedy. By our lifestyle and our eating habits, we are killing ourselves. The nineteenth-century health reformer, Ellen White, opinioned that many people are:

Digging their graves with their teeth. [8]

The primary cause of this self-inflicted epidemic is that we have, to a large degree, severed the connection between food and nutrition. We eat for pleasure, but not to nourish ourselves—and this is the root of the problem. In 1909 Ellen White wrote:

Indulgence of appetite is the greatest cause of physical and mental disability. [9]

Self-indulgence is destroying us as a nation and is the inexcusable cause of the great epidemic of chronic degenerative diseases now sweeping America. It is the cause of our staggering healthcare bill which now exceeds two trillion dollars annually. And yet we know better. We select the best brands of food for our pets while we fill ourselves with foods which are filled with deadly fats, refined sugars, chemical additives and excessive protein; not to mention refined foods which are almost completely void of the essential micronutrients. Nonchalantly we eat grease-dripping-cheese-burgers, wash them down with a can of Pepsi or Dr. Pepper, and relax over coffee and a cigarette—oblivious to the fact that the high fat, sugar, phosphate, caffeine and nicotine lifestyle is slowly poisoning us. And all this is so unnecessary! Eating wholesome foods can be both nourishing and pleasurable.

In the first two sections of this segment, we will hear evidence concerning the causes of heart disease. In the last three sections, we will compare and contrast the drug-based medical approach to the solution of this epidemic with that recommended by the practitioners of nutritional medicine. We must understand the causes *before* we can determine how to cure the problem of heart disease. The causes are both simple and complex. The evidence will demonstrate that switching to a low fat, low protein and high complex carbohydrate diet, rich with the micronutrients vitamins, minerals and enzymes, will not only prevent heart disease but reverse it. But there are other causes. How we respond to stress and whether we have a spiritual anchor are all part of the picture. It is important to understand the causes of heart disease; once you do, you will discover that it is within your power to prevent it. No one else can do this for you. No amount of high-tech surgery or the use of designer drugs of modern medicine can cure you of heart disease. We must simply stop doing what is killing us.

Today we rely on modern medicine to free us from the consequences of our choices. But modern drug-based medicine cannot help you here. It can only treat the symptoms of heart disease while doing nothing to remove the cause. The factors that can prevent or cure heart disease are all under your control. These factors include getting proper nutrition, adopting a correct mental attitude and engaging in healthy social and spiritual relationships. Natural, unrefined food is the best medicine. Dr. William Castelli, medical director of the famous Framingham Heart Study, stated:

It is a sad fact that for most heart attack victims, diet alone would work, if we advocated diet in American Medicine—but we don't. The average patient who comes out of a coronary unit or a cardiologist's office never gets hooked up to a diet program. [10]

Is Dr. William Castelli correct? Is diet alone sufficient to reverse heart disease? When you understand that our diets are the primary means of obeying or disregarding the laws of health, then what Dr. Castelli and others are saying makes capital sense. On the role of diet in disease causation Ellen White wrote:

Disease never comes without a cause. The way is prepared, and disease invited by disregard of the laws of health. Many suffer in consequence of the transgression of their parents ... They should avoid the wrong habits of their parents, and by correct living, place themselves in better conditions.

The greater number, however suffer because of their own wrong course of action. They disregard the principles of health by their habits of eating, drinking, dressing and working. Their transgression of nature's laws produces the sure result; and when sickness comes upon them, many do not credit their suffering to the true cause, but murmur against God because of their afflictions. But God is not responsible for the suffering that follows disregard of natural law ... [11]

Precisely how does an improper diet cause coronary heart disease? In tracing cause to effect, it is often helpful to start with the effect. The mechanism of coronary heart disease is rather simple: the supply of blood to the heart is reduced, and the heart is deprived of oxygen and nourishment. If the interruption of oxygen to the heart is brief, we may feel heart pain. This is often referred to as angina. If the interruption is severe or prolonged—that is, for more than a few minutes—we experience a heart attack. [12]

Simply stated, the heart is essentially a muscular pump. It pumps life-giving blood through a network of arteries to all parts of the body. If these arteries become plugged up, the organs supplied by these arteries become starved of oxygen and nourishment, and they in turn underperform in their function. If the undernourishment is prolonged, those organs and tissues affected simply die. We can all readily understand this mechanism. But what we do not often stop to consider is that the heart itself needs oxygen and nourishment. The heart pumps blood to itself through three major coronary arteries. Coronary simply means *crown-like*; the term was coined to describe the crown-like arrangement of the arteries as they wrap around the heart muscle. From these three coronary arteries descend a vast network of smaller arteries and capillaries that supply the entire heart muscle with oxygen. If a blockage occurs in any one of these coronary arteries, the portion of the heart fed by that artery will malfunction or die, depending on the severity of the blockage.

Ladies and gentlemen the experts tell us that there are three basic causes of coronary artery blockage:

1. Damage to the endothelial lining in the inside of the artery and the attempt of the body to repair the damage with fat and cholesterol bandages.

2. Clumping or sludging of the red blood cells due to excessive saturated fat in the blood.

3. Coronary artery muscle spasm that partially or completely constricts the artery.

Let us consider each of these in detail. Looking at the first cause, we may ask, what causes damage to the endothelial lining of the artery, and how does the body's attempts to repair the damage lead to coronary artery blockages? Arteries are long slender tubes made of muscle tissue. They are in effect *porous* tubular muscles. The inside of this tubing is lined with special connective tissue to make it leak proof, so that it can transport blood. We refer to this inner lining as the endothelial layer. This layer of endothelial cells serves other functions besides making the artery leak-proof to blood. One other vital function they serve is to inject substances into the blood stream that dissolve blood clots. [13] So destruction of this inner lining of the arteries has many dire consequences. The process of heart disease starts with damage to this endothelial layer of connective tissue. The evidence shows that there are several factors that cause damage to the endothelial lining:

1. High blood cholesterol.

2. Excessive dietary cholesterol and saturated fat independent of blood levels.

3. Excess protein.

4. High blood pressure.

5. Nicotine.

6. Coronary artery spasm.

Dr. Julian Whitaker stated that inadequate intake of vitamin C can also contribute to the destruction of the endothelial lining of the arteries. [14]

In this section we will consider the role of cholesterol, saturated fats and proteins in destroying the endothelial lining of the arteries. How does excessive blood levels of cholesterol and saturated fats and protein byproducts damage the inner lining of the coronary arteries, thus leading to heart disease? Excessive amounts of cholesterol and fat particles in the blood stream can tear into this endothelial lining, creating holes through which blood can leak into the interior of the artery muscle and into the surrounding tissue. When damage to the endothelial lining occurs, the body recognizes it as a state of emergency and right away attempts to repair the damage by plugging it with a layer of cholesterol, fatty particles, collagen and other substances. [15] If the damage is repetitive the cholesterol cement builds up, slowly filling the inside of the artery, until after many years of chronic abuse, the temporary patches completely block the inner diameter of the artery thus stopping the flow of blood. During the repair process, the inside of the arteries begin to look like the inside of a corroded rusty pipe. The body's attempt to heal itself in the face of repeated abuse becomes destructive.

It is the shearing action of excessive cholesterol in the blood stream that does the initial damage to the endothelial lining. However the type of cholesterol we eat can also enhance damage to the artery lining. Cholesterol can become oxygenated by the process of frying foods in a frying pan or by deep fried foods such as potato chips. The frying process creates what is called pre-oxygenated cholesterol, a substance toxic to the body. The pre-oxygenated cholesterol chemically damages the endothelial lining, permitting blood to leak out. The leakage of blood then triggers the repair mechanism described above. [16]

In general, if the blood cholesterol level is 150 mg or less, the body can keep up with repairing the damaged inner lining of the artery. When the level is greater than 150 mg, the body's repair mechanism cannot keep up with continuing damage to the endothelial lining and excess cholesterol and fat leak through the inner lining into the interior of the artery muscle. These cholesterol and fatty particles irritate the artery muscles, and a defensive mechanism attempts to engulf these foreign particles. In the process the artery muscles swell and multiply, putting pressure on the endothelial lining. The pressure can tear the lining, thus causing more leaks to appear, and a vicious cycle is created. As more cholesterol and fat leak into the interior of the artery muscle, the inflammation and swelling continues, reducing the inner diameter of the artery, and in turn reducing the flow of blood to the heart. Severe swelling can completely block the coronary artery. [17]

Keeping blood cholesterol below 150 mg is, however, not the total answer to avoiding coronary artery disease. A person could die from coronary heart disease and other cardiovascular disease regardless of the level of their blood cholesterol. That is because cholesterol has an effect on the body independent of blood cholesterol levels. [18] Dr. Richard Shekelle at the University of Texas and Dr. Jeremiah Stamler at Northwestern University issued a joint report on clinical studies of middle aged men in Chicago who were followed for twenty-five years. They found that dietary cholesterol intake increased the risk of death from coronary heart disease more than all other causes of death combined.

Dr. Neil Nedley observed that oxidized cholesterol might be the most important factor that influences heart disease. This type of cholesterol is created when the cholesterol stored in foods is exposed to air and become oxidized by interacting with the oxygen in the air. [19] He reported on research done by Peng and Taylor in Albany, New York, which found that certain oxidation products of cholesterol could damage the lining of arteries in less than twenty-four hours, often doing permanent damage. [20] Peng and Taylor made chemical measurements of different type of foods to determine which stored the most lethal cholesterol oxidation products. By far the winner was dried pancake mix consisting of eggs, milk and sugar. Its chief selling point, a long shelf life, exposed it to increased oxidation. [21] Over a hundred years ago Ellen While wrote about the harmfulness of the free use of milk, sugar and eggs in puddings.

> Especially harmful are the custards and puddings in which milk, eggs, and sugar are the chief ingredients. The free use of milk and sugar taken together should be avoided. [22]

Saturated fat in the blood can also damage the endothelial lining of the coronary artery by depriving it of oxygen. Without oxygen life simply stops. We can all understand that. Many of these endothelial cells begin to die off when starved of oxygen. Eventually large sections of the inner artery lining are destroyed. The mechanism at work here is simple.

Saturated fat is a greasy substance that does not dissolve in water. We all have some experience with the sticky greasy feeling of fat that does not wash away at room temperature. Fat is a pretty inert substance. Excess saturated fat in the blood stream deposits in the inner lining of the artery and acts like a greasy layer of insulation, preventing oxygen from getting to the endothelial cells. [23]

Saturated fat, found primarily in animal products, can also be transformed into cholesterol by the liver, thus contributing to atherosclerosis or hardening of the arteries. Dr. John McDougall observed that this is yet another reason why we should limit the amount of saturated fat in our diets. [24]

Ladies and gentlemen of the jury, saturated animal fat is not the only vilian; the evidence also demonstrates that a diet that includes excess animal protein can contribute to the formation of coronary artery blockages. [25] Mark well that it is animal protein and not plant protein that is the culprit. Dr. Dean Ornish stated that excess animal protein has been shown to raise blood cholesterol levels, while plant protein lowers blood cholesterol levels. [26] Dr. Colin Campbell, also reported that animal protein increases blood cholesterol levels, while a plant-based diet decreases body cholesterol. [27]

Excess animal protein contributes to heart disease in the following way. A breakdown product of protein is homocysteine. High levels of homocysteine can attack and destroy the artery walls and set the stage for the cholesterol/fat repair mechanism that leads to plaque buildup and hence coronary artery disease. [28] Dr. Julian Whitaker stated that a recent Harvard study of 271 patients confirmed that men with high levels of homocysteine levels are 300% more likely to have a heart attack than the rest of the population. [29] Thus a person can have a heart attack from a diet of excess animal-based protein, regardless of their cholesterol level.

Let us now consider the second mechanism for coronary artery blockage: clumping or sludging of the blood. Saturated fat can cause the red blood cells to stick together, thus causing the blood to sludge up. [30] This sludging reduces the amount of oxygen absorbed by the blood and hence the amount available to the cells of the body. Oxygen is carried by the red blood cells by specialized protein molecules. To get the oxygen to the cells, the blood must pass single file through very small or narrow capillaries. Through these small capillaries the blood delivers oxygen and other nutrients to the cells, and receives in exchange carbon dioxide and other waste products from the cells. The carbon dioxide is taken back to the lungs and exhaled. A fatty meal can ruin this delicate process; it thickens the blood, thereby preventing it from flowing with ease through the small capillaries. [31]

It is important to understand the relationship of fat to the blood. The evidence reveals that the body metabolizes fat differently from proteins and carbohydrates. While the liver plays a part in breaking down proteins and carbohydrates so that the amount of these substances that directly enter the blood stream is controlled, there is not a similar control mechanism for fat metabolism. When you eat fat, it is emulsified by the bile acids into tiny droplets that bypass the liver and enter the lymphatic system; from there they directly enter the arteries at the level of the heart. Thus the amount of fat that enters our blood is directly related to the amount of fat we eat! [32]

The heart then pumps this fat all over the body corrupting and gumming up all the arteries with saturated fat. This sticky saturated fat causes the red blood cells to stick together. The more fat in the blood the greater the number of red blood cells that clump together. After a particularly high-fat meal, the blood can literally turn to sludge. Oxygen cannot effectively aerate the blood, and so less oxygen is absorbed and less is available to cells. This process can reduce the amount of oxygen carried by the blood by as much as 30%. [33] The heart muscles and other organs are thus deprived of oxygen.

The problem is compounded by a mechanical one. The clumped-together blood cells cannot pass through the small narrow capillaries. Normally red blood cells must pass single file through the narrowest capillaries to deliver oxygen and take in carbon dioxide. [34] These red blood cells have a slight electromagnetic charge to keep them separated so they can perform this delicate function. When the blood sludges due to the sticking together of these red blood cells by the action of saturated fat, no oxygen can get to the cells fed by these small capillaries. [35] Ever wonder why your thoughts seem so sluggish after a high-fat, cheesy meal? That is where we get the term *cheese brain*. This condition can lead to strokes and other problems. The coronary arteries are also deprived of adequate oxygen and the inner lining is destroyed proportionately. Dr. Timothy Regan at Wayne State University College of Medicine has shown that a high fat meal can reduce the amount of oxygen going to the heart by 20%. [36]

One by-product of plaque buildup in the arteries is high blood pressure. This high blood pressure can further destroy the endothelial lining of the arteries by the shearing force of the blood against the artery walls. [37]

If there are partial blockages in the arteries, due to the initiation of the endothelial repair process, the result is restricted openings for the blood to flow though. Like the nozzle in a garden hose, these narrow junctions increase the velocity of the blood considerably, thus increasing their shearing force. A vicious cycle is set up. As the lining tears and is repaired by the cholesterol bandage, the inner diameter is reduced and the blood pressure rises and so on. Sixty million Americans have blood pressure levels in the danger zone; that is to say blood pressure above 140/90. [38]

Ladies and gentlemen of the jury, let us now consider the phenomenon of coronary artery spasm. As we have stated, the arteries are long lengths of muscular tubing. Like all muscles they can, under certain conditions, go into spasm. A spasm is a process of constriction. When the arterial muscles go into spasm, the diameter of the arteries are constricted, reducing the flow of blood and hence the amount of oxygen available to the heart. [39] If the spasm is mild, the flow of blood is slightly reduced and we may experience angina pain. If it is severe we can suffer a heart attack.

Dr. Dean Ornish and others have noted that several mechanisms can trigger artery spasm or constriction.

1. High fat and cholesterol intake.

2. Nicotine.

3. Stimulants.

4. Excessive exercise.

5. Emotional Stress through a variety of mechanisms.

In this section we will only consider the role of high fat and cholesterol in creating artery spasm. Other causes of artery spasm will be considered in other segments of this trial.

The long-term damage to the body of a high fat and high cholesterol diet is well known. What is not often considered is that a single high fat and cholesterol meal can have immediate harm to the heart and coronary arteries by triggering coronary artery spasm, which can cause sudden cardiac death. Excessive fat and cholesterol in the blood stream can prompt the body to release a hormone called thromboxane which causes the arteries to go into spasm or the blood to clot at a faster rate. [40] Not surprisingly many heart patients often complain of chest pain after a fatty meal.

Seemingly healthy people can end up in the emergency room after a rich Thanksgiving dinner. [41]

Fat and cholesterol buildup in the artery can compound the effect of artery spasm. If there is plaque buildup, artery spasm can cause plaque hemorrhage and bleeding inside of the artery muscles. The bleeding can cause the artery to swell, further reducing the diameter of the inner space and thus reducing blood flow. Spasms can also cause plaque hemorrhage to release blood clots into the arteries which in turn can cause strokes or coronary thrombosis.

Often all these mechanisms occur together. If an artery is already partially blocked, only a small amount of spasm is required to significantly increase the blockage and decrease the flow of blood. Likewise a small blood clot flowing through a partially blocked artery can complete the blockage and bring on a heart attack. A high fat and cholesterol diet can trigger both artery spasm and platelet clumping, which can result in sudden reduction of blood to the heart and hence sudden cardiac death. [42]

Ladies and gentlemen of the jury, there are other lifestyle causes of heart disease such as the excessive use of refined foods such as white sugar, white bread, white rice, and white pasta, as well as harmful substances such as alcohol, nicotine and caffeine. Stress is also an important factor in causing heart disease. A detailed analysis of these causes is not within the scope of this trial. However, a brief mention will be made of the role of refined foods in the following section.

Section 2:

REFINED FOODS: POISON ON OUR PLATES

Ladies and gentlemen of the jury, refined foods are stripped of virtually all natural ingredients. Sixty-four food groups have to be stripped from natural cane sugar to produce the white crystal of refined sugar. It is now not a food but a slow poison. It may be *sweet* to the taste, but it creates a deadly *acidic condition* in the body and blood. To digest white sugar and other refined foods the body has to rob its mineral bank in the bones and tissue. The result is a depletion of vital nutrients from the body and an upset of the blood chemistry. [1] The evidence has shown that micronutrients work in synergy to metabolize our foods. An imbalance in minerals prevents the body from turning even wholesome food substances into nutrients. Ladies and gentlemen there is poison on our plates. America's stomach is full, but she has no nutrition.

Because of our overconsumption of refined sugar, the following brief testimony will focus on this refined food poison, but bear in mind that there is overwhelming evidence that white bread and white rice and pasta are just as deadly to our systems. The recent study by the University of Sydney as reported in the March 11, 2008, issue of the *American Journal of Clinical Nutrition* (actually the first comprehensive study of its kind) linked the consumption of refined white bread with an increase in the risk of heart disease, cancer, and diabetes. Incidentally the study also linked white sugar with an increased risk for these chronic diseases. [2]

On the other hand, (to soften the litany of bad news) a review of the scientific literature by Dr. Harold E. Miller and colleagues and published in the *Journal of the American College of Nutrition* in 2000, reveals that the antioxidants and other phytochemicals in whole grain cereal foods (as wells as in fruits and vegetables) reduce the incident of heart disease, cancer and other chronic degenerative disease. After reviewing the scientific and epidemiological evidence the team of researchers concluded:

> Considerable scientific evidence suggests that whole grains, as commonly consumed in the United States and Europe, reduce risk for chronic disease including cancer and heart disease. Whole grains provide a wide range of nutrients and phytochemicals that may work synergistically to optimize human health. Fruits and vegetables provide protection against age related diseases. It is believed their high content of antioxidant compounds is key to such protection. [3]

Refined foods, especially white bread and white sugar, are adulterating our food supply. Read your food labels, folks. Tons of sugar is added to ordinary food to make it taste good and to addict us to overconsumption. Nutritionist, Dr. Nancy Appleton, explained that ingesting refined sugar creates cravings, which lead to more consumption of sugary foods and so a vicious eating cycle is set up which leads in turn to weight gain. But these cravings are not induced by the naturally occurring sugars in fruits and vegetables. [4]. White Sugar can cause allergy-addiction; weight gain and food allergies are actually related consequences of eating refined sugar. Dr. Appleton explained this connection and then passed on some good advice:

> Sugar is implicated in a long chain of events in the body that leads to weigh gain. The minerals in the body become unbalanced, enzymes don't function correctly, food does not digest properly and allergies occur. Allergies cause addiction, addition causes cravings, and overeating is the result. So forget simple calorie counting. If you want to lose some pounds or keep from gaining unnecessary weight, eliminate sugar and other refined foods—such as white flour, spaghetti, and pizza—from your diet. Get back to the basics: exercise regularly and eat meals that include lots of vegetables, legumes, protein, and grains. [5]

Ladies and gentlemen, the Cartel of defendants profits while we suffer the deadly consequences. CNN reported in October 2007 that there are 400,000 deaths from obesity annually and 12 ½ million of our kids are overweight. It pointed out that in 1997, *four* states reported that 20% or more of their population was overweight. By 2007, *all* states except four reported that their populations were 20% or more overweight.

The consequences for heart disease are frightfully alarming. The evidence shows that there is a lot of research that establishes the link between sugar and heart disease. Dr. John Yudkin stated, over a decade ago:

> A person ... who is taking more than 120 grams of sugar a day is perhaps five or more times as likely to develop myocardial infarction (clotting of the coronary artery in the heart) as one taking less than 60 grams.] [6]

Ladies and gentlemen, refined sugar causes heart disease through a number of mechanisms. Firstly, fructose or fruit sugar raises the level of cholesterol, triglycerides and low-density lipoprotein cholesterol in the blood stream, all of which are associated with heart disease. [7] Refined sugar can also contribute to heart disease by upsetting the mineral balance. All minerals act in synergy, that is, in dynamic relation to each other. When refined sugar changes the mineral relationships some of the minerals occur in excess and become toxic. Toxic minerals can bind to cholesterol, causing it to destroy the arterial lining and precipitate heart disease. [8]

Sugar unbalances the body's chemistry by depleting the body of various minerals during its metabolism. Sugar needs chromium to be metabolized. Since refined sugar has no chromium in its food matrix, the body has to supply chromium in order to digest the ingested refined sugar; other organs and tissues of the body are thus depleted of their chromium and this increases their risk of impaired function. Dr. William Philpott found that people who died from arteriosclerosis have no detectable chromium left in their aortas, while people who died from other causes, such as accidental deaths, have normal levels of chromium present in their aortas. [9]

Refined sugar also contributes to atherosclerosis by upsetting the calcium/phosphorous balance. The normal ratio of these minerals in the body is ten parts of calcium to four parts of phosphorous. The body chemistry requires 2.5 times as much calcium as phosphorous for proper metabolic functioning. [10] But if phosphorous levels fall, the proportion of calcium increases and this excess calcium becomes toxic to the body. The excess calcium can invade the cells and precipitate atherosclerosis, kidney stones, cataracts, arthritis or plaque in the teeth. [11] Researchers have found calcium deposits in advanced atherosclerosis lesions. [12]

Sugar also upsets the calcium/magnesium ratio. This ratio should be 2 to 1. If excess sugar depletes the calcium level, then the excess magnesium is not usable and fails to protect the heart muscle. When the ratio of calcium to magnesium is less than 2 to 1, coronary heart disease and diabetes can result. [13]

But there is also good news for the sugarholic. Dr. Nancy Appleton reports that in her clinical practice she has seen people achieve normalization of their blood pressure, cholesterol levels, and triglyceride levels by removing refined sugar from their diets. [14]

Section 3:

HEART SURGERY: THE BILLION DOLLAR INDUSTRY

Ladies and gentlemen of the jury, our premise throughout this trial has been that in order to determine the proper treatment of heart disease or any kind of degenerative disease, we must start with a clear understanding of their causes. Because heart disease is America's number one killer, we will take a few moments to review what was discussed in the previous sections regarding its causes. There are two primary physiological causes of heart disease:

1. Blockages in the coronary arteries resulting in a reduction of blood flow to the heart.

2. Malfunction of the heart muscles.

These causes overlap. Let us focus on the causes of the coronary artery blockages. Obstructions in the coronary arteries can occur from a variety of mechanisms. There are three primary mechanisms:

First, by damage to the endothelial lining on the inside of the artery and the attempt of the body to repair this damage by fat and cholesterol bandages. Damage to the endothelial layer arises from a variety of causes:

1. High blood cholesterol.

2. Excessive dietary cholesterol and saturated fat, independent of blood levels.

3. Excess protein.

4. Excess sugar.

5. High blood pressure.

6. Nicotine.

7. Coronary artery spasm.

Second, heart disease can result from the clumping or sludging of the red blood cells due to excessive saturated fat.

Third, by coronary artery muscle spasm that constricts the artery partially or completely. We have also seen that spasms can occur from a variety of causes:

1. Excessive cholesterol and saturated fats intake.

2. Nicotine.

3. Stimulants.

4. Excessive exercise.

5. Emotional stress through a variety of mechanisms.

The primary contributing factors in all three of these mechanisms are lifestyle choices that include a high animal fat, cholesterol and protein diet and intemperate habits. We should also note that that these causes are compounded by such intangible factors as stress and social and spiritual isolation.

Ladies and gentlemen of the jury, given these facts about the cause of heart disease, what do you think is the best approach to treating and reversing heart disease? As usual there are two broad approaches:

1. Focusing on the *symptoms* of heart disease and trying to suppress them.

2. Focusing on the *causes* of heart disease and trying to eliminate the causes and the symptoms.

The medical establishment has predominantly followed the first approach. This chapter focuses on evidence pertaining to the superficial and inefficacious remedies of conventional medicine. Doctors and pharmaceutical companies generally treat the symptoms of heart disease through a variety of mechanisms:

1. Bypass surgery to remove the blocked arteries.

2. Angioplasty to squish the fat/cholesterol blockage to open a passage for blood to flow.

3. Drugs to lower blood cholesterol.

4. Drugs to lower high blood pressure.

5. Drugs to remedy irregular heart beat.

Ladies and gentlemen, the evidence will reveal that several problems with these techniques endanger your health and pocket book. They are temporary fixes that suppress the symptoms but do nothing to remove the causes of heart disease. The side effects of surgery and drugs can endanger your health and can at times be deadly. And they are extremely costly.

In this segment of the trial, we will consider the pros and cons of surgical procedures. Bypass surgery and angioplasty are temporary fixes that deal with the problem of heart disease in a superficial manner. Given the fact that the end result of coronary artery blockages was a reduced blood flow to the heart, doctors focused on finding ways of improving the blood flow to the heart. This may seem to be a logical place to start and would have provided lasting benefits if they went to the heart of the problem, but they do not, as you will see. Ladies and gentlemen the stone hard truth is that conventional medicine does not go to the heart of the problem in treating heart disease, because if it did, the profits would dry up. Today heart surgery is well over a $50 billion dollar industry. Citing 1995 figures, Dr. Julian Whitaker stated in July 1999:

> The heart surgery industry is booming. According to American Heart Association statistics, in 1995 doctors performed 1,460,000 angiograms (the diagnostic procedure that starts the ball rolling) at an average cost of $10,880 per procedure. This resulted in 573,000 bypass surgeries at $44,820 a shot, and 419,000 angioplasties (the balloon procedure for opening up arteries) at $20,370 each. The total bill for these procedures is over $50 billion a year. [1]

The pivotal questions are: Were these procedures justified? Were our hard-earned tax dollars justifiably spent in subsidizing this lucrative industry? Did the patients benefit? Dr. Julian Whitaker emphatically states that there are safer, saner, and more effective ways to treat cardiovascular disease:

> There is no, repeat NO, scientific justification for the use of angioplasty and bypass surgery to treat most cardiovascular diseases. Several studies over the past two decades, involving over 6,000 patients with heart disease, have shown that patients funneled into surgical procedures are significantly *worse* than those treated with the noninvasive techniques. [2]

Is Dr. Julian Whitaker correct in his dismal assessment of the benefits of heart surgery and angioplasty? He is not alone in his assessment. Dr. Neil Nedley observed that the great drawback on surgical fixes for heart disease is that they do not go to the underlying causes and have sometimes lethal and serious side effects.

> One of the greatest concerns with these methods (bypass and angioplasty) is that they do not address the underlying disease process. That disease is atherosclerosis, a condition that silently affects blood vessels throughout the body. The disease causes a slow but steady increasing blockage of major arteries. Bypass surgery and angioplasty do nothing to change this gradual accumulation of fatty deposits throughout the body. These high-tech procedures only "buy time" ...

> Although the risk of operative death is now down to about three percent or less in some centers, most people are completely unaware of the *potentially permanent side effects* that can occur from this surgery (bypass surgery). For example, two percent of bypass patients have a stroke and up to 57 percent suffer some kind of neurological complications, often so subtle that the individual's family may have simply written it off as "Dad is just getting older." MRI evaluations have shown that the brain swells within an hour of bypass surgery; the reason may be partly explained by microscopic blood clots that are common during heart surgery ...

The failure of angioplasty done on a single heart blood vessel in the first six months is 35 to 45 percent, and for multiple vessel angioplasties is 50 to 60 percent within the same length of time. Such failures then require another angioplasty, stent placement, or even bypass surgery.

Thus, performing surgery on a person with heart disease has three drawbacks: 1. Provides a temporary fix. Does not correct the underlying cause. 2. Permanent side effects can occur. 3. High cost. [3]

Let us examine the historical and research evidence. In 1946 Dr. Arthur Vineberg invented a procedure for increasing blood flow to the heart, and he gave his name to this procedure. He redirected the internal mammary artery that supplies blood to part of the chest wall by splicing it into the coronary artery downstream of the cholesterol and fat blockage. [4] After thousands of these procedures were performed, controlled scientific studies revealed that the operation was worthless. Dr. Dean Ornish stated that patients who had sham operations in their chest were equally relieved of chest pain as those who had their mammary arteries redirected. [5]

In 1961 the first coronary artery bypass operation was performed using a section of a vein removed from the patient's leg to splice around the blocked artery. The operation was a success and since then cardiac surgeons became the most powerful doctors in many medical centers. [6] Dr. Dean Ornish pointed out that two decades later when the euphoria settled down, doctors in the 1980s began to do randomized controlled studies to assess the effectiveness of bypass surgery. Problems were surfacing that were quite disturbing.

Bypass patients were experiencing heart attacks, strokes, infection and sometimes death during the surgical procedure. Dr. Ornish stated that up to one third of those who had bypass surgery were suffering some transient or permanent neurological damage or loss of IQ. [7] Not surprisingly it became increasingly clear that bypass surgery was only a very expensive and risky temporary fix. Within five years 50% of bypassed arteries clog up and within seven years the number rises to 80%. [8]

Dr. Julian Whitaker cited a 1983 report by the Coronary Artery Surgery Study which was published in the prestigious *New England Journal of Medicine*. In this study a total of 780 patients with significant heart disease were divided into two groups. One-half was treated with surgery and one-half by medication. The outcome was not favorable to those advocating heart surgery—surgical patients did worse than non-surgical patients. Dr. Whitaker observed:

> The results of this study stunned the medical establishment, and should have condemned the heart surgery industry into shame. Patients having surgery fared no better than those on medical therapy. In fact, after ten years, *the majority of the surgical patients were worse than those who avoided the surgery*!

> This study proved that neither bypass surgery nor angioplasty could possibly reduce the death rate, since it was less than 2% per year in the group without surgery. In other words, all those millions of people who were told that they needed immediate surgery to save their lives actually had a 98.4% chance of surviving *without* surgery. [9] [Emphasis added.]

A more recent study of the issue confirmed the 1983 study. A report published in the June 18, 1998 issue of the *New England Journal of Medicine* also demonstrated that patients who underwent surgery did worse. In this study 1,000 patients were randomly selected from across the country. One-half was randomly selected for invasive surgery which included angioplasty or bypass surgery. The other half was treated with conservative measures. The results were startling.

> The in-hospital death for heart attack rates was 214% higher in the surgical group. [10]

Ordinarily if a doctor opts for a non-emergency surgical or medical procedure that was not only unnecessary in light of other more effective options, but left the patient worse off than if the procedure was not performed, then the odds are that he has committed medical malpractice. The heart surgical industry is too lucrative an industry for the medical profession to acknowledge this fact.

Ladies and gentlemen of the jury, let us continue to examine in detail the evidence relating to the problems with bypass surgery. It is a known fact that because bypass surgery does nothing to stop the process of ath-

erosclerosis, the arteries that have received the graft undergo an accelerated degree of atherosclerosis. Dr. Whitaker cited the work of Dr. B. J.
Maurer at the Alabama Medical Center in Birmingham, which showed
that total arterial occlusion was sixteen times more frequent in arteries
that had received bypass grafts than in arteries that did not have grafts.
[11]

Although it had been known for quite some time that grafted arteries
are more prone to cholesterol and fat occlusion, physicians have continued
the surgery, possibly putting their patients at risk. [12] The patients that
were put at greater risk were those that had minimum blockage, less than
50% of their coronary arteries. At the University of Southern California,
School of Medicine, Drs. W. Linda Cashin and David H. Blankenhorn
did a thirty-seven month follow up on eighty-five men who had bypass
surgery. The arteries with 50% blockage before the surgery blocked up ten
times more frequently than arteries of similar blockage that did not receive
the surgical graft. [13]

Evidence shows that one of the gravest drawbacks of bypass surgery
involves the use of the heart lung machine. During bypass surgery the
heart is stopped completely and the heart lung machine takes over the
functioning of these organs. Blood is taken out of the body through a vein
in the abdomen and pumped back in into the body through an artery in
the lower abdomen. This process reverses the normal direction of blood
flow, moving it from the legs to the chest and to the brain. This reversal
of blood flow disrupts cholesterol plaques, sending a stream of clots to
the brain and other organs, creating brain damage often characterized by
gross loss of intellectual ability, strokes, visual disturbances and abnormal
reflexes. [14]

The heart lung machine can also result in autoimmune problems.
When the blood is circulated out of the body into the heart lung machine,
the strange environment activates the protein immunoglobulins that are
part of the body's natural defense mechanism. When the blood is pumped
back into the body, the activated immunoglobulins attack the body, doing
damage to the lungs, liver, kidney and brain, sometimes leaving the patient
severely disabled. [15]

In light of the high cost of bypass surgery and the high risks involved, is
the procedure worth it? Is bypass surgery cost effective? Dr. Dean Ornish
does not think so. He stated that in 1987, 200,000 bypasses were performed
at an average cost of $30,000. This amounted to over 6 billion dollars. [16]

Other observers have noted the trend of rising costs in bypass surgery. In 1990 America was spending more money—approximately $78 billion annually—on treating heart disease, and of this $7 billion went for bypass surgery. By 1998 the annual price tag for bypass surgery topped $26 billion dollars. [17] Is the high price of bypass surgery worth it when the problem can be fixed at relatively low cost—by merely changing ones' dietary habits and lifestyle? You the jury will be able to make this decision after you have considered the evidence for alternative medical approaches.

Ladies and gentlemen, let us now look at the history of angioplasty. In 1977 Dr. Andreas Gruentzig invented a new, less-invasive procedure for unclogging coronary arteries. He inserted a tube with a small balloon at the end of it into the coronary artery. The balloon was inflated at the site of the blockage, squishing the blockage and making room for blood to flow past into the heart. The procedure was called angioplasty and it became a good competitor to bypass surgery because it was less invasive. Within a few years angioplasty was being performed by cardiologists all over the world. [18]

But this procedure too proved to be only a temporary fix. Dr. Ornish stated that one-third of arteries opened by angioplasty clogged up within four to six months. [19] Other problems with angioplasty soon surfaced. Sometimes the coronary artery would rupture when the balloon was inflated, necessitating immediate bypass surgery. Sometimes the patient undergoing angioplasty had a heart attack. The procedure itself could injure the endothelial lining of the artery wall, setting up the patient for the cholesterol/fat repair mechanism and clogging of the arteries years later. [20]

Besides being dangerous to the patient, angioplasty can also be expensive. Over 200,000 procedures were done in 1988, at a cost to $22,000 for a single blood vessel [21] Can we as a nation afford to spend this kind of money merely to suppress symptoms? The cost of prevention and reversal through nutritional modalities and lifestyle changes is negligible compared to this level of expenditure. Considering the lifestyle choices that result in heart disease, it is patently unfair for the average citizen to be taxed in order to pay the medical bills of those who do not exercise prudence or self-control in their food and lifestyle choices.

When Dr. Christian Barnard performed his first heart transplant in 1967 it appeared that a new day had dawned for heart surgery. This was total invasion for the heart. Again the same pattern was seen. Coronary arteries feeding the new heart were becoming clogged up. Hearts were being rejected. A predictable pattern was also seen with artificial hearts: clogged arteries and blood clots in the artificial heart. [22]

Ladies and gentlemen, the contention here is not that we should dispense with surgical procedures for heart disease. That would not be wise or prudent. As an emergency response or when natural cost effective remedies do not work, surgical procedures can mean the difference between life and death. The objective should be to preserve life. America has the finest emergency and acute care system in the world; let us keep it that way. But do not let us use our technology in such a way that it treats only symptoms while ignoring the underlying causes of avoidable diseases, thereby endangering the patient's life and health.

Dr. John McDougall stated that although the American Heart Association has published guidelines for determining when emergency heart surgery is appropriate, they only provide essential reasons *for* heart surgery. First, surgery is indicated if the left ejection factor of the left ventricle is between 35 to 50%. This would indicate a severely weakened heart and these patients may benefit from heart surgery. [23] Second, if there is significant occlusion of the left main coronary artery and there is a weakened left ventricle. [24]

Other doctors take the position that drug therapy should be considered before surgery is considered. [25] But how effective is drug therapy in treating heart disease? That is the subject of the next segment of testimony.

Section 4

DRUG THERAPY FOR HEART DISEASE: A BLESSING OR CURSE?

Ladies and gentlemen of the jury, as with most drug therapies, the initial use of drugs to lower blood cholesterol and reverse arteriosclerosis appeared to be promising. In 1966 Dr. C.R. Ost in Sweden treated thirty-one patients with blockages in the arteries to the legs using large doses of Niacin to lower their cholesterol levels. Angiograms were taken before commencement of drug therapy. After three years follow up angiograms were taken. The results were unexpected: 10% of the patients showed a reversal of the blockages, while 35% had not gotten any worse. [1]

When cholesterol-lowering drugs were combined with a low-fat diet, the degree of reversal of the heart disease became more impressive. Drs. Robert Barndt and David Blankenhorn conducted a study at the University of Southern California in which they put a group of twenty-five patients with severe blockages on a low-fat diet and cholesterol-lowering drugs. After fourteen months 36% of the patients showed impressive reversal and 10% remained stable. [2]

In the mid 1980s, the National Institute of Health recruited 3,806 men for a seven-year study with the cholesterol-lowering drug Questran. This drug binds with cholesterol in the intestinal tract, thus eliminating it from the body. The result is a decrease in blood cholesterol levels. In this study one half of the men were given a placebo. Both groups ate a moderate cholesterol-lowering diet. After seven years the group taking Questran showed an 8.5% reduction in blood cholesterol levels, with a corresponding 19% decrease in the death rate. [3]

But, ladies and gentlemen of the jury, for these marginal results, what are the drawbacks of cholesterol-lowering drugs? Besides being expensive they have serious and sometimes deadly side effects. Take Niacin for example. At low doses it is a nutritious vitamin, but at high levels it acts like a drug and has the quality of lowering cholesterol levels. However, the side effects include liver damage, glucose intolerance, gout, headaches, itching and skin flushing. Fortunately most of these conditions resolve when the drug is discontinued, however long-term use can be dangerous to one's health. [4] Dr. Dean Ornish stated that Lovastatin or Mevacor has side effects that include liver damage and cataracts. [5] As we have seen from the testimony of Dr. Max Gerson, the evidence is overwhelming that impairment of the liver can lead to cancer.

Dr. John McDougall noted that the side effects of Questran (Cholestyramine) include constipation in about one third of patients, abdominal discomfort, gas, nausea and a bleeding tendency in people with low vitamin K. [6] Do cholesterol lowering drugs actually *reverse* heart disease? Dr. Dean Ornish questioned this assumption. He stated that only two studies have demonstrated reversal, while other studies such as the $170 million dollar study by the National Heart, Lung and Blood Institute concluded that cholesterol lowering drugs do not reverse coronary artery disease. [7]

Other drugs in the medical arsenal are deployed to deal with the myriad of other complications of heart disease. To relieve angina or chest pain, doctors often prescribe calcium antagonists, called calcium channel blockers. These drugs interfere with the entry of calcium into the heart muscles, thereby causing them to relax, thus reducing heart pain. However the side effects can be devastating. These range from constipation, overgrowth to the gums, and surgical bleeding to a 60% of increased risk of death. [8] [9] Beta-blockers also reduce heart pain. They do this by reducing the heart muscle's work and subsequent demand for blood and oxygen by blocking the action of heart stimulating hormones. However, interfering with the hormonal function is not good. Dr. McDougall observed that beta-blockers raise triglyceride levels and lower good HDL cholesterol levels, making the patient a candidate for more heart disease. [10] Dr. Lynne Walker noted that Dr. Julian Whitaker contended that the use of beta blockers has resulted in an epidemic of congestive heart failure: between 1979 and 1991 hospital admissions for this disease doubled to 822,000; while the death rate peaked at 60 percent during this period. [11]

Doctors have also turned to various types of blood thinning therapies to treat heart disease. These types of drugs are called anticoagulants. One of these, Warfarin, initially showed promise in reducing death rates after a heart attack. But since its introduction, the side effects have grown to include fatal hemorrhage, which discouraged its use. [12] Another popular blood thinner is aspirin. Although it has reduced the risk of death by 15% for fatal heart attacks, and nonfatal attacks by 30%, it also has side effects, which include hemorrhaging and increased risk of strokes. Dr. Lynne Paige Walker questioned whether these studies are reliable. She noted that the study which showed a 40% reduction of heart attacks in male doctors, actually used Bufferin which contains magnesium, a natural vasodilator that reduces platelet adhesion independently of the effects of aspirin! [13] Dr. Walker also pointed out that the use of aspirin increased a certain type of stroke. [14] There is a tradeoff between reducing clotting and extending bleeding times. The wrong balance sometimes leads to an increase in the risk of cerebral hemorrhage. [15] But most importantly, she concluded, while aspirin may reduce heart attacks, the overall survival from heart diseases has not been demonstrated. [16] The harmful lifestyle eventually catches up with the patient and the grim reaper takes his toll.

The evidence demonstrates that high blood pressure is one of three major health risks for heart disease. High cholesterol and smoking are the other two. Ladies and gentlemen of the jury, while tons of research has shown that dietary changes could eliminate high blood pressure, the routine approach of many doctors for many years was to start the patient on blood pressure medication. [17] However the dangerous side effects of these drugs may outweigh any benefit to the patient. The most common drugs used to lower high blood pressure are diuretics such as Dyazide, Hydrodiuril and Diuril.

Dr. P. K. Whelton at the British Medical Research Council demonstrated as early as the mid 1980s that these diuretics increased the incidence of irregular heart rhythm in his patients. [18] In the process of inducing water elimination, diuretics lower the amount of potassium in the cells to dangerous levels—thus inducing irregular heart beats. [19]

Another danger of hypertensive medication is that it may increase other risk factors for heart disease. This places the patient at a disadvantage and in some cases at extreme risk. Dr. Richard H. Grimm of the Department of Medicine at the University of Minnesota Medical School raised this issue in a 1981 article in the *Annals of Internal Medicine*.

An increase in serum total cholesterol and low density lipo-protein fraction may increase coronary heart disease in patients treated with diuretics. This has special implications for hypertensive persons already at increased risk for atherosclerosis and coronary heart disease. Even a small average increase in these lipid fractions would have considerable public health import because of the millions taking these drugs. [20]

In his study Dr. Grimm demonstrated that patients taking Hydrochlorothiazide for high blood pressure had on average increased their cholesterol by 14.8 mg. Those taking Chlorthalidone had increased cholesterol levels of 18.8 mg. His patients also had an increase in their triglycerides and uric acid content; excessive amounts of the latter can cause arthritis and gout. Concerned by these findings, Dr. Grimm challenged the medical profession to continue research into non-pharmaceutical means of lowering blood cholesterol. [21] Dr. Neil Nedley, in *Proof Positive*, also cautioned against attempts to reduce cholesterol and triglycerides by means of the *statins* class of drugs which include Zocor, Pravachol, Mevacor and Lescol. [22] These statins can cause severe liver damage, as well as inflammation and destruction of the voluntary muscles of the body. [23]

In his 1990 best seller, *Reversing Heart Disease*, Dr. Dean Ornish warned that the side effects of hypertensive drugs can include impotency, fatigue, blood cell disorders and depression, and in some instances may increase mortality. [24] He related a study of 43,000 patients with moderate hypertension performed by the National Heart, Lung and Blood Institute in the 1990s. They were treated for 5.6 years with hypertensive drugs. The researchers concluded that the drugs did not specifically reduce mortality from coronary heart disease. [25]

The evidence also revealed that the hypertensive medication may have *increased* the risk of heart disease. The untreated group had fewer nonfatal heart attacks and fewer fatal heart attacks than the group treated with drugs! [26] Why did this happen? The diuretics had increased the other risk factors for heart disease. Dyazide actually increases blood sugar and LDL or *bad* cholesterol. It also decreases blood levels of potassium and magnesium which increase the risk of sudden cardiac death! [27]

Ladies and gentlemen of the jury, Dr. Dean Ornish complained that the entire healthcare system encourages spending on drugs and surgery, not on health education; [28] but given the fact that surgery and drugs are only temporary fixes and do not reverse the cause of heart disease, why is it that our nation is spending so much money on non-solutions while spending next to nothing on prevention and on nutritional modalities that would cure the problem of degenerative diseases? The answer is simple but frightening. *Disease management has become big business.* Dr. Whitaker indicted the whole system of health care financing.

> Managing disease is a lucrative business. As long as people stay sick, they keep coming back for more. You and I may look at all the zeros in $1,000,000,000,000 and feel the weight of the cost involved. Special interest groups see only the benefits: inside that $1 trillion is a great deal of profit for them. [29]

Everyone at all levels in the chain is indicted. From the doctor who opts for an expensive surgical procedure, to the laboratory companies who do the supporting diagnostic tests, to the hospital who supplies the operation theater and the pre and post surgical care, to the insurance companies that pay for these expensive procedures through the premiums paid by the wage earner. Also indicted are those companies that manage our Medicare and Medical dollars generated by tax levies on the citizen. Everyone takes a cut. Everyone profits but the patient. Managing the symptoms of a disease is not in the best interest of the patient *if* nothing is done about removing the causes of the disease.

Most of the modalities used by modern medicine are not geared toward eliminating the cause of heart disease—atherosclerotic blockage from cholesterol and fat build up. If this were done the need for bypass surgery would diminish considerably. But very few involved in the whole complex chain of dispensing this type of *voodoo* medicine are prepared to recognize the profit motive driving the type of health care we deliver to patients with heart disease. Dr. Whitaker further stated,

> Every step leading to the bypass operation is profitable for those providing the services. The profit motive is at work in almost every endeavor in this country. This in itself is not bad but we are reticent to recognize the profit motive as a force when it comes to the practice of medicine. [30]

Dr. Whitaker keenly observed that there is tremendous profit to be made by keeping the emphasis of our medical system away from prevention. Drug companies are in the vanguard of this struggle. The pharmaceutical industry is the most profitable industry in America. [31] Dr. Whitaker cited an editorial from *Biological Psychiatry*, "*The Addiction to Drug Companies*" that poignantly revealed the influence of drug companies on perpetuating the disease-management orientation of modern medicine.

> The overall influence of the [Health Care] industry is to emphasize drug treatment at the expense of other modalities: psychotherapy, social approaches, nutritional, herbal, and natural remedies, rehabilitation, general hygienic measures, non-patentable drugs, or other alternative approaches. It focuses attention on disorders that are treatable by drugs, and may promote over-diagnosis. It reinforces the practice of dealing with disease by treatment of symptoms, and diverts interest from prevention. [32]

Dr. Colin Campbell also indicted the whole system that puts profit before health. When he lectures on the benefits of a plant-based diet to reverse degenerative diseases, a recurring question posed to him is, if all you say is correct, why have we not heard this before? His answer: He who has the gold makes the rules.

> There are powerful, influential and enormously wealthy industries that stand to lose a vast amount of money if Americans start shifting to a plant-based diet. Their financial health depends on controlling what the public knows about nutrition and health. Like any good business enterprise, these industries do everything in their power to protect their profits and their shareholders ... As far as I know they do not pay scientists to cook the data.

> The situation is much worse. The entire system—government, science, medicine, industry and media—promotes profits over health, technology over food and confusion over clarity. Most, but not all, of the confusion about nutrition is created in legal, fully disclosed ways and is disseminated by unsuspecting, well-intentioned people, whether they are researchers, politicians or journalists. The most damaging aspect of the system is not sensational, nor is it likely to create much of a stir upon its

discovery. It is a silent enemy that few people see and understand. [33]

Ladies and gentlemen, the evidence also reveals that the drug companies profit by systematically, year in and year out, raising prices. Dr. Julian Whitaker pointed out that from 1980 to 1992 the average prescription price went up 300 % from $6.52 to $22.50. [34] Dr. Dean Ornish noted that the cost per patient per year for using the cholesterol-lowering drug Lovastatin was $2,000 to $3,000; and the market is wide open. There are 100 million Americans with elevated cholesterol levels. Treating all of them with Lovastatin, he stated, would cost the nation $200 to $300 billion per year. [35] And this is not even the ceiling for profits. Most high blood pressure patients are expected to use medication for the rest of their lives!

But the drive for profits has not stopped here. Ray Moynihan and Alan Cassels have brought to light a new scandal: The pharmaceutical companies are now *selling sickness* by the fabrication of new diseases to open up yet new channels for the sale of their drugs! In *Selling Sickness: How the World's Biggest Pharmaceutical companies Are Tuning us All into Patients* they wrote in 2005:

> The marketing strategies of the world's biggest drug companies now aggressively target the healthy and the well. The ups and downs of daily life become mental disorders, common complaints are transformed into frightening conditions, and more and more ordinary people are turned into patients. With promotional campaigns that exploit our deepest fears of death, decay, and disease, the $500 billion pharmaceutical industry is literally changing what it means to be human ... the global drug giants are no longer content selling medications only to the ill ... There's a lot of money to be made telling healthy people they're sick ...

> Sometimes a little-known condition is given renewed attention, sometimes an old disease is redefined and renamed, and sometimes a whole new dysfunction is created. [36]

This shameless exploitation is threatening to corrupt medicine, destroy the nation's health and undermine trust in physicians who have become tools of the drug companies.

The unhealthy influence of the pharmaceutical industry has become a global scandal. That influence is fundamentally distorting medical science, corrupting the way medicine is practiced, and corroding the public's trust in their doctors. [37]

Dr. Dean Ornish also pointed out that the influence of the drug companies starts in medical school. By the time the student graduates, they are conditioned to view disease and to practice medicine from the perspective of the pharmaceutical industry. Drug companies spend millions of dollars educating physicians. They are the major advertisers in all medical journals. They fund the clinical trials of their drugs. They sponsor scientific meetings at exotic resorts, often paying for the transportation and meals and entertainment of the physicians. [38] All of this sends a subtle message to the physician: we are your friends—we care—use our services. Which of us would willingly bite the hand that feed us? Being publically traded companies the drug companies are expected to maximize profits. They do this in many other ways than by funding medical schools. All drugs are poisons and have side effects which often lead to new diseases in the patient. The drug companies reap even more profits by creating new drugs to counter the side effects of their drugs and to treat the new crop of diseases. The cycle is endless; the patient is fleeced; his constitution weakened; and our national treasury is raided.

The only sensible approach to treating heart disease is to determine the causes of coronary artery blockages and try to eliminate them. It bears repeating that this does not mean that conventional medical procedures are not necessary. For the severely diseased patient the approach must be an integrative one. There will always be a place for conventional medicine. America has the best acute care delivery system in the world. But we must use it wisely, not in such a way that it perpetuates diseases by ignoring their causes.

When a patient comes into the emergency room with severe chest pain, saying, "Doc, please get this elephant off my chest," I don't just feed him broccoli and ask him to start meditating—I use whatever cardiac drugs, electrical shocks, and surgical procedures are necessary to treat the acute, life threatening condition. [39]

However, the life-threatening emergency opens a real window of opportunity for the physician to educate the patient on the real causes of heart disease and to start the individual on a lifestyle and nutritional program that can make a lasting difference. After all, is not the meaning of the word doctor to teach? For physicians to forsake their oath and do otherwise is medical negligence; for a quick fix provides only temporary relief, while exposing the patient to new sets of problems, even endangering their lives in some cases.

> ... treating only the physical manifestations of heart disease without addressing the more fundamental causes will provide only temporary relief, and the disease is likely to recur. At best, we will trade one set of problems or illness for another. [40]

In the next segment we will consider the true success stories in treating heart disease. The evidence will demonstrate that nutritional modalities coupled with exercise have proven to be the best approach for not only preventing heart disease, but reversing it.

Section 5

WATER & NUTRITION: THE NATURAL PATHS TO VIBRANT HEALTH

Ladies and gentlemen of the jury, what is the best treatment for coronary artery disease? The answer should be obvious now that we know the causes of heart disease and the ineffectiveness of the non-emergency use of surgery and drugs. In this chapter we are concerned with not only treating heart disease, but reversing it. The causes are all lifestyle choices. The major contributing factors are excess saturated fats, cholesterol and animal protein in the diet, seconded and compounded by excessive refined sugar, smoking, stress and dehydration; other intangible but important factors such as social and spiritual isolation must not be overlooked. Adopting a lifestyle that eliminated these causes would not only prevent heart disease, but would actually reverse it.

The evidence has been accumulating for decades. Moving against the current of modern medical practice, a few courageous physicians have established practices utilizing nutritional modalities and lifestyle changes as the *primary* tools for reversing heart disease and other degenerative diseases. These physicians are trying to turn medicine back to the common sense perspective of Hippocrates, the Father of medicine, who recognized that food is the best medicine. Their efforts are beginning to bear fruit. Not only have they helped thousands of patients with heart disease to gain control, and in most cases, to reverse their coronary heart disease, but because of their efforts the medical establishment as a whole is beginning to take notice.

Some of the more recent physicians utilizing nutritional and lifestyle modalities to reverse heart disease are: Dr. Vernon Foster (previous medical director) and his colleagues at Weimar Institute, California; Dr. John McDougall at St. Helena; Dr. Julian Whitaker at Newport Beach, California; Dr. Andrew Weil, director of the department of Integrative Medicine at the University of Arizona in Tucson; Dr. Dean Ornish at the University of California, San Francisco Pacific Medical Center; and Dr. Neil Nedley, graduate of Loma Linda University and present chair of the Medical Education committee at Mercy Memorial Hospital, Ardmore, Oklahoma. The physician who has done outstanding pioneer work in this area is Dr. Dean Ornish. He began his pioneering work on heart disease while still a medical student at Baylor College of Medicine in Houston. By 1990 Dr. Ornish became the first physician to offer to the scientific community documented proof that heart disease can be halted and reversed by simple lifestyle changes in the area of diet, exercise, and stress control. In his ground-breaking study published in the *Lancet* on July 21, 1990, Dr. Ornish randomly divided a selected group of patients with severe coronary artery disease into two groups. Under scientific controls he placed one group on a low fat vegetarian diet with no animal products except low fat dairy and egg whites. This group also stopped smoking, using caffeine and other stimulants, and engaged in moderate exercise and stress reduction techniques. [1]

The other group followed the protocols of conventional medicine which included advice from their physicians to make only moderate changes in diet—i.e., eat less red meat, more fish and poultry, substitute margarine in place of butter, and eat no more than three eggs per week. This second group also exercised moderately and quit smoking. [2] Both groups were given angiograms at the beginning of the study and one year later. At the end of the year the majority (82%) of the patients in group one, those making the more comprehensive changes called for in the Ornish program, had measurable reversal of their coronary artery blockages. Not every blocked artery was reversed, but a majority were. What was also remarkable was that the most severe arteries showed the greatest reversal. Even arteries that had been blocked for years were opened up. In contrast, those in the control group following the advice of their doctors became measurably worse. [3] Because the most severely blocked arteries showed the greatest reversal, the question can be raised whether so much heart surgery is justified.

A number of other important observations can be made from this study. First, it is never too late to begin making changes that can improve one's health and quality of life. Age is not a factor. Neither is the severity of the disease. The degree of improvement was related to how faithfully the patients stuck to the program. The greatest improvement was seen in a seventy-four-year-old patient and in another patient with the most severe blockage. [4]

Secondly, the disease-reversal program must be viewed as a matrix of cooperating modalities. It was not possible to say how much of the improvement was due to each individual component of the program. While each component was an integral part of the treatment, some aspects of the program may be more important to some patients than for others. Beware of looking for a silver-bullet to cure diseases. The body is too complex and the laws that regulate it are interrelated, working synergistically for the benefit of the whole organism. Dr. Ornish noted:

> ... dietary changes may be more important for a person who has been eating a high fat, high cholesterol diet but who is not under much stress, doesn't smoke, exercises, and has a lot of emotional support. Likewise, the stress management techniques may be more important for someone who is in a high-stress job but whose blood cholesterol level is only 150. The point is that while there may be some individual differences, it is the program as a whole that has been demonstrated to begin reversing coronary heart disease in most of our study participants. [5]

Thirdly, the study demonstrated that while cholesterol is a very important risk factor, it is not the whole story. Because of the Framingham Heart Study in Framingham Massachusetts in 1948, which showed that no one with blood cholesterol under 150 developed heart diseases, Dr. Ornish was under the assumption that blood cholesterol levels would have to fall below 150 before reversal could be seen. He was wrong. Patients were experiencing reversal with blood cholesterol levels above 150. Dr. Ornish concluded:

> While there was a direct correlation between adherence to each part of our program (diet, stress management, exercise, and stopping smoking) and the degree of improvement, there was very little correlation between blood cholesterol levels and degree of change in their arteries. [6]

Ladies and gentlemen, this is a very important finding because some doctors place too much emphasis on lowering blood cholesterol levels without considering other risk factors such as the amount of dietary intake of fat and cholesterol and their impact on the body, independent of blood levels. Dr. Ornish stated that one of the patients in the control group used Lovastatin (Mevacor) a powerful cholesterol-lowering drug for one year and actually decreased his cholesterol levels from 248 to 172, yet his coronary artery blockages *worsened substantially* and he had a heart attack at the end of the year. [7]

Fourthly, and significantly, the degree of reversal of blockage from plaque need not be large to improve blood flow. Even a *small* amount of reversal in a severely blocked artery can cause a *great* improvement in blood flow to the heart. For greater accuracy, measurements were made with a Positron Emission Tomography (PET) scan. [8] Why is it possible for a small improvement in the blocked artery to create a disproportionate improvement in blood flow? The reason is that *plaque blockage* is not the *only* cause of decrease in blood flow. *Spasms* in the muscle wall can also decrease the blood flow. A decrease in artery spasm as a result of the elimination of dietary saturated fats would also increase blood flow.

Let us take a clearer look at the nutritional aspects of the therapy through which Dr. Dean Ornish achieved these remarkable results. It is important to understand that this is not a *diet* as that term is normally used. In his program, there were no restrictions in the quantity of food a person could eat. In fact one could eat more abundantly. The nutritional therapy regime is just a *different way* of eating. It is eating more sensibly— *eating for nutrition rather than for pleasure only*. It is eating the foods God designed for human consumption. This common sense approach to eating rearranges the proportions of the nutrients in a meal so as to provide the body with nutrients in the proportions it was designed to handle from a physiological and metabolic stand point.

It goes without demonstration that fats and proteins are building materials. They are not, primarily, fuels to supply the body with energy. Hence they must be eaten in certain restricted proportions. Complex carbohydrates are the primary fuel of the human body therefore they must be eaten in greater proportion compared to fats and proteins. Complex carbohydrates provide the continuous supply of energy that keeps the body active and every organ alive. When you attempt to reverse the proportions of fats and proteins and carbohydrates by eating more building materials (fats and proteins) and less fuel (complex carbohydrates), you force the body to burn the building materials as fuels. The metabolism of excess fats and proteins creates metabolic disorders and initiate disease processes. It must be carefully understood that these studies utilize natural, unrefined complex carbohydrates, not refined and denatured carbohydrates. *Refined* carbohydrates are poisonous to the body in that they are slow poisons due to the fact that they leach essential nutrients *from* the body, thus upsetting its metabolic and immune functions.

Ladies and gentlemen of the jury, the good news for the patient with chronic degenerative disease is that when you correct the proportions of fats, proteins and complex carbohydrates in your diet the disease process begins to reverse in *every* area. Dr. Ornish discovered this to be true also with heart disease. The proportion of nutrients in his Reversal diet provided a greater proportion of carbohydrate fuels and lesser amounts of fats and proteins in the following ratio:

10 % fat (mostly poly and mono unsaturated fats)

15 % to 20 % protein

70 % to 75 % complex carbohydrates

Because of the near elimination of animal products, the patients received only 5 milligrams of cholesterol per day. [9] This diet did not restrict the quantity of food his patients ate; it merely imposed selection guidelines to bring the meal into compliance with the body's nutritional requirements. Broadly speaking, the diet virtually eliminated animal products except for non-fat milk, yogurt, and egg whites. This near elimination of animal products accomplished at least three things.

1. It virtually eliminated dietary cholesterol which is found only in animal products.

2. It drastically reduced saturated fats, the only kind of fat found in animal products

3. It drastically reduced excessive animal protein.

Excessive dietary saturated fat, cholesterol and animal protein are the primary dietary agents in precipitating heart disease. The Ornish Reversal diet also excluded plant foods high in unsaturated fats such as avocados, nuts and seeds. It also *excluded* all oils because they are 100% fat. [10] If you do not have heart disease or have completely recovered from it, then these plant foods which contain a mixture of saturated and unsaturated fats may be used in moderation. Essential fats such as Omega-3 oils are important to maintaining good health. These foods are part of Dr. Ornish's Prevention diet. [11] Dr. Ornish erred in the side of caution in drastically reducing nuts, for in his clinical practice, Dr. Neil Nedley, obtained significant reductions of bad LDL cholesterol with walnuts. [12]

The Ornish Reversal diet is low in animal protein compared to the typical American diet because too much protein is as harmful as too much fat. This is even true in the animal kingdom. Dr. Dean Ornish observed that animals fed on a high protein diet die sooner than animals fed on a low protein diet. [13] High levels of homocysteine, a toxic byproduct of protein metabolism, destroy the artery walls, thus initiating the fat/cholesterol repair mechanism which in turn results in plaque buildup. [14] The evidence is replete that excess animal protein can also raise blood levels of cholesterol which can cause coronary artery blockages. [15] Dr. Ornish's observations are compatible with Dr. Campbell's findings that animal protein increases blood cholesterol. [16]

Excess protein also leaches minerals such as calcium and magnesium from our bones; this process can lead to osteoporosis. [17] Many people fear that if they do not eat animal protein, they will not have enough dietary protein. This is an error born of propaganda from the meat and dairy industry. Dr. Julian Whitaker stated that the real protein problem is this country is not too *little* dietary protein, but protein poisoning from ingesting too *much* protein. [18]

Dr. Dean Ornish pointed out that a plant-based diet can provide all the protein you need. Combining a large variety of carbohydrates such as grains and legumes, beans and rice, provides sufficient amino acids for your body to create a complete protein, so there is no need to worry about getting adequate amounts of protein in our diet. [19] He stated that egg whites also provide a complete protein. [20] (You can discard the yoke, which is full of cholesterol.) The non-fat milk and yogurt in the Ornish diet also provides vitamin B12, the only vitamin you cannot get from a vegetarian diet. Dr. John McDougall however observed that these small concessions to animal products are not necessary because vitamin B12 is manufactured by the bacteria in the small intestine. [21]

Lastly, Dr. Dean Ornish's plant-based diet consists primarily of complex carbohydrates. Complex carbohydrates are basically fruits and vegetables, grains and greens in their natural unrefined state. [22] Complex carbohydrates are the natural fuel for the body. However, if they are stripped of their vitamins and minerals by refinement, they become empty calories that are very damaging to the body. As mentioned, these refined carbohydrates should be dispensed with, for they only leach minerals from the body, thereby upsetting the chemical balance of the body and initiating enzyme dysfunction and metabolic disorders.

Because complex carbohydrates are very filling you never feel starved, but are always satisfied. It is only complex carbohydrates which can adequately satisfy the hunger drive. Complex carbohydrates also add a lot of fiber to the diet. Earlier evidence showed that there are two kinds of fibers, both of which are vitally important to your health. The insoluble fibers provide bulk which speeds up the elimination of waste. This process decreases the risk of developing diseases such as hemorrhoids and appendicitis. The soluble fibers help prevent heart disease by delaying the absorption of glucose and cholesterol, thus keeping blood levels of both at healthy low levels. [23]

In summary, the heart disease reversal diet is a very low-fat vegetarian diet. Dr. Dean Ornish considered this type of diet to be the world's healthiest diet for adults whether they have heart disease or not. [24] Many people have grown up thinking that a vegetarian diet is a wimpy diet and that you need animal products to be well nourished. The opposite is the truth. The excessive use of animal products is the primary reason for our epidemic of degenerative diseases. It is becoming increasingly clear that the way back from disease is to adopt a vegetarian lifestyle, or at least to be very conservative in the use of animal products.

In 1988 the America Dietetic Association (ADA) issued a position paper to correct this misguided view about vegetarianism. Whether intended or not, the finding extols vegetarianism as a tool for reversing degenerative diseases.

A considerable body of scientific data suggests positive relationships between vegetarian lifestyles and risk reduction for several chronic degenerative diseases and conditions, such as obesity, coronary artery disease, hypertension, diabetes mellitus, colon cancer, and others ... Vegetarians also have lower rates of osteoporosis, lung cancer, breast cancer, kidney stones, gallstones, and diverticular diseases.

Although vegetarian diets usually meet or exceed requirements for protein, they typically provide less protein than non-vegetarian diets. This lower protein intake may be beneficial, however, and may be associated with a lower risk of osteoporosis in vegetarians and improved kidney function in individuals with prior kidney damage. Further, a lower protein intake generally translates into a lower fat diet, with its inherent advantages, since foods high in protein are frequently also high in fat. [25]

Gary Null, in *The Vegetarian Handbook, Eating Right for Total Health*, cited the culminating concession of the ADA to vegetarianism, a statement found in the 1988 position paper, and repeated by the ADA's Journal in 1993:

It is the position of The American Dietetic Association that vegetarian diets are healthful and nutritionally adequate when appropriately planned. [26]

For the ADA to conclude otherwise would have been to ignore a huge body of scientific evidence, and to condemn the diets of some of the most brilliant people who ever lived. Prominent vegetarians have included Sir Francis Bacon, Shakespeare, Voltaire, and Benjamin Franklin. [27] But there is more! The list goes on to include Socrates, Plato, Buddha, Leonardo da Vinci, Sir Isaac Newton, Thomas Edison, Vincent Van Gogh, Leo Tolstoy, and Albert Einstein. Notice that the greatest geniuses in science, literature, and philosophy have been vegetarians. Could there be a correlation between these geniuses in their respective fields and their vegetarian diets?

The International Conference on Vegetarian Diets, which met at Austin Texas in November 1997, introduced a vegetarian Food Pyramid Guide that was an alternative to the U.S. Food Pyramid Guide which is a meat-based pyramid. The Conference claimed that until Americans switch from animal-based foods to more plant-based foods, the rate of heart disease, cancer and other degenerative diseases will not decline. [28]

The new food pyramid is a giant step towards the degenerative disease *Reversal diets* of Dr. Dean Ornish and other physicians promoting Wellness diet programs. Except for the freer use of milk, eggs, sweets and plant oils (which are 100% fat), the new pyramid is a good *Prevention* diet. A more stringent regime is however required to *reverse* existing degenerative diseases. The newly devised vegetarian food pyramid is divided into three categories:

1. Foods at the base of the triangle are to be eaten at every meal: Fruits, vegetables, whole grains, and legumes.

2. Foods in the middle of the triangle are to be eaten daily: nuts, seeds, egg whites, dairy and soy cheese, milk, and plant oils.

3. The top of the pyramid are foods to be eaten occasionally: whole eggs and sweets.

Ladies and gentlemen of the jury, the purpose for presenting this testimony is not primarily to convert anyone into a vegetarian. Its purpose is to advance the most recent scientific evidence for *reversing* heart disease. The evidence is abundantly clear and irrefutable that the best diet to reverse heart disease is a *vegetarian* diet. In the mid-1980s Dr. Kaare Norum, Professor of Nutrition at the University of Norway, tried to put to rest the controversy with the meat and dairy industries who deny the link between cholesterol and heart disease. He sent out questionnaires to twenty-one top scientists doing research in the area of arteriosclerosis. [29] Two main questions and their responses were:

Do you think there is a connection between diet and the development of coronary heart disease? Answer: 188 said yes. Only 1 said no. 4 were uncertain. This is a 97% yes response.

Do you think there is a connection between plasma cholesterol and the development of coronary heart disease? Answer: 189 said yes, only 2 said no, 2 were uncertain. Once more, this was 98% affirmative.

Regardless of the propaganda of the meat and the dairy industry, top research scientists the world over link excess cholesterol with heart disease. There is actually no reason to eat cholesterol. Your body makes all the cholesterol it needs from the wholesome fat you eat in plant-based foods. [30] A well-planned vegetarian diet will reverse your heart disease. The choice is ours. Half way measures will not work; nor will eating man-made refined carbohydrates in place of the complex carbohydrates help you. You cannot cheat, for your body never lies. The patients in the control group in Dr. Dean Ornish's 1990 study, who merely cut back on their meat, fish and fowl, had their heart disease worsen. [31] Ladies and gentlemen of the jury, epidemiological studies also show a link between a vegetarian diet and the near absence of heart disease. Nations that consume a low fat, low cholesterol vegetarian diet have low blood pressure, low blood cholesterol and very low rates of heart disease. [32]

The Ornish heart disease Reversal diet is moderate in its use of salt. Excess salt affects the health of your heart to the extent that it causes your blood pressure to increase. The body naturally tries to maintain a precise concentration of salt, so when excess is consumed, your body retains water to dilute the salt and to keep its concentration constant. All things being equal, when you increase the volume of liquid in a closed system, the pressure goes up. Thus water retention can also increase your blood pressure. [33]

Stimulants such as caffeine and alcohol are also excluded in the Ornish heart disease Reversal program because of the damage they do to the heart. Dr. Neil Nedley also reported similar findings in a study of 16,000 adults in Norway. It found that homocysteine, which cuts the arterial lining, is increased in the blood by the consumption of coffee and by smoking. [34] The biggest coffee drinkers had almost 60% more homocysteine than abstainers. [35] Caffeine is a dangerous stimulant. It excites the sympathetic nervous system, stimulating it to produce adrenalin and other stress hormones which provide a nervous rush of energy. Unfortunately this supply of energy is temporary and is followed by an energy crash, bringing you lower than before you took the caffeine—this low feeling leads you to take more caffeine, hence the cycle of addiction. [36]

Stress hormones produced by the stimulating effects of caffeine can cause coronary artery spasm that can injure your arteries and heart muscles. They can initiate irregular heartbeats some of which can be life threatening. [37] Caffeine is found in coffee, colas, chocolate and many popular drinks. Beware of so-called de-caffeinated coffee, which can contain more caffeine than you think. An expose done by WCCO-TV of Minnesota on November 28, 2006, which corroborated an earlier study published by the University of Florida on October 22, 2003, revealed that some outlets were serving almost double the amount of caffeine permitted to be in de-caffeinated coffee by the National Coffee Association, and one outlet's de-caffeinated serving had as much caffeine as a regular cup of coffee! Decaf is not the same as caffeine-free; if it were the customer would not get hooked and sales would drop.

Nutritional physicians discourage alcohol use when trying to reverse heart disease because its use is associated with many health risks. Alcohol has a toxic effect on the heart muscles. [38] Over time this can cause the heart to malfunction. Alcohol is also toxic to the liver and pancreas. [39] Studies have shown that even one drink a day could double the risk of stroke by hemorrhage, when compared to not drinking alcohol at all. [40] Dr. Nedley reported that reducing alcohol consumption reduces blood pressure, [41], thereby reducing the risk of heart attack or stroke. Even moderate drinking has been shown to increase the risk of breast cancer by 50% to 100%. [42] Alcohol also increases blood levels of triglycerides. [43] And when drunk to excess alcohol can cause a number of cardiovas-cular diseases such as high blood pressure, heart failure, stroke and cardio-myopathy, besides causing the well-known alcohol related illnesses which include: cirrhosis of the liver, breast cancer, hepatitis, and diseases of the nervous system, digestive system, urinary system and reproductive system. [44]

Some Wellness programs permit the use of fish because it is a source of Omega-3 fatty acids which protect the lining of the arteries from dam-age from LDL-cholesterol. Dr. Ornish stated that omega-3 fatty acids also reduce other risk factors for heart disease by reducing blood clot for-mation. They reduce coronary artery spasm by decreasing the production of thromboxane, while increasing the production of prostacyclin and tis-sue plasminogen activator. [45] However there are a variety of vegetar-ian sources of Omega-3 fatty acids that are recommended over fish for a variety of reasons. The proportion of Omega-3 fatty acids in fish is too high for human consumption; while the proportion of Omega-3 fatty acids in grains is in the correct proportions for use by the body. The higher amount of Omega-3 fatty acids in fish leads to stroke by hemorrhage. [46] Eskimos have very little heart disease it is true, which is due to their consumption of fish. But they have higher incidences of stroke. [47] So they trade heart disease for stroke. Both fatal outcomes. Fish oil may also cause insulin resistance and hence cause an elevation of blood sugar levels, a danger for diabetics. [48]

Dr. Neil Nedley contended that fish is not a safe food any more. He reported that fish found in mildly polluted water can concentrate toxins up to more than 1,000,000 times more than detected in the water. [49] The toxins in the fatty acids of fish can include pesticides, chlorinated hydrocarbons, mercury and dioxin, as well as PCBs, heavy metals, lead, and petroleum compounds. [50] The bottom line, he stated, is that one can get Omega-3 acids from a variety of plant foods, including linseed oil, English walnuts, almonds, green soybeans, spinach, bananas, sweet potatoes, roasted potatoes, un-peeled apples, cucumber and whole wheat bread. [51]

Ladies and gentlemen of the jury, the evidence will show that Dr. Julian Whitaker has been helping cardiac patients reverse their heart disease since the early 1980s at his famous Whitaker Wellness Institute in Newport Beach, California. He stated that there are two nutritional approaches to reversing heart disease. The first approach is to gradually reduce the amount of animal products consumed until they are eliminated. The second approach, which he has found to be the better of the two, is to immediately immerse the patient in the optimum dietary program to give maximum benefit. He stated that the more drastic program eliminates compromise.

This means making no compromise at the beginning and setting up a detailed, structured program for the patient to follow. I personally believe this latter approach is more successful for two reasons.

First, how many alcoholics do you know who control their habit by drinking moderately, or how many smokers are able to simply to cut down the number of cigarettes? Obviously the avenue for success in these two addictions is simply to stop. Many of our food habits are the same and require the same degree of discipline, particularly at first.

For many of my patients, the disease has already reached such a level of seriousness that one can no longer take it lightly. The diet program that we use at the Institute and that is offered in this book is designed for maximum benefit in the shortest amount of time. As such, it is very powerful in lowering the cholesterol level and producing the other benefits outlined.

The rapidity with which beneficial and significant changes occur is quite astounding to many patients who take this type of dietary regimen. With this rapid improvement, patients who are frightened and debilitated by cardiovascular disease then become enthusiastic and motivated about strict adherence to the regimen.

Of the thousands of patients who have completed this program at the Institute, without exception those who enjoy the most success and get the most pleasure out of their new regimen are those who do not look upon this regimen as a deprivation, but rather as an opportunity to improve their health and enhance their lives. Their continuing good health becomes a hobby—an avocation, and a labor of love. In some cases people will begin to treat themselves as well as they treat their automobiles. [52]

The diet Dr. Whitaker utilizes in reversing heart disease generally avoids all foods of animal origin because they are high in cholesterol and saturated fat and low in fiber. [53] Additionally he advised his patients to eat sparingly of plant foods that are high to moderate in fats such as coconut, fish, low fat dairy, nuts, soybeans seeds, vegetable oils and wheat germ. [54] The patient is encouraged to eat abundantly of high fiber plant foods such as beans, grains, fruits and vegetables. [55]

The Whitaker Wellness Program is comprehensive. It does not involve merely a change in diet, however important this may be. In his best seller *Whitaker's Guide to Natural Healing*, he outlined a seven-step program, which will be briefly outline here:

Step 1 is to adopt a healthy lifestyle. To become and remain healthy we must make healthy choices in our eating and our lifestyle. This means quitting smoking and alcohol abuse of our bodies. We must adopt a positive mental outlook and take responsibility for our lives and health. He stated that people with a healthy lifestyle have a high resistance to disease. [56] He also noted that religious people tend to be healthier. A recent survey by Purdue University psychologist Kenneth Ferraro found that only

4% of people who went to church reported ill health, compared to 9% for those who did not attend. [57]

Step 2 requires the patient to become more active. Dr. Whitaker stated that the physiological benefit of physical activity is equivalent to the most powerful anti-aging and health-promoting medicine. For every hour you exercise you increase your longevity by two hours. [58]

Step 3 involves the use of multiple vitamins and minerals. Although supplementation with these micronutrients is important they are not the main focus of the program. He stated:

All the supplements in the world cannot compensate for an unhealthy lifestyle, poor diet, and lack of physical activity. Supplements are just that—a supplement to the diet, physical activity and lifestyle program. They are not the primary healing factors. [59]

In their proper place, supplementing with micronutrients can improve our health and save the nation millions in health care costs.

As our leaders in Washington are debating methods of cutting our "disease management cost," they would benefit from suggestions on how to prevent these diseases that are costing so much. One way that I see is to encourage Americans to take vitamin and mineral supplements. [60]

These micronutrients costs pennies compared to the exorbitant costs of pharmaceuticals or the cost of treating the diseases.

Step 4 encourages the patient to take a special class of micronutrients called antioxidants. Dr. Whitaker stated that despite the FDA's refusal to acknowledge the health value of antioxidants, conventional medicine is gradually changing its opinion on their usefulness. They protect the body from free radical activity. [61] Free radicals are molecules which are highly reactive, due to the fact that they either have an extra electron or are lacking an electron. Free radicals bind to and destroy body components in a process called oxidation. Thus they are responsible for the initiation of many diseases, including heart disease and cancer. [62] The key antioxidants that help to protect us from disease include selenium, beta-carotene, vitamin E and vitamin C.

Step 5 in Dr. Whitaker's program involves special supplementation with the minerals magnesium and potassium. He stated that these minerals are the most important ones within the individual cells of our bodies. [63] They are electrolytes which conduct electricity and thus are important in maintaining water balance and distribution, acid-base balance, muscle and nerve cell function, heart function and kidney and adrenal function. [64] Because of their intracellular activity, a deficiency in these minerals can result in a host of diseases, including heart disease.

Magnesium and potassium are involved in many cellular activities including energy production, protein formation, and cellular replication. A deficiency of either magnesium or potassium is characterized by a host of symptoms. These include mental confusion, irritability, weakness, heart disturbance, problems in nerve conduction and muscle contraction, muscle cramps, loss of appetite, insomnia and a predisposition to stress. [65]

Although magnesium is found in green leafy vegetables, whole grains, nuts and legumes, Dr. Whitaker advises his patients to supplement with 1,000 milligrams of elemental magnesium daily because it is depleted in processed foods. [66] Magnesium specially helps the heart muscle to contract. Very low levels of magnesium have been found in individuals who suddenly die of heart attacks. [67]

Dr. Whitaker stated that the potassium to sodium ration should be 5 to 1, but most Americans by their free use of salt reverse this ration, consuming twice as much salt as potassium. [68] Although potassium is found abundantly in bananas, legumes and citrus, he recommended 400 milligrams daily, preferably taken with other nutrients such as vitamin C, and the B vitamins. [69]

Step 6 involves the use of an Omega-3 oil supplement. He stated that while a diet high in saturated fats is strongly linked to heart disease, stroke and cancer, a diet high in unsaturated fats and low in saturated fats is associated with a low incidence of these diseases. [70] Omega-3 oil has the essential fatty acid that determines normal cell structure and function: alpha-linolenic acid. Alpha-linolenic acid is a key component of nerve cells, cell membranes and hormone-like substances known as prostaglandins. [71] Linoleic acid, an omega-6 is another essential polyunsaturated fat. The ideal ration of omega-6 to omega-3 fatty acids in our diet should be six or five to one. However, the typical American diet has a ration of 24 omega-6 to 1 omega-3. Dr. Whitaker stated that:

> Reversing this ration can have long-lasting, positive effects on many illnesses, including heart disease, arthritis, stroke, migraine headaches, and other serious and even fatal maladies. [72]

Step 7 outlines Dr. Whitaker's comprehensive dietary program. Of course it is not a diet as the term is commonly used. It is merely a more natural and smarter way of eating. In this program one eats for health *and* pleasure, not for pleasure only, as is commonly the case. Although this is step 7, it is the most important improvement you can make in order to improve your health. The diet is basically a low fat, high complex-carbohydrate one. [73] Dr. Whitaker realizes the power of addiction of unwholesome foods. Sugar and fat are addictive. He stated that if you do not believe this, try giving them up! Dr. Whitaker recommended that we adopt two helpful attitudes as we embark on a healthy way of eating. First, we should realize that there are many delicious, good-for-you foods and food combinations available in a healthy menu. [74] God has designed what is good for us to be also tasty and pleasurable to the palate. Secondly, we should not focus on what we are giving up; rather we should focus on discovering the many great and tasty dishes the new healthful diet will provide. [75]

Ladies and gentlemen, the use of vitamin and mineral supplements is still a controversial matter, even among practitioners of natural medicine. Dr. Neil Nedley argues that we should get all of our vitamins and minerals from plant-based foods such as organically grown fruits, grains and vegetables. [76] He reported on a study by a Swiss researcher, Dr. A. Mozafar, which demonstrated that vitamin B-12, often claimed to be lacking in a vegetarian diet, is amply found in *organically grown* soybeans, barley and spinach, [77] This also goes for the valuable antioxidants needed for good health. These can be obtained in such fruits as strawberries, plums, oranges, red grapes, bananas, apples and tomatoes, and from garlic, kale, spinach, broccoli, beets, red bell peppers and corn, and many more vegetables. [78] His reasoning is partly based on the concept that vitamins and minerals do not act alone. They act in synergy with other vitamins and minerals, so taking them in their natural form and abundant variety is better that taking them separately. [79] Besides, these micronutrients may be also dependent upon the host of yet undiscovered phyto-chemicals in whole foods. [80] Moreover, any vitamin taken to excess may act as a drug in the body. [81] For this reason many nutritional experts are turning to micronutrients preserved in their food matrix and administered not singly but in multiple combinations.

Despite the position of the FDA and the medical Cartel, Dr. Whitaker contended, like his mentor the great Hippocrates, that wholesome, nutritious food is the best medicine:

Over the last twenty years, I have found that a very low fat, high-complex-carbohydrate diet is the most powerful tool in health care. It is useful in preventing disease, and it is useful in treating disease. My experience is the basis of my recommendations. [82]

Dr. Julian Whitaker presented a number of good reasons in support of his recommendation to adopt a vegetarian dietary plan. First, he noted that the human being was not designed to eat flesh. We have teeth for grinding grain and plant foods, not teeth to rip into flesh. Secondly, the bowel of the human is long and convoluted and very unlike the short bowel of carnivores. The short bowel of the flesh eater is designed to evacuate undigested and breakdown products of meat before they putrefy in the bowel. The long bowel cannot do this, so the meat putrefies before it is eliminated. He connected the long bowel of humans with the high incidence of colon diseases in meat eaters. [83]

Dr. Whitaker also stated that there is plenty of epidemiological evidence showing the rise of chronic degenerative disease among populations that were once primarily vegetarian and who turned to heavy meat eating.

The evidence is resoundingly clear. A tremendous array of chronic diseases, which were previously virtually unknown, began to be seen when the usual diets of these populations had been largely vegetarian: heart disease, cancer, stroke, diabetes, and arthritis. Their deviation from a predominantly plant-based diet appeared to be a major factor in the increased incidence of these diseases. [84]

Ladies and gentlemen, for decades the medical establishment ridiculed nutritional doctors such as Whitaker for practicing medicine on the basis of this epidemiological evidence. Now they are not laughing as loud or as long. The medical establishment has finally realized that the threat to America's health is no longer the infectious disease of yesteryear, but the killer epidemics of chronic degenerative diseases, heavily linked to our unwholesome affluent diets. [85] In 1988 Dr. C. Everett Koop, Surgeon General of the U.S., released a report on Nutrition and Health. The report was favorable to the nutritional doctors. Dr. Whitaker made this comment about the Surgeon General's findings,

> Finally, after many years of nutrition-oriented physicians calling out in the wilderness for more attention to the relationship between diet and health, light began to dawn.

> The findings [by the Surgeon General] were convincing. Links were finally established between the typical American diet and many diseases. The diet that is the culprit is the one that our gastrointestinal tract is not built to assimilate. It is the diet that our cousin primates are not choosing. It is the diet through which, by adopting it, our Japanese brothers and sisters are spreading diseases amongst themselves. It is a diet low in plant foods, and high in animal foods and refined sugar. [86]

The common cardiovascular diseases generated by a low plant-food and high meat diet include hypertension, cerebrovascular disease, stroke, angina, heart attack, varicose veins, deep vein thrombosis and pulmonary embolism. [87] Dr. Whitaker stated that study after study have demon-strated that following a dietary change to a low fat, high-complex-carbohydrate diet, reductions in the incidence of these diseases occur; and this type of diet also reverses these diseases. He therefore recommended:

1. Reduce total fat intake to 30% or less of calories. (Many experts say 20% or less is optimal.) Reduce saturated fatty acid intake to less than 10% of calories. Reduce intake of cholesterol to less than 300 milligrams daily.

2. Eat five or more servings per day of a combination of vegetables and fruits, especially green and yellow vegetables and citrus fruits.

3. Increase the intake of fiber and complex carbohydrates by eating six or more servings per day of a combination of whole-grain breads, cereals, and legumes.

4. Maintain protein intake at moderate levels.

5. Balance food intake and physical activity to maintain appropriate body weight.

6. Limit the intake of alcohol, refined carbohydrates (sugar) and salt (sodium chloride). [88]

The diet program prescribed by Dr. John McDougall and others for reversing heart disease generally follows these guidelines. Dr. McDougall's regime is more strictly vegetarian. He recommended the avoidance of all animal products, the elimination of all oils and avoidance of sulfur dioxide and MSG. [89] He also recommended that the heart patient eat sparingly of fruit because of its fructose content. [90] Exercise, of course, plays a key role in all these nutritional programs designed to reverse cardiovascular disease and is recommended by all nutritional physicians.

Ladies and gentlemen of the jury, let us turn our attention to testimony regarding that elixir of life—water. Dr. F. Batmanghelidj has taken a new approach to preventing heart disease. He emphasized the need for proper hydration of the body. He contended that disease is a response to a condition of dehydration existing in the body. He stated that high blood cholesterol and cholesterol production in the cells is a sign that cells of the body have deployed a defensive mechanism for preventing the high osmotic force of the blood from drawing water through the cell membranes. Essentially it is a defense against dehydration. [91]

> Cholesterol is a natural "clay" that, when poured in the gaps of the cell membrane, will make the cell wall impervious to the passage of water. Its excessive manufacture and deposition in the cell membrane is part of the natural design for the protection of living cells against dehydration. In living cells that possess a nucleus, cholesterol is the agent that regulates permeability of the cell membrane to water. [92]

Dr. Batmanghelidj stated that the secret to controlling cholesterol levels is not only to have a well-hydrated cell system in the body, but to drink adequate water before you eat. He observed:

> If we begin to appreciate that for the process of digestion of food, *water is the most essential ingredient,* most of the battle is won. If we give the necessary water to the body *before* we eat, all the battle against cholesterol formation in the blood vessels will be won.

> After a longer period of regulating daily water intake, so that the cells become fully hydrated, gradually the cholesterol defense system against the free passage of water through the cell wall will be less required; its production will decrease. [93] [Emphasis added.]

Dr. Batmanghelidj further stated that it is more important to pay attention to our water intake than to the foods we eat. That is, given a proper nutritious diet, it is adequate water that will keep us healthy and disease free.

> Let us get one thing clear: *Excess cholesterol formation is the result of dehydration.* It is the dehydration that causes many different diseases and not the level of the cholesterol in the circulating blood. It is therefore more prudent to attend to our daily water intake rather than to what foods we eat. With proper enzyme activity, any food can be digested, including its cholesterol content. [94] [Emphasis added.]

Dr. Batmanghelidj backed up his position by citing testimonials from patients who have tried drinking more water and who have reduced their cholesterol levels. You can't fight success. However, given what we know about proper nutrition, when this nutritional information is combined with Dr. Batmanghelidj's emphasis on getting daily adequate water intake, our battle against degenerative diseases will be greatly advanced. Ladies and gentlemen, this evidence highlights the fraud and folly behind cholesterol lowering drugs from which the drug Cartel profits handsomely at our expense!

As long ago as 1905 Ellen White wrote in *Counsels on Diet and Foods*, about the value of adequate water intake in preventing the onset of disease.

> In health and in sickness, pure water is one of Heaven's choicest blessings. Its proper use promotes health. It is the beverage which God provided to quench the thirst of animals and man. Drunk freely, it helps to supply the necessities of the system, and to assist nature to resist disease. [95]

In *Your Body's Many Cries for Water*, Dr. Batmanghelidj warned us against treating the symptoms of dehydration with medication. It is often the case, he stated that *you are not sick, you are thirsty*. [96] While there may be a proper place for medication, Ellen While also warned against the unnecessary use of medication when adequate water, along with fresh air and exercise, could have resolved the problem.

> Thousands have died for want of pure water and pure air, who might have lived ... These blessings they need in order to become well. If they would become enlightened, and let medicine alone, and accustom themselves to outdoor exercise, and to air in their houses, summer and winter, and use soft water for drinking and bathing purposes, they would be comparatively well and happy instead of dragging out a miserable existence. [97]

Ladies and gentlemen, consider soberly the evidence you have just heard. Many of the symptoms of hydration and of poor nutrition are *managed* by the drug industry when these symptoms could be *eliminated* by proper hydration and nutrition! The management of these symptoms by drugs produces even more symptoms to be managed by even more drugs.

Something is wrong with this picture. Is our health and wellbeing being traded and bartered for profits by the medical Cartel? No wonder *they* have declared war on nutrition. They grow rich on our ignorance. Knowledge is power and the road to our independence.

High Blood Pressure

The Physician's Secret Retirement Plan

Section 1:

THE MOST HIGHLY MEDICATED ILLNESS IN HUMAN HISTORY

Ladies and gentlemen of the jury, high blood pressure is epidemic in America. An estimated 60 million people in America have high blood pressure, sometimes called hypertension. It is the most common reason people go to the doctor. [1] Dr. John McDougall observed that more people take medication for high blood pressure than for any illness ever encountered in human history. [2] It is the source of great profits for the pharmaceutical companies and the medical profession.

This is a great tragedy, considering that high blood pressure is preventable and virtually reversible by proper nutritional and lifestyle choices. The evidence will show that the greater tragedy is the medical fraud perpetrated upon millions of people. Dr. John McDougall stated that approximately 40 million people take medication for high blood pressure which provides them with no benefit. [3] The only ones who benefit are the drug companies who make millions off the suffering of countless number of people he added. Dr. John McDougall further stated:

> The evidence to date suggests that the current treatment for high blood pressure is largely a failure for the vast majority of patients. This means millions of people are taking drugs that are doing them no good, costing them money, and subjecting them to potentially serious side effects. Clearly, "the emperor has no clothes." More people receive drug treatment for high blood pressure than for any other disease, but most of these people derive no benefit from these medications. [4]

An examination into the causes of high blood pressure will readily show why drug therapy does not work and why nutritional and lifestyle changes work best to prevent and reverse this disease. Dr. Julian Whitaker is emphatic that for most Americans with high blood pressure, an improper diet is the cause and a change in diet is the cure. [5] Conventional medicine adopts an incorrect pharmaceutical approach to treating high blood pressure because they do not properly appreciate the fact that, strictly speaking, high blood pressure is *not* a *disease* but a *symptom* of underlying disease processes that interferes with the functioning of the circulatory system. [6] Hence the emphasis should not be on the *pressure* of the blood but on the *underlying metabolic causes* of high blood pressure.

Blood pressure is a measure of the contraction and expansion of the heart as it pumps blood through the arterial system. Upon contraction blood is pumped into the arteries, and upon expansion blood is pumped into the heart through the veins. The contraction force is referred to as systolic pressure, the top reading; the expansion phase the diastolic pressure, the bottom reading. [7] Normal blood pressure is 110/70 or less without the help of medication. [8] A blood pressure of 140/90 to 160/110 is considered mildly to moderately high and over 160/110 is regarded as severe. [9]

The primary causes of high blood pressure are a high fat and cholesterol diet, excess animal protein, and an excess use of salt which contributes to low levels of potassium and calcium. [10] The use of stimulants such as cigarette smoking, alcohol and caffeine also contribute to high blood pressure. [11] Let us see how each of these causes operates to create high blood pressure.

Excess dietary fat causes high blood pressure through a number of mechanisms. In one of these mechanisms, saturated fat causes the red blood platelets to stick together, sometimes becoming sludge-like. [12] The heart has to work harder to push this thickened blood through the arteries, thus raising the blood pressure considerably. Accordingly, when fat consumption is reduced, blood pressure falls. [13] High fat consumption can also initiate atherosclerosis, the buildup of plaque in the arteries, which in turn can narrow the arteries and cause blockages, thus raising the pressure in the system. Atherosclerosis commonly strikes vessels in the head and neck that carries blood to your brain. [14] The word atherosclerosis comes from the words *athero*, which refers to the mushy or fatty material deposits in the arteries and *sclerosis*, which means hard, and refers to the tough fibrous material the body uses to insulate the fatty deposits. [15] The buildup of plaque can result in both high blood pressure as well as coronary artery disease. [16] It has been observed that 40% of people with high blood pressure also have cholesterol levels above 240 mg/dl. [17]

Arteries are tube-like muscular organs that expand and contract. [18] Excessive cholesterol can damage the arterial endothelial lining causing fat and cholesterol particles to infiltrate the artery wall, making it less elastic. This reduces the ability of the artery to expand during the contraction cycle of the heart, thus increasing the systolic blood pressure. [19] Dr. McDougall pointed out that high fat and cholesterol intake can cause high blood pressure through yet another pathway. Fat and cholesterol can trigger the release of prostaglandin hormones which can cause the muscular walls of the blood vessels to contract, reducing their diameter and raising the pressure needed to push the blood through these constricted arteries. [20]

Excess protein can also increase blood pressure. The type of protein ingested is important. Animal protein increases blood cholesterol levels. [21] While excess animal protein has been shown to increase blood pressure, plant proteins lower it. [22] Dr. Frank Sacks found that substituting animal protein into the diet of vegetarians raised their blood pressure. [23] Dr. Ian Rouse of the Department of Medicine, University of Western Australia, discovered that placing meat eaters on a vegetarian diet lowered their blood pressure. [24] Animal proteins release homocysteine, a toxic substance, as a byproduct of protein metabolism. Homocysteine is linked to damage of the endothelial layer of the artery. [25] This initiates the process of atherosclerosis, resulting in both high blood pressure and heart disease.

It is well known that excess sodium salt in the blood raises the blood pressure. [26] The sodium draws excess water from the surrounding tissues into the blood stream, raising the volume of blood and hence its pressure within the arteries. [27] Although sodium is an important electrolyte, we do not need near the quantity normally consumed. Dr. Julian Whitaker estimated that we use twenty to thirty times the amount of sodium necessary for bodily functions. [28] Several studies show that merely cutting back on salt usage will reduce the blood pressure for many people. [29] Dr. Nedley reported that societies that ingest little or no salt have no hypertension. [30] Dr. McDougall stated that about 30% of people with high

blood pressure are salt sensitive and can benefit from reduced salt intake.
[31]
   Because high blood pressure has other causes besides high salt intake,
reducing salt intake may not work for many people with high blood pressure. Other nutritional tools must be implemented. [32] For the vast majority of people sodium salt is not as damaging as fat and cholesterol. Studies
of people following a vegetarian diet that includes generous amounts of
salt reveal no high blood pressure problems. [33]
   A low potassium intake is also an important index for high blood pressure. Dr. Naosuke Sasaki studied people in two Northern Japanese towns
where large amounts of salt were consumed. While many of the people in
one town had high blood pressure, those in the other town did not. The
difference was due to the generous amounts of potassium used by the
people of the town which did not have a high blood pressure problem.
[34] Dr. Graham A. MacGregor at the Blood Pressure Unit, Department
of Medicine, Charing Cross Hospital Medical School, London, England,
was able to lower the blood pressure of twenty-three hypertensive patients
using 2.3 grams of potassium. He recommended that people with high
blood pressure substitute potassium salt for regular sodium salt. [35]
   Low calcium levels have also been linked to high blood pressure. Dr.
David A. McCarron, Associate Professor of Medicine of the Oregon
Hypertension Program in Portland, Oregon, demonstrated that reducing
the calcium intake is associated with high blood pressure. [36] He also
showed that significant decreases in consumption of calcium, potassium,
vitamin A and vitamin E were all associated with increases in blood pressure. [37] This study, however, demonstrated that low calcium intake was
the most constant factor in hypertensive individuals. [38]
   Excess insulin helps to produce high blood pressure, and this is one
of the complications of using insulin to control adult onset diabetes. The
insulin activates the sympathetic nervous system to trigger the release of
the hormone norepinephrine in the blood which normally operates to
raise the blood pressure under stress. [39] Excess insulin also increases
high blood pressure through different pathways. Insulin stimulates the
proliferation of smooth muscle cells in the arteries and encourages connective tissue growth. The inner diameter of the blood vessels is reduced,
and high blood pressure and heart diseases is the result. [40]
   High insulin levels can also upset the chemical balance of minerals
in the cells, leading to high blood pressure. Insulin adversely alters the

sodium pumps in the cell membranes which increase the flow of sodium into the cells. The cells can go into a cramp, a condition known as vasospastic activity, which in turn can cause high blood pressure. [41] Insulin results in too much calcium flowing into the cells which in turn can result in vasospasm and high blood pressure. [42]

Cigarette smoking is a major factor in causing high blood pressure. [43] A single cigarette can cause blood pressure to rise for thirty minutes to an hour, and continuous smoking throughout the day results in elevated pressure throughout the day. [44] Smoking can also result in permanent high blood pressure. Smoking oxidizes LDL cholesterol and causes the onset of atherosclerosis, a risk factor for both high blood pressure and heart disease. [45]

While moderate use of alcohol can lower blood pressure, excessive use of alcohol is associated with high blood pressure. [46] But what is moderate and what is excess? Dr. Nedley reported that just an ounce or two a day of alcohol is enough to raise blood pressure significantly. [47] Dr. Neil Nedley stated that from his medical experience, eliminating alcohol has become a necessary element in reducing the blood pressure of his patients. [48] Caffeine use is also associated with high blood pressure. [49] Dr. Nedley reported that just one cup of coffee per day, or the equivalent in cola drinks, raises the diastolic and systolic blood pressure five to six points. [50] Thus consuming caffeinated drinks just before or during exercise can turn a health activity into a potentially serious and even deadly cardiovascular event. [51]

Certain degenerative diseases such as artery disease, diabetes and kidney dysfunction can also produce high blood pressure. Diabetes is a major risk for developing atherosclerosis and hence hypertension. [52] Diabetics have twice the risk of suffering a heart attack or stroke than non-diabetics. Diabetes is a serious disease. It contributes to the destruction of blood vessels throughout the system and thereby increases the likelihood of suffering from kidney disease, blindness and other illnesses. [53]

The destruction of the kidneys by high fat and high protein diets can lead to high blood pressure. The mechanism is simple to understand: Fat and cholesterol can cause atherosclerosis plaques to form in the kidneys, thus blocking the arteries and diminishing the functional size of the kidney. [54] High protein diets can wear out the kidneys by calling on it to filter out excessive amounts of uric acid. When kidney function is diminished, the body cannot filter out excess toxic materials including excess sodium in the blood. The sodium draws extra water into the blood, increasing its volume and pressure. [55]

Ladies and gentlemen of the jury, Dr. F. Batmanghelidj took a new and refreshing approach to the cause of high blood pressure. He stated that high blood pressure is essentially the result of an adaptive process to a gross body water deficiency. [56] In other words, you are not really sick, you are thirsty! He stated that when the body is short of water, it carries on essential functions by drawing away 66% of water volume from inside of the cells, 26% from outside of the cells and 8% from blood volume. [57] During this adaptive process the body shuts down capillaries in less active areas of the body. The closing of capillary beds, however, offers resistance to the circulating blood, which in turn requires an increased force behind the circulating blood. The result is increased blood pressure. [58]

High blood pressure results in many medical complications. It is one of three major risk factors for developing heart disease and strokes. [59] Elevated cholesterol and smoking are the other two. [60] Dr. McDougall observed that people with high blood pressure are seven times more likely to suffer a stroke, four times more likely to have a heart attack and five times more likely to die of congestive heart failure. [61] In a similar vein, Dr. Nedley warned that high blood pressure, America's silent killer, can result in stroke, congestive heart failure, heart attack, atherosclerosis, aneurysm, kidney disease, diseases of the retina, blood vessel rupture and weakening of the memory and decreased mental ability. [62] Severe chronic high blood pressure can cause the hemorrhage of small blood vessels, thus precipitating visual impairment and blindness, headaches, convulsions, vomiting, paralysis and coma. [63] High blood pressure is a serious medical condition, and it must be taken seriously.

Section 2

DRUGS: THE PROFIT PIPELINE

Ladies and gentlemen of the jury, the evidence is very clear that high blood pressure is not a disease, rather it is a symptom of underlying diseases. Hence lowering the blood pressure by the use of drugs treats only the symptom of the underlying diseases. Drugs do nothing to arrest the causes of high blood pressure. Predictably, drug therapy for high blood pressure will not work because it treats only the sign and not the cause of the problem. [1] On the other hand, voluminous research has shown that dietary changes can eliminate the symptoms as well as the causes of high blood pressure. Yet the routine practice of many physicians is to immediately start the high blood pressure patient on drugs, and usually without recommending any dietary changes. [2] In light of the fact that high blood pressure medications do not benefit the vast majority of patients, you the jury must decide whether the conventional treatment of high blood pressure without dietary reform is medical malpractice and reckless profiteering at its worse. What is even more egregious is that the evidence shows that high blood pressure medication can do positive harm, aggravating the cause of the disease itself and increasing the rate of mortality. [3] Dr. Julian Whitaker observed:

> In fact, a large scale government funded study called the Multiple Risk Factor Intervention Trial (MRFIT) found that the mortality rate was actually *higher* in a group of hypertensive patients that received aggressive treatment compared to a group of hypertensive patients that received no treatment or less aggressive approaches.

> Another study by Dr. Anders of Helgeland, of Oslo, Norway,

demonstrated that the incidence of *sudden death* among patients with mild hypertension who were treated with hydrochlorothiazide was *three times* that of the control group not treated with the drug. [4] [Emphasis added.]

These serious findings indict the use of certain drugs to treat high blood pressure. Dr. Lynne Paige Walker observed that the Multiple Factor Intervention Trial is even more disturbing than even Dr. Whitaker reported. She stated that both the treated and the non-treated group modified their diets and lifestyles. While the modified diets in the non-treated group resulted in a 21% reduction in coronary heart disease, the treated group had an increase in death rate! [5] Thus the drugs themselves interfered with the beneficial action of diet and lifestyle changes! [6] The drugs fought against nature's own healing action! Dr. Walker also reported that in the 1980 Oslo study in which 800 men were divided into two groups, 400 hundred receiving the hypertensive medication, and 400 put in a control group, the incident of sudden death was not only greater in the treated group, but death from *all* causes was 11% more in the treated group. [7] Are the benefits of hypertensive medication greater than the side effects? Not if you are dead. Dr. Walker sadly noted that modern pharmaceutical medicine has forgotten Hippocrates' very first principle of medicine, in their pursuit of profits: First do no harm. [8]

Ladies and gentlemen, a review of the drugs commonly used to treat hypertension can be very enlightening and sobering. The drugs most commonly used are classified as diuretics. These drugs promote water elimination on the assumption that reducing the amount of water in a closed system, the arterial system, would reduce the pressure in the system. Diuretics do cause the kidneys to excrete more water from the body and this lowers the fluid volume of the blood, thereby lowering blood pressure. [9] The thiazide diuretics commonly used are Dyazide, Hydrodiuril and Diuril. While they do promoted elimination of water from the body, their side effects are devastating to the body.

To begin with, the excessive elimination of water often washes out vital minerals from the body that are important to cellular function. Such loss of minerals can result in changes in heart rate and heart failure among other serious medical complications. [10] The thiazide diuretics have been shown to cause irregular heart rhythms. [11] Dr. Walker explained that among the minerals that diuretics wash out is potassium which is vital to maintaining the heart's electrical activity. [12] Irregular heartbeats often result when the blood potassium level is reduced below normal. Dr. Brian Holland studied twenty-one patents that had thiazide-induced low blood potassium levels; he found that seven of them (33%) developed irregular heartbeats. [13]

Dr. Neil Nedley also observed that lack of water can cause dehydration of red blood cells, making them less flexible and inducing in them a greater tendency to clot. [14] Hematocrit levels can rise thus increasing the risk of heart attacks and strokes. [15] Dr. Walker noted that the loss of potassium by diuretics can even exacerbate the problem the medication was given for in the first place! [16] Potassium helps prevent strokes, the dreaded scourge that hypertensive drugs are supposed to counteract! The loss of potassium translates into greater incidents of stroke. [17] To help us further understand the widespread disruption of the physiological and metabolic processes of the body by washing out potassium, let us consider the testimony of Dr. James Marti as found in his *Alternative Health Medicine Encyclopedia.*

> Potassium is important for the proper functioning of muscles, including the heart. Potassium is a crucial regulator of the amount of water in cells, which determines their ability to function properly. It helps in the transmission of nerve impulses, is a buffer for body fluids, and catalyzes the release of energy from carbohydrates, proteins, and fats. Potassium may also help prevent high blood pressure. [18]

Thiazide diuretics can also adversely affect the metabolism in other ways. They can cause elevations of blood sugar levels and uric acid levels, thus causing or exacerbating diabetes and gout. [19], [20] Thiazides also raise cholesterol and triglyceride levels thus increasing the risk for heart disease, and hence high blood pressure. [21] In the long term the very drugs used to lower blood pressure, become key factors in creating high blood pressure. Thus the patient is on drug support for life and the physician's retirement plan is guaranteed. But this is blood money, for diuretics can cause biochemical derangements that result in weakness, confusion, palpitations and dangerous arrhythmias, even doubling the rate of sudden death. [22] Researchers are coming to the conclusion that diuretics may be the reason for the high mortality rate for people treated with these drugs. Dr. Kaplan noted the effect of diuretics on the coronary arteries of the heart in his textbook, *Heart Disease: A Textbook of Cardiovascular Medicine:*

> [T]he presence of diuretic-induced biochemical derangements has been offered as a potential explanation of the lack of coronary protection. [23]

Besides their dangerous side effects, diuretics often *fail* to reduce blood pressure. Dr. Jan Drayen of the University of California at Irvine College of Medicine stated that many patients were *non-responders* to diuretics. That is a polite way of saying that the drug failed to reduce the blood pressure, even increasing it in some cases. [24] Fifty percent of fifty patients in one of his studies were classed as non-responders. [25]

Dr. Neil Nedley also observed that treating high blood pressure with drugs is a failure and even dangerous. While this practice may have been excusable many years ago, he contended that our knowledge of the side effects of these drugs compels us to alter course.

> A common answer [for hypertension] would be to take medication prescribed by a doctor. Not many years ago, this seemed to be the only answer. We now know that this is usually not the best answer. There are several reasons for this:
>
> 1. Every drug has multiple potential side effects—including effects on quality of life that often go unnoticed by the mediation user.
>
> 2. High blood pressure, even if controlled by medication (and not lifestyle), causes a slow deterioration of brain matter which weakens the patient's ability and intelligence. Uncontrolled high blood pressure causes the same problems.
>
> 3. Less than half of those who take drugs lower their pressure below 140/90.
>
> 4. The cost of the drugs.
>
> 5. Lowering blood pressure with medication is not equivalent to lowering blood pressure naturally. [26]

In his assessment the treatment appears to be worse than the disease! Moreover the medication may exacerbate the disease, requiring more treatment in an endless cycle with no one benefitting but the doctor and the drug companies. While diuretics may lower blood pressure by increasing sodium excretion, the body often counters this action by increasing the production of the enzyme renin and the hormone aldosterone, which decrease sodium loss. The result is increased blood pressure. [27] Dr. Nedley reported that people taking antihypertensive drugs have *higher* rates of heart disease than people who have identical blood pressure without medication. [28] Ladies and gentlemen, Dr. Whitaker is emphatic that diuretics present *a clear and present danger* for those taking them. [29]

Ladies and gentlemen of the jury, it is high time that we the people take appropriate steps to stop this medical malpractice being practiced upon us by conventional rationalistic medicine. One day the public will wake up. It is now your duty as a national jury to arouse them to their predicament. Then there will be a very high price to pay for the years of abuse and exploitation we have been subjected to by the medical Cartel.

The more recent drugs used to combat high blood pressure include beta-receptor blockers, calcium channel blockers and angiotensin-converting enzyme inhibitors (ACE inhibitors). [30] Dr. Walker stated that it was the concern about the harmful side effects of diuretics that prompted the Joint National Committee on Detection, Evaluation and Treatment of High Blood Pressure to propose beta-blockers as the first step in hypertensive treatment. [31] But the new treatment became just as harmful or even worse. Beta-blockers block the effects of adrenaline on certain beta-receptor cells found in the heart, lungs, blood vessels and other tissues. The theory behind beta-blockers is that when a person is under stress the nervous system releases excess adrenaline which binds to the receptors in the heart and causes the heart to pump blood with greater force, thus raising the blood pressure. Beta-blockers prevent this natural physical reaction from occurring, thereby *theoretically* keeping the heart rate down and the blood pressure down. [32]

But, ladies and gentlemen of the jury, the evidence shows that interfering with this natural process can have *disastrous consequences* that far outweigh the transient gain beta-blockers may provide. Here is the problem created by beta-blockers: beta-receptors in the arteries cause the arteries to expand to allow more blood to flow to the heart and other tissues; at the same time beta receptors in the lungs simultaneously open air passages and allow more oxygen to pass to tissues. [33] Because beta-blockers block this sequence of physical reactions, people taking them often complain of chronic fatigue and feelings of weakness and exhaustion, especially during excitement and exercise. [34] Essentially, they are being starved of oxygen. But that is not all!

Dr. Nedley reported that beta-blockers such as Propranolol can reduce the hormone melatonin in the body. [35] This exposes the patient to some awful risks, for melatonin is a natural antioxidant which reduces the very toxic hydroxyl radical, and can protect us from certain carcinogens, herbicides and radiation [36] Decreasing the level of melatonin can also adversely affect the immune system for melatonin helps the body to produce white blood helper T cells. [37] Calcium channel blockers have the same adverse affect on melatonin levels. [38]

Other side effects of beta-blockers include dizziness, diarrhea, constipation, hallucinations and Raynaud's phenomenon (cold hands and feet). [39] Beta-blockers also decrease good HDL cholesterol, elevate blood triglyceride levels, sugar levels and can worsen asthma. [40] Heart function can become so depressed with beta-blockers that the blood can back up in the lungs causing the person to drown in their own blood. [41] Beta-blockers can weaken the heart and induce heart attacks in people at risk. [42] Ladies and gentlemen it is a perilous thing to interfere with the delicate chemical and metabolic processes of the body in an attempt to manage the symptoms of disease! The chemical processes of the body are so intricately interrelated that attempts to micromanage it can result in upsetting the delicate balance with disastrous consequences. Introducing drugs such as these into the delicately balanced chemical machinery of the body is, in many respects, much the same as introducing a virus into a finely tuned computer; one or more systems may malfunction (disease is initiated) or the system may crash (death ensures). But this disruption of the body's chemical and physiological processes is exactly what keeps the drug companies rich, for they have a drug for every side effect they induce!

Let us look at the testimony regarding calcium channel blockers. Their function is to prevent the uptake of calcium along electromagnetic channels within the cell. The diminution of calcium in the cells of the blood vessels prevents them from constricting. [43] When blood vessels constrict, blood pressure is raised. When they dilate blood pressure is lowered. But is this form of treatment worth the risks? Dr. McDougall stated that the list of side effects of calcium channel blockers is daunting: gastrointestinal disorders, excess potassium in the blood, headaches, edema, liver dysfunction, flushing, constipation and heart block, a disorder in which the coordination between the atrium and ventricle is disrupted! [44]

To reduce blood pressure, drug companies have introduced the drug know as ACE (angiotensin-converting enzyme) inhibitors in an endeavor to prevent the blood vessels from constricting. The blood vessels are dilated and this lowers the blood pressure. [45] But again the list of side effects are not inviting, they include: cough, shortness of breath, hypotension, dizziness, diarrhea, angioedema in which the face, tongue and airways swell, headache, vomiting, skin rashes, loss of taste and kidney failure, which can result in the condition treated: high blood pressure! [46] Patients using ACE inhibitors can experience sudden cardiac death if they use certain potassium-salt substitutes. [47] ACE inhibitors can also degrade the immune system by depressing the white blood count. [48]

Section 3

NUTRITIONAL CURES: DEFLATING HIGH BLOOD PRESSURE

Ladies and gentlemen of the jury, it is obvious to all but the medical profession and drug companies that a less life-threatening approach should be used in treating high blood pressure. Copious amounts of research reveal that when you remove the dietary and lifestyle causes of high blood pressure, the patient gets better. Dr. John McDougall cited a 1986 British study that divided fifty-eight people with mild hypertension into two groups. One group was placed on a lacto-ovo-vegetarian diet and the other on a meat diet. Those on the vegetarian diet showed a 5 mm Hg drop in their diastolic pressure. The researchers concluded:

> On treating subjects with mild hypertension, changing to a vegetarian diet may bring about a worthwhile fall in diastolic blood pressure. [1]

Although a lacto-ovo-vegetarian diet (a vegetarian diet that diet includes milk and eggs) has plenty of cholesterol, fat and sodium, it has less of these ingredients than a diet that includes meat, hence the significant improvement in blood pressure. The evidence shows that a pure vegetarian, one excluding eggs, milk, and cheese, diet would have shown greater improvement in blood pressure. A lacto-ovo-vegetarian diet may reduce some chronic degenerative disease, but may not prevent others.

When British researches treated people with either a low fat diet, a low sodium diet, a high fiber diet or all three combined, they found that none of the individual approaches worked as well as all three combined.

[2] This revealed the multifaceted cause of high blood pressure; hence, the cure must also be multifaceted.

Ladies and gentlemen of the jury, the evidence is clear and forceful, yet very simple to understand—to reduce high blood pressure, we must simply reverse its causes. It is that simple. Let us look at each of these causes and consider the effect on blood pressure as the causes are reversed. Researchers have found that weight loss is one of the most powerful treatments for reducing high blood pressure. Numerous studies show that weight loss by itself reduces blood pressure and allow people to go off medication. [3] The *Archives of Internal Medicine* published a study in which persons who had lost ten pounds during a six-month period reduced their diastolic blood pressure by 11.6 mm Hg. [4] The researchers concluded that effective weight loss that was ten pounds and greater lowered blood pressure as effectively as low dose drug therapy. [5]

Dr. Neil Nedley stated that the news for those who are overweight and have high blood pressure is even better. You do not have to reach your ideal weight to eliminate the high blood pressure. He stated that just *initiating* the weight loss program and shedding as little as five pounds will substantially reduce your high blood pressure. [6] Of course, to continue the steady downward trend of the blood pressure, the weight loss program must continue until your ideal weight is reached. [7] But since excess weight is just one (though major) factor in high blood pressure, other lifestyle changes must be adopted. Researchers have found that weight loss combined with other modalities can be even more effective. A study in the *Journal of the American Medical Association* found that combining weight loss with sodium restriction was more effective in reducing high blood pressure than weight loss alone. [8] The study also demonstrated that weight loss with sodium restriction was more effective than stress management alone or nutritional supplements alone. [9]

Dr. Neil Nedley placed salt very high up on the list of causes, if not the major cause of high blood pressure, and reported impressive reductions in blood pressure by reducing sodium salt content. He reported that twenty patients with an average blood pressure of 161/101 mm were placed on a moderately reduced salt diet of less than 3,000 mg/day. After one year their average systolic pressure was lowered by 19 points and diastolic pressure was lowered by 14 points. [10] The blood pressure of sixteen of these twenty patients was controlled by simply reducing their salt intake. [11] What is the necessary minimum salt intake for human beings? Dr. Nedley believes it is 250 mg/day; but the average American takes in 4,000 mg/day! [12]

An interesting question is, which element is the active ingredient in sodium chloride salt? Is it the sodium or the chloride? The answer may surprise you. The evidence shows that it is neither. [13] Dr. Nedley reported that it is the combination of sodium with chloride that does the damage. In animal studies neither excess sodium alone nor chlorine alone caused an elevation in blood pressure. [14]

Moderate aerobic exercise that involves the heart and the lungs is another effective modality for lowering blood pressure. [15] The moderate exercise must involve at least a brisk thirty-minute walk three or four times a day or its equivalent. [16] When exercise is combined with weight loss and sodium restriction, the improvement in blood pressure is even more impressive. [17] Dr. John McDougall observed that in study after study, exercise alone or in combination with salt restriction and weight reduction effectively lowered blood pressure and eliminated the need for medication. [18] Scientists studied the effects of weight loss, exercise and sodium restriction in people between the ages of 65 and 80 and found that patients with mild hypertension could eliminate their blood pressure medication altogether. [19] Of course people with high blood pressure should always start an exercise program with the knowledge of and supervision of their physicians.

Since caffeine has been found to raise blood pressure—one cup a day has been shown to raise the systolic pressure by 5 to 6 points—Dr. Nedley recommended that caffeine intake be reduced or stopped. [20] He stated that one ounce of alcohol has been show to raise blood pressure significantly. He therefore recommended that the use of alcohol be eliminated in a program for reducing high blood pressure. [21] Smoking is another bad habit that causes high blood pressure. Just one cigarette can raise the systolic pressure by 10 mm of mercury for 30 minutes or more. [22] Of course one cigarette alone will not permanently raise blood pressure, but many smokers have a series of cigarettes that result in a sustained elevated blood pressure. [23] Since all of these chronic degenerative diseases have common lifestyle causes, it is not surprising that the same lifestyle change impacts a variety of degenerative diseases. The program advocated by Dr. John McDougall for achieving a healthy heart and maximum weight reduction has been found to help 90% of hypertensive patients discontinue their medications and improve their overall health and vitality. [24]

Dr. F. Batmanghelidj maintained that the evidence is overwhelming that one of the most effective cures of high blood pressure is simply drinking more water. Because a primary cause of high blood pressure is the shutting down of capillary beds due to dehydration of the body, he felt that the remedy must be re-hydration which will re-open closed capillary beds and so reduce the pressure required to pump blood through the circulatory system. [25] He stated that the symptomatic treatment of high blood pressure with diuretics by pharmaceutical medicine borders on absurdity.

> Essential hypertension should primarily be treated with an increase in daily water intake. The present way of treating hypertension is wrong to the point of scientific absurdity. The body is trying to retain its water volume, and we say to the design of nature in us: "No, you do not understand—you must take diuretics and get rid of water!" [26]

Dr. Batmanghelidj stated that water is the best diuretic. This seems like a paradox, but understanding how the body functions resolves the mystery. He argued that if people with high blood pressure increased their daily water intake, they would not need to take any diuretics. [27] He cautioned that the patient with heart failure complications should remain under a physician's guidance to make sure water intake is increased gradually to avoid excessive fluid collection in the body. [28] Drinking more water flushes excess sodium salt out of the body, reducing another cause of water retention and high blood pressure. He stated that the retention of sodium in the body is a defensive mechanism of the body to retain more water. [29]

Dr. Lynne Paige Walker agreed with Dr. Batmanghelidj that lack of adequate hydration of the body is one of the primary causes of high blood pressure, and hence the *re-hydration* of the body is a reliable path to the reversal of high blood pressure. [30] Dr. Walker reported on patients that refused medication and simply drank more water and achieved blood pressure levels within safe and normal limits. [31] She noted that those patients who began a regime of increased water intake dispensed with all hypertensive medications. [32]

What is the primary cause of high blood pressure? Obesity? Too much salt in the diet? Dehydration? Dr. Walker stated that modern medicine simply does not know. Thus they call hypertension that is unlinked to known chronic degenerative diseases, essential hypertension. [33] [34] A recent massive study called INTERSALT appears to reveal that salt is not the prime culprit. [35] This led Drs. Walker and Batmanghelidj to say that the importance of drinking adequate amounts of pure water cannot be over emphasized. While proper nutrition is a key factor in preventing and curing chronic degenerative diseases, Dr. Batmanghelidj argued that water is of primary importance. Ranked in order of importance, Dr. Batmanghelidj would put water above nutrition, for without adequate water the body cannot adequately use its nutrients.

But water is not the silver-bullet cure for high blood pressure, for adequate water is part of proper nutrition. While nutrients provide the materials of repair for the body, water provides the *energy and materials* to effectuate the repair mechanism of the body, a mechanism that is itself water based. Both Drs. Batmanghelidj and Walker noted that clinical research on the importance of water in preventing and curing degenerative diseases, revealed the utter bankruptcy and absurdity of modern pharmaceutical medicine. [36]

Dr. Walker pointed out that high blood pressure can have many specific causes, such as too much refined sugar or salt which both clog the arteries thus increasing the pressure needed to pump blood though narrow arteries. [37] These abuses can lead to the one of two primary reasons for high blood pressure: a recognized chronic degenerative disease such as diabetes or clogging of the arteries. [38] But simply reversing these specific causes can remove the harm and lower the blood pressure. [39] Similarly deficiencies in calcium, magnesium and potassium have also been linked to increased blood pressures, supplying these with fresh fruit or supplements can reverse the condition. [40]

But Dr. Walker emphasized that a well balanced whole-foods diet, which includes adequate water intake, is simply the best overall approach to the problem of high blood pressure, for it does not depend upon diagnosing the exact cause in each individual. Nature's pharmacy simply goes to work and supplies everything the body requires. She stated that this was born out in a 1997 landmark study reported in the *New England Journal of Medicine*, which found that high blood pressure can be lowered by diet without the side effects of drugs. [41] Dr. Walker stated that "the study was hailed as demonstrating the most significant improvement in life expectancy of any dietary intervention to date." [42] Thus, ladies and gentlemen of the jury, it should be medical malpractice to treat the symptoms of thirst and the consequences of dehydration and poor diet with pharmaceutical poisons that compound the problem and do irreparable harm as well.

Osteoporosis

A Raging Epidemic

A BONE TO PICK WITH THE DAIRY INDUSTRY

Ladies and gentlemen of the jury, osteoporosis is a disease of the skeleton frame that has reached epidemic proportions in America. [1] More than 44 million people in the United States are affected in various stages by this disease; 10 million individuals have the disease and 34 million have low bone density, indicating that the disease process has long since commenced, thus placing them at risk for the full blown disease. [2] It is one of the most common bone diseases of Western societies. [3] This epidemic is causing a colossal drain in scarce financial resources. As of 1985 America was spending 4 billion dollars a year in the diagnosis and care of osteoporosis. [4] Bone loss causes an estimated 1.3 million fractures annually in the United States. [5] Dr. Neil Nedley reported that 70% of all fractures in Americans over forty-five years of age are due to osteoporosis. [6] The cost of caring for osteoporosis related hip fractures alone was over $10 billion dollars in 1998. [7] The National Osteoporosis Foundation, previously cited, placed the cost of all osteoporosis-related fractures at $19 billion in 2005 and by 2025 it expects the cost to rise to 25.3 billion.

Osteoporosis literally means porous bones. The disease of osteoporosis is characterized by loss of bone mineral, especially calcium and magnesium, which leaves the bone porous, fragile and weak. [8] In the spine it manifests in a crumbling of the body posture as the weakened vertebrae fail to support the weight of the upper body. We are all familiar with the stooped posture of the elderly. This forward stoop places pressure on internal organs, impairing their function. [9] The more bone material that is lost from the skeleton frame the greater the risk of fracture. Not surprisingly, fractures of the hips, backbone and wrists are common in people suffering from osteoporosis. [10] Porous bones can become so weak that a mere cough can break a rib. Riding over bumpy roads can fracture a backbone, and the weight of a woman's body can cause her hip to fracture. [11] Because of this epidemic of osteoporosis, one third of all American women, and one sixth of all American men will fracture their hips in their lifetime. [12] Between 12 and 20% of those who fracture their hips will die, and 50% will lose the ability to live independently. [13]

But osteoporosis is not just a disease of the elderly. Women are most often affected by this disease due to a decrease in estrogen production in post-menopausal life. One in four post-menopausal women suffers from osteoporosis. [14] Over 25% of sixty-five-year-old women in America have lost over 50% of their bone density. [15] In women over sixty-five years of age, about 40% have suffered from one or more osteoporosis-related fractures. [16] Since 1985, 15,000 women were dying each year from osteoporosis. [17] The evidence is grimmer yet. By 1987 osteoporosis was responsible for more deaths in women than cancer of the breast and cervix combined! [18] Of course the situation is much worse today. Dr. Nedley reported that presently one in three women in the world over fifty have osteoporosis. [19] Dr. Walker noted that as of 1998, 60,000 women were dying within six months of sustaining osteoporosis fractures. [20]

But ladies and gentlemen the evidence is overwhelming that the disease of osteoporosis does not only affect women. Osteoporosis is not a disease of menopause. The latter condition may be a risk factor, but it is not a cause. There are many countries in the world where osteoporosis is rare among women as well as men. Osteoporosis is virtually unknown in the African Bantu women. [21] However, when they immigrate to America and follow the Western diet, they sustain the disease as much as other women in America. [22] Whereas in America, the disease affects women in their fifties and sixties, it begins to manifest itself in men only after age seventy-five. [23] Men do not pass through a period of rapid decrease in reproductive hormones so they are more shielded from this disease than women. Also the greater physical activity of men may protect them against bone loss until activity declines with advancing age. [24]

Some experts have tried to shift the responsibility for osteoporosis to heredity. However, Dr. John McDougall correctly pointed out that the fact that Bantu women in Africa do not get osteoporosis but American Bantu women do, rules out heredity as a causative factor. [25] It also rules out calcium deficiency in the American diet as a causative factor. These Bantu women get only 240 to 450 milligrams of calcium a day from their diet of grains, fruits and vegetables. This is about one third of the calcium intake of America women. [26] Bantu women typically bear ten children and wean them at ten months; despite this drain in their calcium resources, they do not get osteoporosis. So what is there about the American diet and lifestyle that has caused an epidemic of osteoporosis?

Dr. Julian Whitaker stated that the high protein character of the meat-based diet of Americans is the most significant cause of the loss of bone minerals such as calcium and magnesium. [27] Dr. Neil Nedley agreed that excessive dietary protein is the chief villain. [28] Because of the misleading propaganda from the meat and dairy industries regarding the need for protein in our diet, America has gone overboard on protein. Let us therefore notice what levels of protein is adequate or excessive in one's diet. Dr. John McDougall contends that 20 grams of protein a day is adequate to support an adult's protein needs. [29] When dietary protein exceeds 47 to 50 grams a day, a negative calcium balance is created in the body. The body is losing more calcium that it is absorbing. [30] The typical American diet includes an astonishing 150 grams of protein per day and this excessive protein creates a continuous drain of body calcium. [31] Americans are eating way too much protein, and it is resulting in not only in osteoporosis but a host of other degenerative diseases.

How does excess protein cause bone mineral loss? Unlike its ability to store fats and carbohydrates, the body has no mechanism for storing excess protein. The excess protein must be broken down and eliminated from the body. Some of the protein break-down products are nitrogen urea, uric acid, sulphur, phosphorus and creatinine. These products produce an acid condition in the blood. An acidic condition in the body is lethal to our health, so the body proceeds to neutralize the excessive acid by drawing on the calcium already in the blood. [32] This depletes the blood calcium levels, and so the body proceeds to draw calcium from the bones to replace the calcium lost from the blood. While calcium is drawn from other body tissues, the bones serve as the main calcium bank. [33] The blood level of calcium takes precedence over the bone level of calcium because the blood calcium is needed for vital functions such as controlling muscular contractions, including the heart muscle, for blood clotting, transmission of nerve impulses and other essential functions. So when the blood calcium levels fall, the body draws from its store of calcium in the bones. [34]

The calcium drawn from the bones is excreted through the kidneys into the urine. This loss of calcium is not compensated for by the absorption of calcium from the diet through the intestines. The net result is that more calcium is lost through the urine than is absorbed by the body. This creates a negative calcium balance in the body. [35] To repeat, the body breaks down protein into amino acids which pass through the intestinal wall into the blood stream. Excess amino acids not utilized by the body are metabolized in the liver into urea, a powerful diuretic, which washes out a lot of minerals from the body. [36]

Excess dietary protein causes calcium loss through other pathways. Proteins are weakly acidic themselves. These weak protein acids, along with the amino acids that they are broken down into, enter the blood stream, creating an acidic condition of the blood. To neutralize this acidic condition in the blood, the body dissolves bone material in order to release phosphorus and calcium into the blood. The alkaline phosphorus neutralizes the acidic proteins and amino acids and the calcium ions associated with the phosphorus are set free and are then excreted by the kidneys. [37] Excess protein also directly interferes with the kidney's ability to absorb calcium into the body. Proteins are made up of combinations of over twenty different amino acids. Some of these amino acids have an adverse affect on the tubules of the kidneys, thereby preventing the reabsorption of calcium that enters these tubules. [38]

Ladies and gentlemen of the jury, the evidence is very clear that the proteins obtained from meat, and not those obtained from vegetables are the main problem. Amino acids are normally composed of carbon, hydrogen, oxygen and nitrogen. Three of the twenty amino acids also incorporate sulphur in their structures. It appears that animal proteins have a higher content of these sulphur containing amino acids, such as the amino acid methionine, than plant proteins. [39] Meat contains five times the amount of methionine than beans and twice as much as in grains. It is these sulphur-based amino acids that are responsible for much of the adverse effects of protein from a meat-based diet. [40] Dr. Neil Nedley also agreed that it is the acidic effect of these sulphur containing amino acids that is responsible for bone loss. [41]

The link between high animal protein intake and osteoporosis is supported by other epidemiological evidence. The Eskimos eat large quantities of meat from fish, walruses, seals and whales. Because of their arctic habitat they get very little vegetables and fruit. Their meat diet provides

200 to 400 grams of protein daily. What effect does this large protein intake have upon their skeleton frame? Both Eskimo men and women show substantial loss of bone material. Eskimos over the age of 40 have an average of 10 to 15% less bone than Caucasians in America. [42] The bones of Eskimo women are on average ten years older than the bones of the American woman of the same age. Dr. McDougall stated that it is remarkable that the Eskimos are very active physically, yet show so much bone loss. [43] This can be only accounted for by their high protein diet.

Dr. Nancy Appleton emphasized the prominent role refined sugar plays in the onset of osteoporosis and other degenerative diseases. The acidic condition created by the ingestion of excess refined sugar causes a fall in blood calcium levels and this leads to a variety of health problems besides osteoporosis. [44] Although the symptoms of calcium deficiency vary from person to person, these symptoms can include heart palpitations, insomnia, nervousness, arm and leg numbness, rheumatism, arthritis, menstrual cramps, premenstrual cramps, menopausal problems, nervousness, finger tremors, backaches, bone pain and plaque on the teeth. [45]

For years the researches funded by the National Livestock and Meat association and the National Dairy Council have maintained that meat and dairy do not cause calcium loss because meat also contains high phosphorous levels. These so-called research findings are biased and are in clear conflict with the evidence. Dr. McDougall stated that in most independent experiments a meat-based diet has been shown to produce a negative calcium balance in the diet. [46] Other studies have shown that there is an increase of 23% or more in calcium excretion when tuna and other meats are added to the diet. [47] Another experiment specifically designed to demonstrate the effects of phosphorus on calcium metabolism in humans showed a 28% increase in calcium loss when a low protein intake was raised to a high protein intake, while maintaining high levels of phosphorus. [48]

Ladies and gentlemen of the jury, let us more fully explore evidence relating to the second major cause of calcium loss in the tissues and bones: refined sugar. [49] The same effect is caused by refined white rice and bread, from which all of the food value is stripped. The American diet matches gram for gram its protein and sugar intake. Yet the average American is ignorant of the fact that both excess sugar and animal protein promote the secretion of calcium from the body. [50] Because the effects of refined sugar on the body is manifested after decades of using it, people do not readily see the connection between sugar and disease. Nevertheless, nutritionists like Dr. Nancy Appleton have argued that sugar is the main dietary culprit in precipitating a host of degenerative diseases, including osteoporosis. [51]

The metabolism of refined sugar and other refined foods create an acidic condition in the body and various minerals are drawn from the bones and tissue to neutralize these acids. Minerals are absolutely important to many bodily functions. Besides giving rigidity to the bones and teeth, minerals serve other vital functions. They are essential in activating enzymes that regulate important metabolic functions. Minerals determine the balance between acidity and alkalinity in the blood. [52] Minerals also take part in the transmission of nerve impulses. [43] By depleting the body's mineral content sugar unbalances the body chemistry, thereby interfering with the internal functioning of the body. [54] *Sugar so unbalances the body chemistry that even nutritious foods cannot provide the nutrition they otherwise would.* [55] Enzymes, which are absolutely dependent upon minerals to function, cannot assist in the digestion of the food we ingest if we deplete the mineral content of the body.

Sugar intake depletes calcium, as well as phosphorus, the very minerals which are essential for making strong bones. [56] When sugar is eaten, the blood calcium temporarily goes up as a result of the flow of calcium from the other tissues; but at the same time its rate of excretion also goes up. [57] When the excretion of calcium continues unabated, the blood level of calcium eventually falls. This causes the parathyroid hormone to be released, which breaks down more bone material in an effort to restore the level of calcium in the blood. [58] Eventually the calcium depletion of the bones makes them fragile and osteoporotic.

How much refined sugar is harmful? Dr. Nancy Appleton stated that as little as two teaspoons of sugar can change the mineral rations in the body. [59] Since minerals work only in relationship to each other, (a process called synergy), disturbing the mineral ratio can have a damaging effect on the body. Refined sugar disturbs the relationship between calcium and phosphorus, which are two of the most important minerals in the body. [60] The body's ability to absorb and utilize calcium directly depends on the amount of phosphorus available in the diet. [61] The normal ratio of calcium to phosphorus is 10 units of calcium to 4 units of phosphorus. [62] Since calcium works synergistically with phosphorus, decreasing the phosphorus level decreases the amount of functioning calcium. If there are only 2 units of phosphorus in the body chemistry then only 5 units of calcium will function.

Ladies and gentlemen, please note carefully that Dr. Appleton contends that if only 5 units of calcium are functioning, then the other 5 units will be *toxic* to the body. [63] Toxic, non-functioning calcium can cause kidney stones, arthritis, hardening of the arteries, cataracts and plaque on the teeth. [64] Toxic calcium also leads to osteoporosis by a pathway now familiar to us: The ingestion of refined sugar lowers the phosphorus in the blood thereby decreasing the amount of usable calcium in the body; because the disassociated calcium can be toxic, the body attempts to eliminate it through the urine, thereby creating a negative calcium balance in the body. [65] Bones become weak not only from a loss of calcium. Whenever calcium is drained from the bones, it is also pulled across the cell membrane, pulling protein molecules along with it. The loss of both calcium and protein from the bone undermines its structural integrity. [66]

Refined sugar is of course not the only acid forming food. Meat, eggs and fish are the most acid forming of foods. [67] Combining excess use of refined sugar with a meat diet is doubly harmful and precipitates degenerative diseases with greater certainty. Osteoporosis is essentially a result of a defensive mechanism of the body to remain healthy. If our blood becomes too acidic, we would die, so in defense of itself, the body draws calcium from the bones to neutralize the acid and restore the pH balance. [68] Unlike meat and dairy foods, most fruits and vegetables generally leave an alkaline ash. So ingesting these foods do not require the body to deplete calcium in order to maintain the neutrality of the blood. John Robbins cited the alkaline quality of fruits and vegetables as one reason why vegetarians are relatively immune from osteoporosis. [69]

To confirm that a negative calcium balance can occur in the presence of high levels of phosphorus, researchers in one experiment raised the phosphorus intake of a group of women to 1400 mg while keeping the calcium intake stable. The researchers found that all the women in the study experienced a negative calcium balance. [70] The key factor was found to be the calcium/phosphorus ratio. The lower the ration, the greater the bone calcium loss. The higher the ration the less bone loss takes place and the stronger the skeleton becomes. [71] In contrast to animal foods, the calcium in vegetables, greens and fruits exists in a higher calcium / phosphorus ration and therefore the calcium is much more available to the body than the calcium in animal products such as milk and cheese. [72] Carbonated soda drinks with their high sugar and phosphorus content similarly creates a negative calcium balance and corresponding bone loss. [73]

Dr. Julian Whitaker stated that stimulants such as caffeine and nicotine and their depressant cousin, alcohol, also deplete calcium from the bones and leads to osteoporosis. [74] Dr. Nancy Appleton pointed out that just three cups of caffeinated coffee can cause the excretion of as much as forty-five milligrams of calcium. [75] Do not be fooled by the sales gimmick of the soft drink peddlers, who entice you to continue to use their products by advertizing *sugar free* and *caffeine free* on their labels. Soft drinks may be sugar free and caffeine free, but nevertheless they still contain phosphoric acid which invariably disrupts the calcium/phosphorus ration and causes calcium loss from the bones. [76]

Ladies and gentlemen, a myriad of poor dietary and lifestyle habits lead to osteoporosis. Many studies have shown the link between cigarette smoking and bone loss. Three quarters of the women who develop osteoporosis are or have been smokers. [77] Excess sodium in the diet also causes loss of calcium in the urine, thereby contributing to osteoporosis. [78] Certain medications can contribute to bone calcium loss and hence osteoporosis. These medications include the blood thinner Heparin, all diuretics, aluminum-containing antacids, convulsant medications, corticosteroids used over long periods, and large doses of the thyroid hormone. [79]

Ladies and gentlemen of the jury, now that we have examined the causes of osteoporosis, let us turn to the treatment of this disease. Once again, we will see that nutritional modalities are shunted aside by the medical, pharmaceutical and animal products industries. In failing to educate the American public as to the true causes of osteoporosis, the medical profession must be held accountable for the untold suffering and death of millions of people from this wide spread and disabling but preventable disease.

GOT MILK? A TREATMENT THAT COMPOUNDS THE PROBLEM

Ladies and gentlemen of the jury, you have seen that the evidence is very clear that the immediate cause of osteoporosis is the loss of calcium and phosphorous and other minerals from the bones. We have also seen that the cause of bone demineralization is excess dietary animal protein, other animal products with acidic residues, refined sugar and refined foods, drinks containing caffeine and phosphoric acid, nicotine, and alcohol. Coupled with inactivity, these are all lifestyle and dietary choices. In light of these facts what is the best course of treatment for the disease of osteoporosis? As usual there are two approaches.

1. Treatment of the symptom.

2. Reversal of the causes by eliminating both the symptoms and disease.

The correct approach may seem logical to a dispassionate observer: simply avoid doing the things that produce the disease. But incredible as it may seem, the medical profession, backed by the National Livestock and Meat Board and the National Dairy Council, totally ignore the causes of osteoporosis and opt for treating the symptom of osteoporosis: lack of calcium in the bones. The evidence will show that in so doing, they inadvertently help to perpetuate a gigantic fraud upon the American people, to the detriment of their health and in many cases, their lives.

The national Dairy Council is the foremost spokesman for the erroneous view that bones lose calcium only if there is not enough calcium in our diets. This position is directly related to the sale of their products. Predictably, the solution they propose is to drink more milk. [1] Profits, not your health, is the motivating factor. There are several obvious problems with this approach. Calcium is not the central issue. An epidemiological study by the eminent Dr. D. M. Hegstead found that *osteoporosis is higher in countries that consume higher amounts of calcium!* [2] This seems like a paradox until you examine the food context in which the calcium is consumed—animal products. Because of the presence of large amounts of animal protein, the calcium in the food is unavailable to the body. [3] We have reviewed evidence that Eskimos have the highest calcium intake, 2,500 mg daily, but because they get it in the form of fish the high protein content makes it unavailable to the body. The result is that Eskimos have 10 to 15 times more osteoporosis that white Americans of the same age. [4] Dr. Neil Nedley concluded:

> These studies and others like them indicate that osteoporosis, contrary to popular opinion, is not related to a *lack of calcium in the diet*. The bigger problem seems to be excessive calcium losses as a result of *consuming too much protein*. We would not expect the American dairy industry to advertise this. After all, they have worked for years to convince us that drinking more milk and eating more cheese and yogurt would help us prevent osteoporosis.

> The fact is this: if your diet is high in protein, you can eat all the calcium that the dairy association has to offer and you are still likely to increase your risk of thinning your bones and perhaps facing a hip fracture later in life. *Excess protein leads to decrease of calcium even when calcium intake is liberal.* [5] [Emphasis added.]

Ladies and gentlemen of the jury, study well this testimony from Dr. Neil Nedley. Your health and that of America which you hold in your hands, depends upon correctly understanding this salient fact: *Excess protein leads to decrease of calcium even when calcium intake is liberal.*

Dr. Julian Whitaker was therefore correct when he stated that calcium deficiency and bone loss are merely *symptoms* of a larger dietary problem. [6] Treating the symptoms will *not* remove the causes. Dr. Whitaker also contended that the focus on calcium reflects conventional medicine's single-agent approach, carried over into the area of natural therapies. Instead of a drug, doctors want to prescribe a single vitamin or mineral. This approach he stated misses the point. The leading dietary player in the drama of osteoporosis is not calcium but the *entire unbalanced and improper diet with its excesses,* Dr. Whitaker emphasized. [7]

Simply adding calcium to a high animal product diet has been shown to be ineffective in preventing bone loss. There is plenty of scientific evidence to support this position. A study published in the *British Medical Journal* in 1984 suggested that calcium intake is, in fact, completely irrelevant to bone loss. In that study a number of post-menopausal women were divided into three groups.

* One group consumed 550 mg of calcium;

* Another group between 550 and 1100 mg of calcium;

* And the third group in excess of 1100 mg of calcium daily.

Ladies and gentlemen the results were unsettling. At the end of two years there was no difference in bone demineralization among the three groups! To the surprise of everyone, except of course the nutritional doctors, the bone loss was exactly the same as that found in women taking no calcium supplements at all in their diets. [8]

The solution chosen by the Dairy Industry—increased milk intake—actually aggravates the problem. John Robbins has pointed out that the National Dairy Council has spent tens of millions of dollars to make us think that osteoporosis can be prevented by drinking more milk and eating more dairy products. [9] But the evidence suggests otherwise. World Health Statistics show that osteoporosis is more common in exactly those countries where dairy products are consumed in the largest quantities: the United States, Finland, Sweden and the United Kingdom. [10] Dr. John McDougall observed that these countries also have the highest rates of osteoporosis-related hip fractures compared to countries with the lowest intake of dairy. [11]

In a study sponsored by the Dairy Council, women were given an extra three eight-ounce glass of low fat milk every day for a year, yet they showed no significant increase in calcium balance. [12] The conclusion drawn by the researchers was that the extra 30% increase in protein intake during the milk supplementation caused a negative calcium balance and hence bone loss. [13] Dr. John McDougall stated in 1985 that the recommendation of the National Institutes of Health that women supplement with 100 to 1500 mg of calcium daily did not help the women—it helped only the manufacturers and distributors of calcium supplements who have made millions. [14]

Ladies and gentlemen of the jury, once again the evidence is overwhelming—treating the symptoms of a disease is *big business*. And when that symptomatic approach is inefficacious, it is up to you as a national jury to label it as *big fraud*. When it is aided and abetted by the medical profession, it is gross medical malpractice and should be so recognized by the courts. Both the medical profession and the meat and dairy industries should be held responsible for the colossal drain of our financial resources in treating this most preventable disease. This is your task. Will you shrink from it, or stand up and be counted?

Dr. John McDougall noted that these recommendations for additional calcium are based on conflicting studies. In most published studies about calcium, the correlation between dietary calcium intake and bone density has been weak or non-existent. The bottom line is that people who consume more calcium in their diets have not been found to develop stronger bones than people who have low-calcium diets. [15] Despite the propaganda of the milk peddlers, studies show that an intake of 150 to 200 mg of calcium is adequate to meet the needs of most normal people, even during pregnancy and lactation. [16] Most of the world population ingest between 300 to 500 mg of calcium which is much less than the 800 mg being recommended in the United States, and our incidence of osteoporosis is higher than in these undeveloped countries. [17]

Until recently the only FDA approved drug for osteoporosis was estrogen therapy. [18] Dr. C. Christensen of Golstrup Hospital in Denmark did a study involving forty-three women who were post-menopausal. They were placed on 2000 mg of calcium daily, a daily estrogen replacement regime, or a placebo for two years. He found that the calcium did no more than the placebo to retard bone loss, while the estrogen group had positive results. [19] Again, the evidence showed that calcium intake had no effect on bone loss. But did estrogen really help? Estrogen may slow down the process, but does not replace bone mass [20], and this is also a vital goal of any therapy for osteoporosis. Dr. Walker stated that the disclosure on all Premarin packages (the most popular prescription drug for administering estrogen) concedes that "There is no evidence that estrogen replacement therapy restores bone mass to a pre-menopausal levels." [22]

Dr. Walker also noted that researchers have found that within four years of discontinuing estrogen replacement therapy (ERT), there is no detectable difference in bone mineral content between women who have never taken the drug and those who began treatment but gave it up. [23] Prolonged use of estrogen after menopause is ineffective. The *American Journal of Medicine* conceded " ... administration of this hormone six years or more after menopause may be no longer effective." [24] Dr. Walker noted that the more recent FDA approved drugs, alendronate (Fosamex) a non–hormonal product, and salmon calcitonin nasal spray (*Miacalcin)* have proven not to be very effective. [25]

Other single-bullet approaches to treating osteoporosis have also been ineffective. Supplementation with vitamin D and fluoride have not been shown to be effective. [26] This result was surprising considering that fluoride is supposed to be one of the most effective simulators of new bone growth. Dr. McDougall observed that bone tissue formed under the influence of large doses of fluoride appears to have less strength, as evidenced by the increased rate of fractures. [27] Fluoride supplements have significant side effects. What the fluoride industry does not let you know is that about 40% of the patients treated with fluoride developed significant side effects such as vomiting, bleeding stomach ulcers, and joint pains. [28]

Ladies and gentlemen of the jury, the bottom line is that calcium supplementation will not work so long as the person continues to ingest excessive animal protein. The evidence is overwhelming that the more animal protein ingested the greater the incidence of osteoporosis. [29]

Got milk? is not a remedy but a cause of the problem.

Section 3

SORRY, AIN'T GOT NO MILK (OR SODA): REPAIRING POROUS BONES

Ladies and gentlemen of the jury, the only rational approach to preventing and reversing osteoporosis is to correct the imbalances of animal protein and refined sugar in our diets. Dr. Julian Whitaker stated that the minute a patient is placed on a low animal protein diet, their body begins to hang on to more calcium. [1] The same is true for the ingestion of refined sugar. Dr. Nancy Appleton contended that osteoporosis can be reversed if the mineral balance of the body is not upset by the ingestion of refined sugar. [2] Thus, eliminating *both* meat and dairy products and refined sugar from your diet will ensure you do not develop osteoporosis, and it will begin to reverse it if you have the bone disease.

Remember that the solution is not just lowering *excess* protein. The true villain is *meat* protein. Animal protein tends to be much more concentrated in methionine, the sulphur based amino acids, and these are very active in depleting calcium from the bones. [3] Dr. Neil Nedley reported that the high sulfur component of meat protein coupled with the fact that excess animal protein is broken down into urea adequately explain the loss of bone mass when animal protein is ingested. The mechanism is simple: urea and other waste products act as diuretics and wash out minerals from the body. [4]

All of these mechanisms may be partial explanations. Whatever the case, it is well established that a meat and high protein fare increases the risk of osteoporosis. [5]

John Robins reminded us that animal products are also high in acid residues which also contribute to leaching calcium from our bones. [6] John Robbins also pointed out that vegetarians who eat as much as 150% of their protein requirements show much less osteoporosis than meat eaters. [7] So the evidence is clear that it is not plant-based proteins, but animal-based proteins that are the causative agents for osteoporosis. Dr. Whitaker also noted that it is a fact that vegetarians at any age have much stronger bones than those who eat meat because of their lower animal protein intake. [8] In March 1983 the *Journal of Clinical Nutrition* reported the results of the largest study ever to be undertaken about the effects of a vegetarian diet on bone health. The researchers in the United States found that by the age of sixty-five, male and female vegetarians have a much lower bone loss compared to male and female meat eaters. [9]

We often associate osteoporosis exclusively with bone loss in the vertebrae and hips and larger skeletal structures. Osteoporosis manifests itself in more subtle forms, all of which can be corrected by nutritional modalities. Dr. Nancy Appleton stated that periodontal disease (pyorrhea) and gum disorders are forms of osteoporosis of the mouth. [10] She recommended that to combat osteoporosis of the mouth one has to stop consuming those items which cause calcium to become deficient and/or toxic, such as ice cream, tea, coffee, cigarettes and products containing aluminum. [11]

In place of milk with its high protein content, one can eat plenty of other foods that have rich calcium stores. There is as much calcium in a glass of carrot juice as in a glass of milk, and it is much more absorbable because of its ideal calcium/phosphorus ratio. [12] Other calcium rich foods include all soy products, nuts, kale, broccoli, collards and other leafy green vegetables. [13] Dr. Neil Nedley noted that collard greens have more calcium that non-fat milk, [14]; the vital truth is that the calcium in the plant food matrix is much more readily absorbed by the human body than the calcium in milk, 60 to 80% of which is un-absorbable by the human body. [15] Foods such as baked beans may have less calcium per unit of measure than milk [16] but can provide your body with more calcium. [16] Dr. Neil Nedley observed that one reason for the absorbability of calcium from plant-based foods is that they have less phosphorous, thus creating the ideal calcium to phosphorus ratio. [17]

Dr. Lynne Paige Walker stated that while the increased bone loss of elderly women is generally thought to be from loss of estrogen, new research have show that progesterone may be the missing catalyst in elderly women. [18] She reported on an eight-year study conducted by Dr. John R. Lee which was featured in the *International Clinical Review* in 1990. The study showed that natural progesterone not only retarded age-related bone loss but actually reverses it! [19] Within three years bone density was brought back to safe levels in 100% of patients treated, something not even estrogen could do. [20] Thus it seems that the FDA was recommending the wrong drug to cure the problem of osteoporosis!

Some researchers believe that exercise is the only natural way to significantly increase bone mass after one has stopped growing. Both muscles and bones strengthen under the stress (not distress) of exercise. [21] Dr. Andrew Weil has observed that weight bearing activities such as running, aerobics and weight lifting increase the uptake of calcium in the bones. [22] The effect of exercise has been shown to not only reverse bone loss but to actually increase bone mass. One study looked at post-menopausal women who exercised moderately for just one hour, three times weekly. With just this small amount of exercise bone loss was prevented and bone mass increased. [23] Other studies have shown that exercise is the major determining factor in the density of bones. They also show that inactivity increases the rates of secretion of both urinary and fecal calcium. [24]

The evidence is consistent with the position taken by Dr. Julian Whitaker that there is a place for vitamin and mineral supplementation in reversing osteoporosis, so long as these are made to supplement not substitute for, a whole-foods plant-based diet. Again, micronutrients preserved in their food matrix are superior to chemically derived micronutrients. Dr. Whitaker noted that women with osteoporosis have been shown to be lower in bone magnesium that people without osteoporosis. [25] He stated that magnesium supplementation is associated with increasing the effectiveness of a form of vitamin D that facilitates the proper utilization of calcium. [26] The research done by Dr. John Lee also supported this. Dr. Walker reported that besides treating the women with progesterone, Dr. John Lee placed them on a low protein diet, fortified with vitamins and calcium and other minerals along with exercise. [27] With the proper diet, calcium and magnesium supplementation is important.

Vitamin B6, folic acid, and vitamin B12 all play a significant role in converting the sulfur-based amino acid methionine into the more usable product cysteine. If methionine is not properly converted into cysteine, then homocysteine levels can increase in the body. We have seen that homocysteine is toxic to the artery lining, but it also plays a role in the development of osteoporosis. [28]

The mineral silicon is responsible for cross-linking collagen strands in the bone matrix. It therefore can contribute greatly to the strength and integrity of the connective tissue matrix of the bones. Silicon is also needed for bone remodeling. [29]

New evidence shows that boron is an important trace element in fighting osteoporosis. Dr. Whitaker stated that just 3 mg of supplemental boron every day has been shown to reduce calcium excretion by almost half. [30]

Of course, the emphasis must not be in merely achieving adequate mineral and vitamin supplementation. Proper nutrition and hydration is essential. Dr. F. Batmanghelidj correctly emphasized the importance of adequate water intake. A great number of chronic degenerative diseases, including osteoporosis are caused by chronic dehydration. The micro-nutrients discussed above in the treatment of osteoporosis would not be available to the body if it is dehydrated. Dr. Batmanghelidj stated that the new scientific truth that Western medicine must appreciate is that:

Water, the solvent of the body, regulates all functions, including the activity of the solutes it dissolves and circulates. [39]

What about estrogen-replacement therapy for post-menopausal women as a form of treatment for osteoporosis? Because of the risk of increased cancer of the breast, Dr. Whitaker recommended *natural* estrogen replacement. [40] Foods such as soy products have estrogen-like substances known as phytoestrogens. These have an estrogenic effect on women. [41] Hence they can make up for the natural reduction of estrogen production in post-menopausal women.

Ladies and gentlemen of the jury, in closing, I would remind you that the best treatment for osteoporosis, like any other chronic degenerative disease, is to adopt a lifestyle and plant-based, whole-foods diet that conforms to natural law; and this includes drinking adequate amounts of water and obtaining plenty of exercise.

ADMISSIONS:

Indicting the Defendants by their Own Statements

Section 1

THE SCOPE OF THE ADMISSIONS MADE BY THE DEFENSE

Ladies and gentlemen of the jury, in the trial of a case, the plaintiff (the defendant also has this privilege), is allowed to submit a list of statements with a request that the defendants admit that these statements are true. If any of these statements in the plaintiff's Request for Admissions are admitted by the defense to be true and accurate statements, then these Admissions are submitted at trial as *proven facts*. This means that the plaintiff does not have the burden of *proving* these facts during the course of trial, for they are deemed *admitted* by the defense to be *true*. We will adopt and adapt a similar procedure during this virtual trial.

Because the real defendants are not available for us to submit a Request for Admissions, we will use their out of court statements in their publications and public statements, as admissions against their own interest and treat them as admitted facts during the course of this trial. A *statement against interest,* is any public or private statement by a defendant which admits the truth of an allegation, and it can be used against him or her, as though it were made in a court of law and under sworn testimony.

The allegations in this trial cover a broad range of issues. The issues that divide nutritional physicians and scientists, from pharmaceutical physicians and scientists, have arisen over the last three hundred years, so we must look at the medical and scientific evidence from a historical perspective. The basis of this dispute is over the true nature of science, and hence of medical science.

The admissions concerning the nature of science and medicine will deal with the following questions:

* Is modern rationalistic science a throwback to Dark Age pseudo-science?

* Is rationalistic science false science because it is based upon opinion and false assumptions and not upon the facts?

* Is empirical science true science because it is based on facts and not on biased opinions and unverified assumptions?

* Has false science corrupted modern medicine?

* Has official science and medicine, that is, science and medicine under the control of governmental agencies and the medical establishment, departed from the principles of true empirical science?

* Does medicine do more harm than good in treating chronic degenerative diseases when it is based on the false rationalistic science?

* Is fraud and dishonesty undermining modern science and medicine?

The Admissions also concern issues about the true nature of chronic degenerative disease and their proper treatment.

* What is the true nature of disease, is it a dysfunction of the entire organism or is it caused by an external agent, such as a germ?

* Can the body heal itself or are we dependent upon external chemical agents to preserve its health?

* Is the use of pharmaceutical medicine in the treatment of chronic degenerative diseases based on false science ?

* Does the current scientific and medical treatment of chronic degenerative diseases constitute medical fraud?

* Are chronic degenerative diseases such as cancer, heart disease and high blood pressure metabolic and physiological dysfunctions

of the body, the result of poor nutrition and lifestyle abuses such as smoking and alcohol use?

* Is a well-balanced nutritional program, as advocated by Hippocrates the Father of medicine, the best method of preventing and reversing chronic degenerative disease?

* Is the use of pharmaceutical drugs to treat chronic degenerative diseases bad medicine, making the treatment worse than the disease?

* Is America's so-called war on cancer and on other chronic degenerative disease a failure?

The Admissions also concern the industrial and governmental entities which control modern medical science and their motives.

* Is medicine under the control of the petro-chemical industry?

* Is there a profit motive over-riding patient safety?

* Has the FDA created a monopoly for drug-based medicine and a hostile environment for nutritional medicine?

* Has the Food and Drug Administration (FDA) abandoned its role in preserving the health of American?

The following Admissions are to be used as *proof* of the facts that you, the people of America, would have had to prove in this trial, but are now deemed to be as admitted. In presenting this testimony sufficient historical and contextual commentary is provided with each category of Admission so as to put them in the context of the issues raised in this trial.

ADMISSION: DRUG MEDICINE IS BASED ON FALSE SCIENCE

Ladies and gentlemen of the jury, rationalistic science upon which ancient and modern medicine is based is not true science, but metaphysical speculations passing off as science.

The failure of rationalistic science must be viewed from a historical perspective, for it is only as we understand why science in the Dark Ages prior to Sir Francis Bacon failed, that we can understand the failures of modern medical science. Many top scientists and physicians warn us that much of science and medicine today has reverted to the irrational methodology of the Dark Ages in which authority and politically correct opinions were given precedent over facts. Many years ago Dr. Julian Whitaker warned us in his best seller, *Dr. Whitaker's Guide to Natural Healing*, that the Allopathic monopoly of medicine is taking medicine back into a new Dark Age where not even doctors had freedom of medical thought.

> We are rapidly marching towards an Allopathic Dark Age in which information not even remotely related to facts is "generated" to serve Allopathic medical dogma. Doctors will become even more like robots, exhibiting no signs of independent thought. [1]

The dispute between pharmaceutical medicine and nutritional medicine today is identical to the seventeenth-century dispute between the false rationalistic science and medicine of the Dark Ages and the empirical science and medicine introduced by Francis Bacon, who was both a scientist and a physician. In Bacon's day *politically correct* public policy overruled the *facts* of science and medicine. It is the same today. Consider the following admissions by Dr. Irwin Bross, one of America's leading epidemiologist in the twentieth century, and author of several books on the subject:

In Official Science ... *official policy* has priority over facts and scientific principles. [2]

Lying to the public about safety is habitual in Official Science ... [3]

Official Science has also acted vigorously to destroy normal science *when the findings are contrary to government policy.* [4]

Ladies and gentlemen of the jury, throughout this trial we have seen that pharmaceutical medicine today does not take *all* of the facts relating to chronic degenerative diseases into consideration when devising a treatment plan. Drug-based medicine only tries to *manage* one or more *symptoms* of a disease, while disregarding most of the facts relating to the nutritional and lifestyle cause of the disease and the nutritional prevention and cure of the disease. Pharmaceutical medicine is interested only in a quick chemical fix, not of the disease, but of the manifestations of the disease. This was precisely the modus operandi of the rationalistic physicians of Francis Bacon's day.

Dr. Irwin Bross tried to warn America that there was a *civil war* [5] taking place between *official science* and what he called *normal science.* The conflict within science and medicine today was actually begun by Sir Francis Bacon who opened the first volley against the *official science* of the Dark Ages.

Sir Francis Bacon (1561–1626) has been recognized as the Father of modern science. But few realize that he was also proficient in medicine. He rebelled against the follies of the scientific and medical establishment of his day. He regarded the so-called *scientific* conclusions of the rationalistic and naturalistic worldview of the Dark Ages, to be a form of insanity.

The specious meditations, speculations, and theories of mankind are but a kind of insanity, only there is no one to stand by and observe it. [6]

Why did Francis Bacon conclude that the so-called scientific conclusions of the scientists and physicians of his day were delusions and a form of insanity? Because, he contended, they were based on *opinions* and *traditions* and not on the *facts of nature*. In his treatises that ushered in the modern world, *The Advancement of Learning* and *Novum Organum*, Francis Bacon contended that there is a false and a true method by which men can attempt to derive natural laws from the particulars of nature: by hastily considering only a *few facts* or by carefully taking into consideration *all* of the facts.

> There are and can exist but two ways of investigation and discovering truth. The one hurries on rapidly from the senses and particulars to the most general axioms, and from them, as principles and their supposed undisputed truth, derives and discovers the intermediate axioms. This is the method now in use. The other constructs its axioms from the senses and particulars, by ascending continually and gradually, till it finally arrives at the most general axioms, which is the true but unattempted way. [7]

Consideration of only a *few facts* was the cardinal sin of Dark Age science and medicine, and it has once again become the cardinal sin of modern scientific medicine. It is this weakness that converts true empirical science and medicine into false rationalistic science and medicine. The evidence will show that many modern scientists and physicians have recognized the fact that there is a false science and a true science and that medicine is only of value to a society to the extent that it is influenced by true empirical science. Unfortunately much of modern pharmaceutical medicine is based upon the false rationalistic science, particularly in its attempts to treat chronic degenerative disease with poisonous drugs with devastating side effects.

Francis Bacon argued that there is a superficial similarity between these two scientific methods in that they both start with the particulars of nature; but this is the extent of their similarity. There is a vast difference between these two methods. One stops short of being science, and the other is true science. Bacon made the point that the rationalist scientists and physicians of his day based their theories or axioms on hastily drawn conclusions from a *few* of the facts, while empirical scientists and physicians took *all* of the facts into consideration.

> Each of these two ways begins from the senses and particulars, and ends in the greatest generalities. But they are immeasurably

different; for the one merely touches cursorily the limits of experiment and particulars, whilst the other runs duly and regularly through them; the one from the very onset lays down some abstract and useless generalities, the other gradually rises to those principles which are really the most common in nature. [8]

Giving priority to the *facts* instead of the *opinions* of scholars and authority figures in the Church and government was the revolutionary idea that Sir Francis Bacon introduced; it led to modern science and to all of the scientific advances that exists in the modern world. The new methodology impacted medicine as well as every other scientific discipline. But it was heresy to the existing scientific and medical establishment then; and it is still heresy to the scientific and medical establishment today, Dr. Irwin Bross contended. [9]

Ladies and gentlemen of the jury, because the evidence is very clear that modern drug-based medicine has largely reverted to the unscientific methodology of the Dark Ages, it may be useful to see what Sir Francis Bacon, speaking as a physician, had to say about medicine in his day. Sir Francis Bacon chided the rationalistic physicians for exalting theory over practice; as a result, he admitted, the empirical physicians and even old women (with their old wives tales regarding herbal remedies) were more successful in treating their patients than were the drug-peddling physicians. Noting the inefficacy of established medicine in his day, he stated satirically:

[O]ld women and empirics are often more successful with their cures than learned physicians, because the latter religiously hold on to their medicines, even when they are not appropriate to the particular disease. [10]

This remarkable observation very closely describes the situation today. Today, those physicians who respect and obey the laws of nutrition and who recognize the healing power God implanted in nature are often more successful in preventing and curing chronic degenerative diseases than physicians practicing pharmaceutical medicine. Francis Bacon advised the physicians of his day to return to the empirical fact-finding methods of Hippocrates. He argued that medicine was inefficacious in his day because it departed from the principles of empirical medical science advocated by Hippocrates.

The first is the discontinuance of the ancient and serious diligence of Hippocrates, which used to set down a narrative of the special cases of his patients, and how they proceeded... this discontinuance of medical history I find deficient ...

They be the best physicians, which being learned incline to the traditions of experience, or being empirics incline to the methods of learning. [11]

Sir Francis Bacon as a physician, was influenced by the pioneering work of the Swiss physician Theophrastus Bombast von Hohenheim, known to history as the great Paracelsus (1493–1541). He is regarded by many as the Father of modern medicine. Anticipating the modern scientific revolution introduced by Sir Francis Bacon, Paracelsus attempted to reform medicine by turning it away from the *speculations* of rationalistic science, to an empirical study of the *facts*.

What a doctor needs is not eloquence or knowledge of language and of books, illustrious though they may be *but profound knowledge of nature and her works* ... If I want to prove anything, I shall not do so by quoting authorities [the Schoolmen] but by experiment and by reasoning thereupon ... I do not believe in the ancient doctrine of complexions or humors ... It is because of these doctrines that so few physicians have correct views of disease, its origins and its course ... Farewell and come with a good will to study our attempt to reform medicine. [12]

On another occasion Paracelsus stated:

From his own head a man cannot learn the theory of medicine, but only from that which his eyes see and his fingers touch ... [13]

Paracelsus argued that if the physician did not base his medicine on knowledge derived from sense perception, he would establish it upon false rationalistic science which he labeled *pseudo-science*. With biting sarcasm he derided the sophists, (rationalistic physicians) as *pseudo-scientists*.

Your eyes which take delight in experience are your masters; for your own fantasies and speculations cannot advance you so far that you can boast of being a physician. Nor can you acquire the art of medicine by sophisms, or after the manner of the sophists, those *pseudo-scientists*, who imagine that their own wisdom reaches as far as the end of the earth and the sea and all elements. [14]

Paracelsus aptly described medicine in the twentieth and twenty-first centuries. His redefinition of disease by basing it upon all the *symptoms of a disease,* and not on *esoteric opinions and theories* of the rationalistic physicians was a masterstroke of genius. He liberated medicine from the exclusive preserve of the elitist Medical Deity who kept the people captive to their harmful nostrums.

When Paracelsus related disease to a violation of the ordinary laws of nature, laws that were discovered by sense perception, it became possible for common folk to reason from cause to effect and discover the causes of their maladies and the appropriate herbal or nutritional remedy. Coulter stated that in doing this, Paracelsus abolished the *invisible empire* of esoteric medical knowledge (note the ominous parallels with the claims of today's medical establishment that the lay person cannot understand medicine).

By shifting the focus of medicine to the formal cause of the disease Paracelsus at one stroke abolished that invisible empire which was the exclusive preserve of the medical profession. [15]

The reaction of the Church-run medical establishment of his day was predictable. The medical profession, blinded by their rationalistic pseudo-science, reacted with vehemence. Their monopoly over medicine and hence over people's lives were threatened by the empirical medicine of Paracelsus. They referred to the teachings of Paracelsus as *insane delusions.* [16] Ladies and gentlemen of the jury, note carefully that the protests of the seventeenth century Medical Deity to the Hippocratic medical science being reintroduced by Paracelsus has a strangely familiar ring to it. It is not unlike the wails and denunciations by today's conventional medicine to the new alternative medicine that seeks to prevent and cure degenerative disease by natural and nutritional means free from the blight of drugs. The evidence shows that modern nutritional medicine is Hippocratic medicine in its finest form.

The following passage cited by the medical historian Harris Coulter typifies the reaction of the medical profession of Paracelsus' time. It demonstrates how blind men can become to truth when they hold on to a false worldview:

The indignation of the latter [medical profession] at this blow [Paracelsus' redefinition of disease which abolished the invisible empire of authoritarian medical knowledge] to their interests is seen in the comments of Thomas Erastus (1523–1583) who called Paracelsus a "beast" and a "grunting swine" and said that he abolished the knowledge of the ancients, replacing sane teaching by insane delusion, the certain by the uncertain, the comprehensible by the incomprehensible, truth by false names and doctrines, the useful by the useless, and salubrious by pestilential poison. [17]

The bottom line of their extreme protests was the same today: loss of profits from the sale of drug medications and the threat to their monopoly over the practice of medicine. Nevertheless, under the painstaking work of Paracelsus and Bacon, medicine began to improve, especially when it followed closely the empirical revolution that was taking place in science.

But, ladies and gentlemen of the jury, after the painful birth of modern empirical science, it was not long before rationalistic theories based upon false metaphysical opinions about the nature of the universe began to creep back in and challenge the empirical science of the early modern age. The retreat back into Dark Age science started with Rene Descartes (1596–1650) and has come down through the centuries in the form of an internal civil war in science. From then on rationalistic science and empirical science existed side by side until the end of the nineteenth century when, under the influence of the resurgent metaphysical worldview of evolutionary theory, rationalistic science completely subverted and eclipsed empirical science. The civil war between the two forms of science turned into a rout for empirical science.

Bertram Russell in his *History of Western Philosophy* stated that beginning with Descartes, Western philosophy [and the science accompanying it], de-emphasized the *facts* and emphasized *human opinion* generated by pure thought.

From Descartes to Kant, Continental philosophy derived much

of its conception of the nature of human knowledge from mathematics but it regarded mathematics as known independent of experience. It was thus led, like Plato, to minimize the part played by perception, and over emphasize the part played by pure thought. [18]

Minimizing the role of perception and over-emphasizing the role of pure thought is the first step in abandoning the modern scientific methodology introduced by Sir Francis Bacon, and therefore a step backwards to Dark Age science. Descartes' rejection of the empirical focus on facts had an adverse impact upon scientific methodology. Dr. Stanley Jaki, in the *Origin of Science and the Science of its Origin*, noted that the French philosopher d'Alembert blamed Descartes for the stagnation of French science. [19] French science began to stagnate because it followed Descartes who abandoned the principles of empirical investigation introduced by Sir Francis Bacon. [20]

Rene Descartes was not only an influential scientist of the old rationalistic school, but he was also a physician; he soon introduced rationalistic thinking into medicine. Harris Coulter cited the seventeenth century French medical writer Sprengel, who criticized the false model of medicine that Descartes inspired.

It must be admitted that the theory of Descartes destroyed the spirit of observation and greatly contributed to the erroneous idea that calculating the movement of atoms could give medicine a truly mathematical certainty. [21]

Descartes followed the path of autonomous humanism that Aquinas had opened the door to when he postulated that man's intellect had not fallen at the biblical Fall of man. Russell noted that Descartes studied Aquinas' works as closely as he did the Bible, so the influence of Aquinas' autonomous humanism upon Descartes could be inferred. [22] Like Aquinas, Descartes placed undue emphasis on the ability of man's unaided intellect to arrive at truth. This emphasis on the power of reason unchecked by experimentation is clearly seen in Descartes' medical teachings. Despite the great advances empirical science was making, Descartes held that sense perception and experience are unreliable compared to man's reasoning power [23], and therefore medical practice must be based upon a comprehensive theory of physical and physiological causes. [24] Thus

Descartes rejected the empiricism that was responsible for all of the great advances in science.

It was not simply that Descartes wrongfully emphasized theory over practice. The revolution he was presiding over went far deeper. He rejected the fundamental principle that the data of sense perception must be the *acid test* of the truthfulness of a theory. He taught that because the *mind* was capable of arriving at truth by the power of shear thinking, *sense perception* could not be the basis for verifying a scientific or medical theory.

All things that we *perceive* very clearly and very distinctly are true. [25]

By *perceive* he did not refer to that which was *observed through sense perception*, but to that which is arrived at by the process of mental abstraction. This attempt to construct reality through the power of the human imagination and intellect was a throwback to the Dark Ages of pseudo-science. Descartes is clearly and deliberately re-introducing the moribund rationalist theory of knowledge which held that only human reason could verify or validate a scientific or medical theory.

Ladies and gentlemen of the jury, having abandoned true empirical science for the false pseudo-science of rationalism, Descartes' influence in medicine was predominantly bad. He inspired the mechanical-chemical model of medicine, and viciously attacked the concept of vitalism in medicine. We have seen that the concept of vitalism came from Hippocrates who believed in the ability of the body to heal itself. To replace the healing mechanism in the body, Descartes invoked the idea of an immortal soul which resided in a chemico-mechanical material body. He got this idea from Pythagoras and Plato who taught that the material body was evil but the immortal soul was good. Commenting on Descartes' attack on vitalism in medicine, Coulter wrote:

> Rationalism in medicine, on the contrary, is deterministic and seeks to eliminate any source of autonomy in the organism by dividing up the vitality into: 1) a physical or chemical process and 2) the immortal soul ...

Descartes is the prototype of this attack on vitalism. He identifies "life" with the immoral soul which at the same time provides the subject

with rational guidance through its single point of contact with the body—
the pineal gland. The body otherwise functions as a machine centered on
a mechanico-chemical process in the heart. [26]

By placing the spark of life in an immortal soul, Descartes separated
life and the healing processes of nature from the human body which he
viewed as nothing more than a mechanical and chemical entity. It cannot
be over emphasized how crucial Descartes' rationalistic pseudo-science
was to the development of modern chemical-based medicine which still
denies or at least diminishes the role of nature in healing chronic degenerative diseases. It is this denial of the existence of vital healing forces
within the human organism which separates pharmaceutical medicine
from nutritional medicine.

After Rene Descartes, the first seventeenth-century rationalistic physician of significance was the German-born Frenchman, Francois de la
Boe Sylvius (1614–1672). He founded the chemical school of medicine,
often referred to as the Iatro-chemical school. [27] His chemical model of
medicine was based on rationalistic theories and not on the data of sense
observation. He reformulated the age-old rationalistic concept of treating
diseases by substances contrary to their symptoms. His chemical model
reduced medicine to a clash between acids and alkalis. [28] He taught
that disease was to be overcome, not by supporting the vitalist forces of
the organism so that its immune system could heal the sick organism, but
by the external intervention of the physician. Thus his view of disease
conformed to the theory that disease was more or less an *external entity*
that could be identified and destroyed by chemical means. He ignored all
the evidence which showed that disease was an internal dysfunction of
the organism. Coulter noted that this approach to medicine had much in
common with twentieth-century pharmaceutical medicine. [29]

Ladies and gentlemen of the jury, Harris Coulter observed that the
chemical-based model of medicine that Sylvius advocated wrecked havoc
among the peoples of Northern Europe where he practiced. [30] When
medicine is based on esoteric and unverifiable assumptions that are not
allowed to be corrected by the experience of the physician, it becomes the
minister of death and not of life. This was true of seventeenth-century
rationalistic medicine, and it is equally true of pharmaceutical medicine of
the twentieth century. This type of false medicine can be more devastating
to a population than the horrors of war itself. Today more people die from
bad medicine in one year than are killed in ten Vietnams. Yet the modern

physician, blindly clinging to his rationalistic theories that are far removed from common sense or empirical data, is strangely numb to the untold suffering he is doing to his patients by his pharmaceutical nostrums.

The historical evidence amply reveals the damage done through the centuries by drug-based medicine. When criticizing the chemical model of medicine advocated by Francois de la Boe Sylvius, Sprengel cited this telling admission:

> Any disinterested and impartial person will have to agree that this School [the chemical model of medicine] did more harm than good; removing medicine even further from the path of observation and representing supernatural principles as sensory objects, introducing pernicious methods based only on arbitrary hypotheses. One could go so far as to say that the opinions propagated by the chemical School have been more devastating than certain wars, so far was the treatment of diseases based on these hypotheses contrary to good sense and reason. [31]

Can you imagine such an admission, medicine inflicting more damage than war? Ladies and gentlemen of the jury, what a stark *indictment* of the chemical model of medicine that is based on the false rationalistic medical science. It cannot be over-emphasized that when medical theory is separated from the evidence of the senses, medicine becomes the handmaid of death and not of life. Lest anyone accuse Sprengel of being an extremist in his opinion that seventeenth-century rationalistic medicine inflicted more damage than benefit to the patients it purported to help, let him consider the admission of a physician who was considered *the most eminent* physician of the seventeenth century.

The Dutch physician Hermann Boerhaave (1668–1738) was without peer in his day. He once received a letter from China hailing him as the *most famous physician in Europe.* [32] Although his practice was eclectic, in that it combined elements of empirical and rationalistic medicine, Boerhaave made an incredible admission about the medical profession dominated as it was through the centuries by the pseudo-science of rationalist drug-based medicine.

> If we compare the good which a half dozen true sons of Aesculapius have accomplished since the origin of the medical art upon earth with the evil which the immense mass of doctors of this profession

among the human race have done, there can be no doubt that it would have been far better if there had never been any physicians in the world. [33]

We cannot just write off these harsh indictments of drug-based medicine to "bad medicine, long ago abandoned." The truth is, the errors in medical thinking that led to these horrors in the seventeenth century are still with us today. For similar reasons, Dr. Robert Mendelsohn medical professor at the University of Illinois Medical School and director of Chicago's Michael Reese Hospital, called twentieth-century modern medicine the "Church of death." [34] The havoc wroth by today's pharmaceutical medicine is a thousand times worse than was inflicted by the seventeenth-century school of pharmaceutical medicine. The wealth of allied industries and the monopoly granted them by state and federal governments ensure their greater ability to inflict harm upon the American populace.

Whereas Hippocratic medicine emphasized the importance of taking a history of the patient and the disease process, Sylvius and other Rationalists tended to disregard the patient's disease history, applying instead an analytical process to arrive at the proper chemical remedy. Any facts that disagreed with their chemico-pharmaceutical theories of medicine were dutifully disregarded. [35] Coulter wrote:

Sylvius like other Rationalist thinkers, converted disease and cure from a historical process into an analytical one and, by the same token, denied the value of medical history itself. Sprengel remarks that ... the noblest of the arts [medicine] became the plaything of the chemists' imagination, and they regarded all their predecessors with contempt. [36]

Medical historians admit that Sylvius' chemical-based and drug-based medicine was irrational.

Sylvius' medical practice was based on the applications of acids or alkalis in such irrational ways that it destroyed the health of many Northern Europeans. [37]

Other rationalistic physicians like George Cheyne and Frederick Hoffman, both of whom applied the mechanical model to the human

organism, taught that drug-based medicines acted physically or mechani-
cally. Hoffman, taught that:

> The operation of drugs is wholly mechanical and can be best
> explained by size, shape, and laws of motion. [38]

Ladies and gentlemen of the jury, the mechanical model for applying drug
doses proved to be so disastrous that the physician Thomas Sydenham
(1624–1689) in England and the physician Giorgio Baglivi (1668–1707)
in Italy advocated a return to the scientific empiricism of Hippocrates
in medicine. They were both influenced by John Locke's empiricism in
science which was in mortal combat with the rising tide of Cartesian
Rationalism in medicine. Thomas Sydenham was an intimate friend of
Locke, and his *Art of Medicine* was once thought to have been written
by Locke. Baglivi modeled his medical science after Sydenham whom he
called the *profoundest observer after Hippocrates*. [39]

While Locke was making a sweeping demolition of the rationalistic
theory of knowledge, Sydenham and Baglivi were devoting themselves to
a general condemnation of the philosophical basis of rationalism in medical science. [40] In a striking admission, Sydenham charged that the false
doctrines of rationalism were speculations that had, "As much to do with
treating sick men as the painting of pictures with the sailing of ships."
[41]

At the opening of the eighteenth century, the medical views of the
German Professor of Medicine, Georg Ernst Stahl (1660–1734), revealed
the influence of the biblical worldview (made popular by the Reformation
and Francis Bacon), on the development of medical science and the
practice of medicine. Harris Coulter stated that Stahl was guided by
Hippocratic-Empiric principles and the doctrines of Pietism in religion
in seeking to reform the science of medicine. [42] Stahl actually started
out on the rationalistic path blazed by Sylvius and Willis but soon discovered that the chemico-mechanical model of medicine was providing false
answers in the treatment of medicine.

> I then recognized the falsity of any application of the chemical
> sciences to the theory of diseases. Furthermore, I could not explain
> by mechanical laws the extraordinary and sudden changes due to
> the passions, which give rise to actions in the various parts of the
> body which are quite different from those resulting naturally from

their mechanical conformation—these being so obviously caused by a disorder of the vital movements that it seemed absurd to accept the involvement of any material cause. Thus I felt the need to reconstruct medical theory on a firmer basis than chemistry and mechanics. [43]

Stahl's abandonment of the mechanico-chemical model of medicine was not due to any ignorance on his part of chemistry or the other sciences. He was held to have mastered the disciplines of chemistry and medicine. [44] Theophile Bordeu who was perhaps one of the greatest figures in French medical history, regarded Stahl as one of the greatest geniuses in medical history. Referring to Stahl's attempts to cleanse medical practice of the harmful influence of the chemical drug-based model of medicine, Theophile Bordeu stated this was the, "dream of Stahl ... the dream of one of the greatest geniuses medicine has ever known." [45] This is the one constant feature one will encounter again and again in the history of medicine, that from Paracelsus in the fifteenth century to Dr. Max Gerson in the twentieth century, the greatest and most brilliant physicians have embraced the empirical medicine of Hippocrates. Similarly the brightest and most brilliant minds from Sir Francis Bacon, Sir Isaac Newton, Clark Maxwell to Albert Einstein and Linus Pauling (who was the only scientist of the twentieth century to be ranked with Einstein) have embraced empirical science and rejected opinion-based rationalistic science.

The end of the eighteenth century and the beginning of the nineteenth century witnessed the finest expression of empiricism in medicine in modern times in the work and doctrines of Dr. Samuel Hahnemann (1755–1843). This medical genius indicted the drug-based medicine of his day which made suppressing the symptoms of disease the focus of medical care, just as it is today. He made the telling admission that the *symptomatic treatment of disease* had achieved universal contempt.

> In all times the Old School physicians, not knowing how else to give relief, have sought to combat, and if possible to suppress by medicines, here and there, a single symptom from among a number in a disease—a *one-sided* procedure which, under the name of *symptomatic treatment*, has justly excited universal contempt because by it not only was nothing gained, but much harm was inflicted. A single one of the symptoms present is no more the

disease itself than a single foot is the man himself. [46] [Emphasis added.]

Today medicine, particularly in the area of chronic degenerative diseases, treats the single symptom, like the tumor in cancer and the sugar level in diabetes, while ignoring the vast array of symptoms that tell of a metabolic dysfunction of the *entire* organism. Medical Rationalism was attractive to the physician because it purported to simplify the nature of disease and hence the nature of the remedy. It provided the physician with a few theoretical concepts that were simple to understand and simple to apply, regardless of the fact that these remedies did not work to remove the *cause* of disease. This tendency led to the neglect of the majority of symptoms associated with a disease, because listing all the symptoms made treatment too complex to understand or implement. Hahnemann further admitted:

The Old School physician gave himself very little trouble in this matter in his mode of treatment. He would not listen to any minute detail of all the circumstance of his case by the patient; indeed, he frequently cut him short in his relation of his sufferings, in order that he might not be delayed in the rapid writing of his prescription ...

"What do we care," say the medical teachers and their books, 'what do we care about the presence of many other diverse symptoms that are observable in the case of the disease before us, or the absence of those that are wanting? *The physician should pay no attention to such empirical trifles;* his practical tact, the penetrating glance of his *mental eye* into the hidden nature of the malady, enables him to determine at the very first sight of the patient what is the matter with him, what pathological form of disease he has to give it, and his therapeutic knowledge teaches him what prescription he must order for it. [47] [Emphasis added.]

Ladies and gentlemen of the jury, this is simply unbelievable! The Allopathic physician would dismiss the *facts* as empirical trifles, and in their place he would use his *mental eye* to discern the disease and its proper treatment! This admission leaves no doubt that medicine had retreated into the misty canyons of Dark Age medicine. Hahnemann contended

that true scientific medicine must turn away from metaphysical speculations and re-focus on the data of sense perception to discover the true
nature of the disease and the appropriate medicine to combat the disease. Following John Locke, the champion of empiricism, Hahnemann
argued that empirical medicine makes the patient's symptoms the vehicle,
through which true science can learn about disease and health,

> Now, as in a disease ... we can perceive nothing but the morbid
> symptoms, it must ... be the symptoms alone by which the disease
> demands and points to the remedy suited to relieve it—and,
> moreover, the *totality* of these its symptoms, *of this outwardly
> reflected picture of the internal essence of the disease, that is, of the
> affection of the vital force*, must be the principal, or the sole means,
> whereby the disease can make known what remedy it requires—the
> only thing that can determine the choice of the most appropriate
> remedy—and thus, in a word, the totality of the symptoms must
> be the principal, indeed the only thing the physician has to take
> note of in every case of disease and *to remove* by means of his
> art, in order that the disease shall be cured and transformed into
> health. [48] [Emphasis added.]

Hahnemann stressed the importance of discovering the *totality* of the
symptoms because this was required by true empirical scientific methodology in order to accurately diagnose the disease. The symptoms provided
the raw data from which the empirical physician, as scientist, could reason inductively to arrive at reasonable theories about the disease and the
appropriate remedy. On the other hand the rationalistic physician, following the path of pseudo-science, reasoned deductively from hastily drawn
up hypotheses derived from only a *few* symptoms of the disease. It is the
nature of pseudo-science to propose a theory and search for data to justify
its position.

True science applies to all theories the acid test of *conformity to the
data of sense perception*. This is what makes it *empirical* science. What
Hahnemann was fiercely fighting for was the establishment of true empirical science as the guide to medical learning. To do this he had to show
the folly and harm of rationalistic pseudo-science as it was being applied
to medicine in his day. Ladies and gentlemen mark this thought well,
the proud rationalist physician fiercely resisted this empirical approach

because it opened the door of natural healing and of medicine to the layman. Empirical medicine was the great leveler, and the haughty physician
selling his sophisticated and poisonous drugs would have nothing of it.
[49]
  Hahnemann criticized the use of drugs in high doses which was prevalent in his day. Not only were the drugs ineffective because they were
wrongly selected on the basis that their symptoms had to be the *opposite* of
the disease symptoms, but they did positive harm in such quantities. This
made the disease more difficult to cure and often resulted in death. Again
Hahnemann admitted that drug treatment exacerbated the disease, making it more difficult to cure.

> By such large doses of the ... medicine ... he creates new morbid
> states which are often more difficult to cure than the original
> malady, and which often enough terminate in death. [50]

Unwittingly Hahnemann accurately described modern drug-based medicine, but he had no idea that the amount of deaths today would dwarf
those in his day.
  Ladies and gentlemen of the jury, Dr. Claude Bernard (1813–1878),
the champion of animal experimentation, did more, perhaps, than any
physician to implant the rationalistic philosophy and science of Descartes
into medical practice. Showing his disdain for empirical medical science,
he contended that the *speculations of the medical scientist can outweigh the
facts.* This concept became the guiding light of his scientific methodology
in medicine. He once stated:

> There are facts that one can't believe because the mind has the
> certainty that things are different. [51]

This is a powerfully arrogant statement, but a true expression of rationalistic science and medicine: *disregard the facts if they do not fit in with your
sincerely held theories!* It is a total rejection of Sir Francis Bacon's empirical
science, which demanded the opposite, that the facts become the criteria
by which all theories are judged for validity. The suppression of unwel-
comed facts was a rejection of the empirical science of Francis Bacon
for the rationalistic science of the Scholastics of the Dark Ages; and it

came to dominate science and medicine in the twentieth and twenty-first centuries.

Ladies and gentlemen of the jury, allow me to remind you of the differences between true science and pseudo science; ancient Dark Age science, and the modern science generated by the intellectual Revolution of the seventeenth century. Phillip Frank, author of the book *Philosophy of Science: The Link Between Science and Philosophy,* wrote succinctly of this difference.

> The difference between ancient and modern science was ... the criterion by which a discovered principle was recognized to be valid. The method of "verification" is different now; more weight is given to the agreement of the results with observed facts than to the agreement of the principles with a world picture that has been accepted for what we called ..."philosophical" reasons. [52]

In the empirical process agreement of theory with the observable facts is paramount; there is no place for metaphysical speculation or politically correct policies. One does not throw out the facts because they disagree with a favored theory, as is being commonly done today in science generally and in medical science. It was this intellectual revolution that brought us out of the Dark Ages, and it is the abandonment of this procedure that will throw us back into the murky depths of the Dark Ages. The choice is ours.

The neo-rationalistic, pseudo-scientific Cartesian methodology, a throwback of the Dark Ages, has become the methodology of modern pharmaceutical medicine. This is the true tragedy of modern science and medicine. This fact explains the torrent of harm and even death inflicted upon patients today. The corrective measure of products liability claims in the courts of law cannot even begin to keep up with the damage being done to patients by poisonous drugs with deadly side effects. The highest awards in these claims are imposed when the pharmaceutical companies knowingly suppress prior knowledge of harmful effects. Unfortunately, many physicians have been caught up in the false scientific methodology without being aware of undisclosed studies pointing to the harmfulness of the drugs they use. The average physician is merely the tool of the petrochemical industry which educates them and supplies them with endless drugs.

Empirical physicians, on the other hand, insisted then as they insist now that *true science* must be based on the data of sense observation and consequently that medical theory must conform to *all* the facts. In the treatment of diseases this data largely comes from the patient's symptoms. Therefore, the physician must make a careful note of *all* of the patient's symptoms to accurately diagnose the disease and hence the proper course of treatment. This is the essence of the dispute between modern nutritional medicine and drug-based medicine today. Which approach is right? The evidence of history has demonstrated that science and medicine has flourished under the empirical tradition. This is true from the days of Hippocrates to the present time. We also know that rationalistic science and medicine has led to setbacks in science and to some horrendous medical disasters.

Ladies and gentlemen of the jury, the scientist who was most responsible for bringing the rationalistic ideas of Descartes into full fruition, thereby thrusting science back into the Dark Ages of Scholasticism in which speculation passed off for science, was Charles Darwin. Modern evolutionary theory was a resurrection of ancient Greek religious thinking which was evolutionary in its foundation. Historian of science Charles Singer admitted the religious and unscientific foundation of Darwin's theory.

> Kolliker and other critics claimed that the "chance" element in Darwin's scheme was but a veiled teleology. Natural selection had been elevated to the rank of a "cause" leading to an "effect" ... In Kolliker's view, Darwin was dealing with the "might" and "maybe" *and not with any theory that could be tested by experience.* Here Kolliker was right. Evolution was perhaps unique among major scientific theories *in that the appeal for its acceptance was not the evidence for it,* but that any other proposed interpretation of the data seemed wholly incredible. [53] [Emphasis added.]

When a strongly held religious or philosophical belief causes one to reject the evidence of one's senses, then one has moved from *science* to *metaphysics*. The *might* and *maybe* is not science, but metaphysics; plainly speaking it is religious speculation masquerading as science, for these metaphysical theories cannot be tested by the facts of experience. Despite its avowed religious basis, the theory of evolution was accepted as *scientific* by the rationalistic scientists and subsequently by almost the entire modern age. In every aspect of human endeavor, in science, philosophy, medicine, biology, economics, religion and literature in general, the idea of evolution is triumphant because it provides a *religious substitute* for believing in a *Creator* to whom man is accountable.

In the nineteenth century, evolutionary theory became one of the leading factors for the acceptance of the mechanical concept of the world. [54] Yet, despite the fact that modern science has almost completely discarded the mechanical model of the world, the idea lives on in modern medicine.

Evolutionary theory *denies* the existence of the Creator. Pharmaceutical science *ignores* the Creator and tries to *replace* the healing mechanism he imprinted in nature and in the human organism with the *chemical manipulation* of the organism. They both try to be the Savior of mankind. Hans Ruesch, in his widely acclaimed book, *The Naked Empress or the Great Medical Fraud*, stated:

A doctor gains renown not by admitting that Nature alone is *suprema guaritrix*—the number one certified Healer—but by asserting his ability to present himself as the supreme healer, the Savior of the patient's life. [55] [Emphasis added.]

Ladies and gentlemen of the jury, once again we remind you that the evidence shows without a reasonable doubt that rationalistic medicine, based on a false rationalistic science, is *not* true medicine and is ineffective in curing chronic degenerative disease. There is no such thing today as *real science* in medicine. Based on *false science*, much of modern pharmaceutical medicine is harmful and useless. Dr. Irwin Bross admitted this when he stated in 1994:

Most of the money spent on the U. S. Health care system—approaching a *trillion* dollars a year—was actually being wasted on payments for medical services that *were useless, counterproductive, or outright medical fraud*. [56] [Emphasis added.]

In the twentieth century Allopathic medicine which is largely based on the pseudo-science of rationalism, tends to discard many of the facts regarding the nature of chronic degenerative diseases. It focuses upon a few of the facts and hastily applies a pharmaceutical remedy to fight one or more symptoms of the disease, while ignoring the underlying nutritional causes of the diseases. And to compound the problem, the medical establishment uses the long arm of the law to prevent physicians from using nutritional modalities to cure the problem in certain diseases. Houston and Null published their investigative findings about the unscientific aspect of the American Cancer Society's war against *unproven* cancer remedies.

> It seems odd that an organization supposedly devoted to encouraging research, by definition the study of the unproven, should use unproven as a pejorative and promote the cardinal error on science of confusing *unproven* with *disproven*. If unproven avenues are blocked what remains is what is already known and progress is foreclosed. [57] [Emphasis added.]

In 1997 Dr. William Campbell Douglass, II, in *Bad Medicine* lamented that *bad medicine* based on *bad science* injuries millions of Americans. He turned the tables upon the National Cancer Society and upon established medicine; whereas they consider their drug remedies to be *proven* cures and nutritional cures *unproven* remedies, Dr. Douglass asserted that it is drug remedies that are the true *unproven* cures for chronic degenerative diseases like cancer.

> [T]he bulk of this report focuses on what I consider to be the very worst of bad medicine—needless, dangerous, and expensive drugs. Each year millions of Americans become seriously ill because of *unproven drug therapies* and the dangerous interaction between prescriptions drugs and over-the-counter medications. [58] [Emphasis added.]

Ladies and gentlemen of the jury, the medical establishment can classify their *unproven* drug cures as *approved and acceptable medicine* because they have the *power* to do so. But their decisions are not based upon empirical facts. In defense of their inefficacious drug-based medicine, many Allopaths desperately defend their drug-based medical model by declaring war upon the very foundation of true science: *consideration of all of the facts, and allowing those facts to verify or disprove their theories.*

Dr. Irwin Bross admitted that giving priority to fads over facts is a mistake establishments are prone to make because they have so little regard for facts. [59] Incredibly, one physician admitted the unscientific nature of Allopathic medicine by boasting that one *cannot judge by the results*.

In nothing is a wholesome skepticism more necessary than in judging of the effects of medicines by the *progress and results* of the cases in which they are employed ... [60] [Emphasis added.]

If one cannot use the results of Allopathic therapeutics to gage the correctness of the medical doctrine, what else *can* one use? The writer's position defies logic and scientific commonsense. Rejecting the data of sense perception as the final authority on the correctness of any theory, the writer adopts the fall back position of rationalism—that a medical theory is correct *because* it is rationalistically correct. Today we would recognize this as the illogic of politically correct thinking. Ladies and gentlemen of the jury, mark this well, the unscientific and unreasoning attitude of Allopathic, drug-based medicine is*: regardless of the facts, our medical therapeutics is proper because our theory of reality is right!*

The unscientific position of nineteenth century, Allopathy can be seen in the position taken by another physician of the day. He would have *his* concept of the truth judge the facts. This admission reveals that his position was the *inverse* of the empirical scientific methodology advocated by Francis Bacon.

Can we not sometimes—do we not, and very properly, judge of the truth or falsity of a doctrine by other circumstances—the general character of those who believe, the relations which it bears to known and long-established truths, and the character of the observations and reasoning by which it is attempted to be sustained? In this way we often see enough at the very threshold of an investigation to satisfy us without going any further. [61]

This admission clearly reveals that Allopathic medicine had by the mid to late nineteenth century, abandoned the Scientific Revolution of the seventeenth century and had reverted to the scholastic traditionalism of the Dark Ages. In 1888 the *New York Times* stated that the American Medical Association (AMA) forbad Allopaths from consulting with physicians who did not rely on drug cures, even if it meant the death of the patient to do so:

The AMA says that if a patient's life cannot be saved except by such a consultation, then the patient must die, and no doctor who will allow a homoeopathist to help him can be recognized by the association. [62]

Let the patient die before you consult a physician practicing alternative medicine. This is an unbelievable admission by the highest authority in established medicine. This was precisely the modus operandi of Dark Age science and medicine. Political correctness, which was also ecclesiastical correctness in mediaeval times, placed tradition over the value of life. We see modern medicine doing the same thing today. It condemns thousands to die rather than allow alternative medicine to save their lives. How blind men can be when they fall in love with their theories while ignoring the facts that undermine these theories.

Dr. Irwin Bross, that famed epidemiologist of the last century sarcastically admitted,

Today we think of a scientific tragedy as a hypothesis or theory killed by a fact. [63]

Section 3

ADMISSION: INSTANCES OF FRAUD AND BIAS IN SCIENCE AND MEDICINE.

Ladies and gentlemen of the jury, unbiased investigation has revealed frequent instances of scientific fraud in modern medicine, particularly in the treatment of chronic degenerative diseases. Past Professor of Medicine and Director of Chicago's prestigious Michael Reese Hospital, Dr. Robert Mendelsohn, made this startling admission:

> Fraud in scientific research is commonplace enough to keep it off the front pages. The Food and Drug Administration has uncovered such niceties as overdosing and under-dosing of patients, fabrication of records, and drug dumping when they investigate experimental drug trials. Of course, in these instances, doctors working for drug companies have as their goal producing results that will convince the FDA to approve the drug ... Since all the "good ol boy" researchers are in the same boat, there seems to be a great tolerance for sloppy experiments, unconformable results, and carelessness in interpreting results. [1]

Dr. Ernest Borek, a University of Colorado microbiologist admitted:

> Increasing amounts of faked data or, less flagrantly, data with *body English* put on them, make their way into scientific journals. [2]

Dr. Irwin Bross admitted that, "Fabrication of basic data is the cardinal sin of modern science." [3] This is inevitable under orthodox science and medicine. An unbiased scientific investigation into effective remedies for chronic degenerative disease will reveal that nutritional medicine produces the best results, and therefore, to maintain the primacy of pharmaceutical medicine, the scientific studies have to be rigged. This goes on more than one imagines. In support of this position, Dr. Richard W. Roberts, director of the National Bureau of Standards made this frightening admission; frightening, because life and death medical decisions and political decisions that affect public policy often ride on these false scientific findings.

Half or more of the numerical data published by scientists in their journals is unusable because there is no evidence that the researcher accurately measured what he thought he was measuring or no evidence that possible sources of error were eliminated or accounted for. [4]

Commenting on how these defective scientific findings affect the practice of medicine, Dr. Mendelsohn admitted:

Since it is almost impossible for the average reader of scientific journals to determine which half of the article is unusable and which is not, you have to wonder whether the medical journals serve as avenues of communication or confusion. [5]

Dr. William Campbell Douglass, II, related the story of how millions of Americans were duped into believing that aspirin could prevent heart attacks. The study was rigged. The evidence showed that the use of pure aspirin produces absolutely no effect in lowering the incidence of heart attacks. This is an established fact. It was published by the British in a sensational report not long ago. [6] What the American study did was to mix magnesium with the aspirin to produce Bufferin, and it was this compound that was used in their study. [7] But it is well know that magnesium *alone* dilates the blood vessels and also aids in the absorption of potassium by the body's cells thus acting as an anticoagulant. Potassium also prevents heart beat irregularities. Magnesium thus acts as a blood thinner and as an agent in preventing the blood cells from sticking together. [8] But you cannot patent magnesium, so it had to be mixed with a profit-making buffering material of no intrinsic value!

Incredibly, all of the benefits of magnesium were assigned to aspirin.

Was this simply to allow the drug companies to sell their ineffective product? You decide. After the British study came out with this sobering news that aspirin alone had no effect on reducing heart attacks, a similar study was undertaken in California. That study showed that aspirin can actually increase the odds of having a heart attack as well as kidney cancer! [9]

Ladies and gentlemen of the jury, many honest scientists and physicians report that the peer review process and scientific publications have been corrupted to support only politically correct science and medicine. Can we trust modern medical and scientific experts today, especially those in governmental agencies? Many scientists and physicians do not think so. In *The China Study*, Dr. T. Colin Campbell blew the whistle on many of his peers involved in scientific and medical research. Exposing their real motives, Dr. Campbell admitted:

> There are some in very influential government and university positions who operate under the guise of being scientific "experts" whose real jobs are to stifle open and honest scientific debate. Perhaps they receive significant personal compensation for attending to the interests of powerful food and drug companies ...

> The vast majority of scientists are honorable, intelligent and dedicated to the search for the common good rather than personal gain. However there are a few scientists who are willing to sell their souls to the highest bidder. They may not be many in number, but their influence can be vast. They can corrupt the good name of institutions of which they are a part, and, most importantly, they can create vast confusion among the public, which often cannot know who is who. [10]

Dr. Campbell further admitted that "science is not always the honest search for truth." [11] Ladies and gentlemen, the evidence suggests that scientific and medical decision making is now a well orchestrated political process and has precious little to do with truth in the scientific and medical fields. [13] Dr. Bross admitted that the peer review process which had worked well in normal science when scientists were honest, has now become the conduit for scientific fraud to shield the deadliest myth in science and medicine and history: *that low level radiation is harmless and not an agent for causing cancer.* [14] Experts reviewing the work of experts is now a recipe for fraud and corruption. Peer review now protects professionals from the review of the lay public. Dr. Bross argued that *the only viable solution to end fraud and corruption in official science is for the lay public to evaluate the activities of professionals.* [15]

Dr. Bross admitted that a corrupt peer review process and rigged scientific studies are only some of the ways the scientific and medical establishment use to steer medical research away from nutrition and prevention into the race to discover newer and smarter drugs to control the symptoms of disease they dare not cure. Exclusion of information and propaganda are other weapons used to preserve the establishment's monopoly on science and medicine. Dr. Bross cited an example of this bias involving the journal *Science*. While many scientific journals have published epidemiological and other studies exposing the fact that cancer can be triggered by low doses of so-called harmless radiation, *Science* refused to publish these studies. [16] This bias in deselecting medical material to publish is replete in the area of preventing, reversing and curing of chronic degenerative diseases. Today the scientific and medical establishment use the term *controversial* to degrade and destroy any scientific finding that disagrees with the accepted policies and protocols. But scientific validity should be based on conformity to the facts, not on whether the finding is controversial or not. [17]

Section 4

ADMISSION: THE SYMPTOMATIC TREATMENT OF DISEASE IS A FAILURE

Ladies and gentlemen of the jury, the evidence is overwhelming that the symptomatic management of chronic degenerative disease is based on the false medical and scientific assumption that disease is caused by an external agent.

Empirical science and medicine hold that disease is a result of a metabolic dysfunction and physiological impairment of the *entire* being; therefore it advocates the strengthening of the immune system so that the organism can heal itself with minimum assistance of medication. This was the guiding light of Hippocratic medicine. But the pseudo science of the medical establishment views disease as caused solely by external agents or conditions which can be targeted and eliminated by *silver-bullet* drug weapons. *The same policy is employed in the treatment of chronic degenerative disease: eliminate the symptom not the cause of the disease.*

The following admissions reveal the bankruptcy of the symptomatic treatment of chronic degenerative diseases. Dr. George Vithoulkas admitted in 1992 that the concept that disease is caused by an external agent is one of medicine's greatest illusions.

The conviction that disease is caused by bacteria is probably one of our greatest illusions. All therapeutic research today is based on this tenet; it has produced a continuous wave of new products, new medicines, at a quite incalculable cost in time, effort, health, and money. But it is based on a wrong assumption, and directed towards the wrong target ...

In homoeopathic practice, the contrary is the case. It is not at all
a question of killing bacteria but of bringing the whole human
organism into a state where it is impossible for bacteria to thrive in
it—in other words, to reduce the patient's susceptibility. [1]

As early as 1880, Boston physician Fred Moore admitted the defects of
basing medicine on pathology—it combats the *results* of diseases and not
their *causes*, he argued:

The radical defect of all therapeutics based upon pathology is that
it deals with the results of disease, and not with its cause ... it is
illogical and opposed to all experience to presume that a cause is
destroyed because its effects are neutralized. [2]

But this is precisely the methodology employed by pharmaceutical medicine in the treatment of chronic degenerative disease today: They seek to
eliminate the symptom and not the underlying cause of the disease. The
patient is still diseased and the remedy often causes other disease states to
appear. Dr. Fred Moore went on to admit that this type of symptomatic
treatment of disease is the whole basis of Allopathic therapeutics which
draws on theories from pathology, physiology and chemistry. These theories, he admitted, are "brilliant, attractive, and specious," but counterfeits,
for when they are submitted "to the touchstone of experience, they prove
to be only counterfeits." [3]

Dr. James Tyler Kent, the leading authority on Homoeopathy at the
beginning of the twentieth century, admitted in his *Lectures on Homoeopathic
Philosophy*, in 1900, that removing the cancerous mass is to remove only
the symptom of an underlying and ongoing disease process.

Yet today removing some of the symptoms of the disease and not
its cause is the modus operandi of allopathic medicine. Removing
a diseased organ or a cancerous mass is not to remove all of the
symptoms, for the diseased organ is only a symptom of a deeper
dysfunction of the body's health, the disease will only manifest
itself in some other way. [4]

Dr. James Kent explained that it is painfully obvious that the totality of
the symptoms can only be removed by eliminating the cause of the disease.
[5] Dr. George Vithoulkas underscored this point well.

There is no such thing then as a "local disease;" one may use this expression only to mean that a particular part of the body is more especially affected, but not that one organ suffers independently of the others ... For instance, in the case of a patient suffering from asthma, constipation, and rheumatic pains, today's allopathic physician will prescribe three different medicines, one for each ailment (and each one probably a combination of several drugs as well)—whereas the homeopath would prescribe a single remedy to cure the single disease which is showing itself in three aspects. [6]

Dr. Max Gerson—the twentieth century physician that many, including the great Albert Schweitzer, considered "the most eminent genius in the history of medicine" [7]—also underscored this concept that an underlying disease state may manifest itself in a cluster of diseases, requiring but a single, nutritional remedy.

Thus, the development of disease, its course and healing process, do not depend so much on the type of tissue or organ involved, but more on the general healing power of the entire organism, united or centralized in all its metabolic processes for the most part concentrated in the liver.

Contrary to this concept, our textbooks and journals have separated different diseases and even cancers as malignant tumors of the nose and paranasal sinuses ... etc., There are of course, differences in the type, development, complications, prognosis, etc., but the basic idea must be maintained that the defense and healing power is an essential part of the whole body and must be restored, whatever organ or organs may be involved or whatever cause the malignancy may have had. I repeat: *In general, the recovery from a malignancy means the restoration of the whole body from a kind of degeneration.* [8] [Emphasis added.]

Consistent with this concept of viewing disease in its totality and not as isolated, local symptoms, Dr. Gerson cited an example by defining cancer as a degenerative disease.

> Cancer is a chronic, degenerative disease, where almost all essential organs are involved in the more advanced cases ... [9]

If we ignore this fundament fact about the nature of disease, we move away from science into the old rationalistic pseudo-science. Dr. Gerson stated that to ignore the concept of totality in disease is to ignore God's law and *abandon* science.

> No wonder we are all sick ... and science is no longer science when it attempts to violate God's natural law. [10]

> Cancer, the great killer, will be prevented and can be cured, if we learn to understand the eternal laws of totality in nature and in our body. [11]

Primarily using faulty logic as their guide, the rationalistic Allopaths rejected the concept that the *totality of disease* must be taken into consideration; hence their failure to include *all the patient's* symptoms (not just the local symptoms) in diagnosis. Allopathic medicine therefore directed medicine into some harmful and fatal practices. For example, in excising the local cancer mass, much emphasis is placed upon getting clear margins while the truth is that the entire system is diseased and susceptible to a manifestation of the symptoms elsewhere. The Allopathic application of medicine to the treatment of chronic degenerative diseases is like blind men groping in the dark, while professing to have great light. Blindly they treat only a few *symptoms* and not the *cause*. Dr. Max Gerson admitted:

> Medical science has eliminated the totality of the natural biological rules in the human body, mostly by dividing research and practice into many specialties. Doing intensive, masterly specialized work, it was forgotten that every part is still only a piece of the entire body.

> In all textbooks, we find that single biological processes have been studied and overestimated statements made about them. *The symptoms of a disease have become the main problem for research, clinical work and therapy.*

The old methods which sought to combine all functional parts in a body into a biological entity, have been pushed aside almost involuntarily, in the clinic and especially in institutions of physiology and pathology ...

The opinion of the best cancer specialists is, as Jessie Greenstein stated, *"Emphasis must be laid on a direct study on the side of malignancy itself."* [12] [Emphasis added.]

Focusing upon the site of the malignancy, the tumor, and not upon the diseased organism as a whole, is predicated upon the assumption that the body *cannot* heal itself but needs some chemical intervention. Ladies and gentlemen of the jury, the testimony of all the best minds in medicine is that the body can heal itself if we cooperate with the divinely imprinted laws.

Most clinicians, long dominated by the surgical tradition, are reluctant to accept or use the concept that the healing capacity of the body, as well as its resistance to cancer, can be augmented. [13] Studies show that when body defenses are good, virulent organisms are more easily overcome by the judicious use of antibiotics. Chemotherapy and radiology in the treatment of cancer, and antiviral agents in the treatment of AIDs are also more effective when body defenses are good. [4]

Allopathic medicine holds that there is no such thing as the *natural* ability of the organism to heal itself. This is the line that separates the pharmaceutical treatment of chronic degenerative diseases from alternative and nutritional remedies. In pharmaceutical medicine, the physician, playing God, becomes the healer. In nutritional medicine, God, working through His imprinted laws, is the healer. This attitude of drug-base practitioners is clearly seen in the arrogant statement of Dr. Benjamin Rush regarding man's ability to substitute his wisdom for the vital healing power that God has placed in nature.

The time, I hope, will soon come, when the *rejection* of the powers of nature in acute and chronic disease, and greater simplicity in pathology and the materia medica, will enable us to reverse the words of Hippocrates, and to say, Arts brevis, vita longa. That is, our short, or speedily acquired art, prolongs life. [15] [Emphasis added.]

It is incredible that Rush argued for abandoning the primary principle advocated by Hippocrates in the practice of medicine, that nature heals, and substituting for it the skill of the physician using drug-treatments. Harris Coulter cited a nineteenth century author who attributed the following statement to Rush:

> As to *nature*, I would treat it in the sick-chamber as I would a squalling cat—open the door and drive it out. [16] [Emphasis added.]

In opposition to Dr. Rush's belief that nature is incompetent to heal, health educator Ellen White wrote that the physician should teach the people that there *is* restorative power in nature, not in the harmful drugs being then administered to the sick.

> Let the physician teach the people that restorative power is not in drugs, but in nature. Disease is an effort of nature to free the system from conditions that result from a violation of the laws of health. In case of sickness, the cause should be ascertained. Unhealthful conditions should be changed, wrong habits corrected. Then nature is to be assisted in her efforts to expel impurities and to re-establish right conditions in the system. [17]

The conflict between the rationalist and empirical schools over the concept that nature alone heals is as old as Hippocrates. It is a battle between lawlessness and lawful obedience to the divinely imprinted laws in nature. It is a cosmic battle being played out in the field of medicine. The dispute over the role of nature in the healing process took on new dimensions in the nineteenth century which saw the triumph of the mechanical concept of nature and of man. It was debated in the context of the religious dispute over a mechanistic evolution versus a fiat Creation. The combatants saw that if one conceded a *vital life force in living organisms*, this truth would undermine the validity of the mechanical model in science and medicine.

Dr. William Cullen understood this when he admitted that to accept the concept of a healing vital force in nature, "would at once lead us to reject all the physical and mechanical reasoning we might employ concerning the human body." [18] At the end of the nineteenth century, Ellen White wrote that God implanted the *vital force* of life in man at Creation.

God endowed man with so great vital force that he has withstood the accumulations of disease brought upon the race in consequence of perverting habits that has continued for 6,000 years. This fact of itself is enough to evidence to us the strength and electrical energy that God gave to man at his creation. It took more than two thousand years of crime and indulgence of base passions to bring bodily disease upon the race to any great extent.

If Adam, at his creation, had not been endowed with 20 times as much vital force as men now have, the race, with their present habits of living in violation of natural law, would have become extinct. [19]

Ellen White appears to be contending that it is *electrical energy* imparted to the body by God, at Creation, that is the foundation of the *vital force* in man. The impairment of this electrical/vital force opens the road to disease. This concept removes the theory of disease from the mechanical and chemical model of man proposed by the rationalistic pseudo scientists, to a vitalist model, as advocated by the empirical scientists. It is interesting that a contemporary of Ellen White, Dr. Max Gerson (1881–1959), wrote that disease and its treatment are not a matter of biochemical symptomology, but the impairment of the *electro-magnetic energies* in man. It is unknown whether Dr. Max Gerson ever met Ellen White or read her voluminous works. She was and still is the most prolific female writer in American history, so it is possible that he was aware of her works. But perhaps, without realizing it, Dr. Max Gerson was in complete agreement with Ellen White's concept of disease and its treatment. In criticizing the chemical-drug model in use in the treatment of disease, he stated:

The general approach to the treatment of patients with degenerative disease should have as its purpose the overcoming of the biochemical abnormalities which are more or less responsible for the development of the disease.

I am convinced that the problem of chronic disease is not one of biochemistry, chemistry or the symptoms we observe in and on the body. Rather, it is produced by deeper-lying forces which cause "deficiency of energies." Physicians observe biological symptoms and work only with them.

The real acting forces behind the visible chemical changes are physical energies, expressed by Einstein as the "electro-magnetic field." To a certain degree, this is closely connected with the electrical potentials which are lowered in cancer, according to almost all investigators ... and also according to the observation of Dr. Rudolf Keller ...

Here the disease starts, but not the symptoms ... We know now that what we have inherited is not a set of chemical substances, but a "pattern of dynamic energies, which directly distribute and ionize the minerals, hormones and enzymes, etc., for harmonic cooperation within the living cells and tissues, where they belong and in which way they have to act and influence the growing tissue." [20]

Ladies and gentlemen of the jury, Dr. Max Gerson made an extremely important point: *the disease process starts long before the symptoms appear.* This fact shows the folly of hoping to effectively treat the disease by attacking one or more symptoms. You may chemically manage the symptom at great cost to the integrity of the immune symptom, but you will never cure or reverse the underlying metabolic dysfunction that gave rise to the disease. The disease is more than the totality of the symptoms. Dr. Gerson quoted Paracelsus on the healing powers of nature.

Diet must be the basis of all medical therapy, yet diet should not be a treatment in itself. But it will enable Great Nature to develop and fully unfold its own healing power. [21]

Ladies and gentlemen through the decades, honest-hearted Allopaths have admitted the inefficacy of Allopathic medicine, especially in the area of managing the symptoms of chronic degenerative diseases such as cancer.
The admissions started in the nineteenth century. The success of homeopathy forced many Allopathic physicians to admit the inefficacy of their remedies. After examining the published claims, one writer stated:

The fact must be admitted that, ever and anon, diseases that have long resisted the big guns of Allopathy and even gained ground in spite of their raking fire, have quietly retreated under the milder auspices of homoeopathy. [22]

William Cobbett (1763–1835), English radical statesman and journalist who lived in Philadelphia for two years, founded a monthly journal to expose the details of the horror stories coming out of orthodox practice. He was sued by Dr. Benjamin Rush for stating that Rush's therapeutics were:

[O]ne of those great discoveries which are made from time to time for the depopulation of the earth. [23]

Truth was and still is an absolute defense against defamation. Other Europeans traveling in America were aware of the dangers of American medicine. Harris coulter cited an 1850 source that stated:

The nation as a whole began to realize that something was wrong with the general condition of its health, that these unkind criticisms on the part of foreign observers had a basis in fact. [24]

To the credit of the medical profession, there were some practitioners who revolted against the influence of the excessive practices of Dr. Benjamin Rush. A Boston physician, Dr. Elisha Bartlett recognized the irrational theories and practice of orthodox drug medicine and called a spade-a-spade in the following harsh words in 1826:

In the whole vast compass of medical literature there cannot be found an equal number of pages containing a greater amount and variety of utter nonsense and unqualified absurdity. [25]

This is a devastating admission by an Allopathic physician against their own system of medicine. The following graphic account of death by mercury poisoning was captured in the 1849 edition of the *Eclectic Medical Journal,* and constitutes a telling admission of the failure of drug medicine in its attempt to eliminate symptoms and not strengthen the immune system:

A lad named Rout, sixteen years of age, died at Covington, Ky., last week from the effects of mercury, administered ten weeks ago by a physician, to alleviate typhoid fever. The *Commercial* says: "In a few weeks purple spots made their appearance on each side of his face, followed by mortification and sloughing of the parts, the usual result of mercury poisoning when thus manifested. For several weeks the poor sufferer laid thus, the poison gradually augmenting its awful work, until the whole jaw, with the exception of a small portion of the chin, was exposed to view from the loss of surrounding flesh. The upper and lower lips were entirely gone, and the appearance was presented of a skull covered with flesh, excepting the teeth and jaws—a most pitiable sight. On the right side of the face the mortification extended to the eye, scalp, and ear, and had the youthful sufferer lived but a few days longer, he would have lost his right eye, ear, and all the flesh on the side of the face and head. But fortunately for himself and friends, death kindly came to his aid and relieved him of his misery. It is impossible for words to convey an impression of the loathsome, sickening spectacle presented above". [26]

To a candid observer the mercurial drugs were killing the patient. But the response of the physician was to administer more poison to cure the patient! The following article is taken from the *Transactions of the Rhode Island Medical Society* and was written by Dr. Henry Bowditch in 1886. It also provided a graphic admission of the failure of drug medicine.

... Calomel and other mineral drugs were abused to a fearful extent and to the infinite injury of mankind. Look at the poor wretch lying on one side for perhaps days unable to swallow even liquids without torture and with his tongue swollen to three or four times its usual size, protruded far beyond the lips intensely sore, while from its lips a constant string of adhesive and stinking mucus was discharging into a spittoon below it. Can you wonder that the stalwart irregular Thompson should have proclaimed even from the housetop: "All this is too horrible to be tolerated." [27]

Lest one dismisses those admissions to bygone times of a darker age, P. Joseph Lisa stated in *The Assault on Medical Freedom* that the Congressional Office of Technology has admitted that Allopathic, drug-based medicine which is enforced through the FDA and National Cancer Institute, is overwhelmingly ineffective today.

> [E]ven the United States government has reported that *only* 15% to 20% of allopathic medicine is effective. A report by the Congressional Office of Technology Assessment said that the rest of allopathic medicine is basically a hit-and-miss situation, that allopathic medicine's effectiveness lies in emergency medicine (trauma) and neonatal. The rest of it (80% - 85%) according to the study *is not effective*. Yet America is paying out hundreds of billions of dollars for something that is only 15% to 20% effective. [28] [Emphasis added.]

Dr. Robert Mendelsohn, professor of medicine at the University of Illinois Medical School, spoke with some authority when he admitted in 1979 that the present orthodox and so-called *proven* methods of treating cancer are irrational and will one day be recognized as such.

> The entire field of orthodox oncology will disappear as well as chemotherapy, surgery and radiation for cancer as irrational and scientifically unsupportable. [29]

In *Bad Medicine*, Dr. Douglass made the following admissions about the effects of drugs deemed safe by the FDA:

* Each year 61,000 older Americans develop drug-induced Parkinsonism.

* 32,000 hip fractures are caused by drug-induced falls.

* 163,000 Americans develop drug-induced memory loss or impaired thinking.

* More than 243,000 over the age of 55 are hospitalized each year because of adverse drug reactions.

* More than 2 million older Americans are addicted to minor tranquilizers and/or sleeping pills. [30]

Dr. Douglass admitted that the grim harvest of woe and death from prescription drugs is much worse, but we will never know the true tragic tale this side of eternity. One reason is that many doctors assign other reasons for death, rather than implicate drugs. Furthermore no autopsies are performed in the majority of cases. Dr. Douglass further admitted:

As you can see, prescription drugs can raise havoc in many ways. In fact, adverse reactions and addiction are all too common, especially in people over age 50. And often the result is death, but the death certificate may read *heart attack* or *stroke* because autopsies are seldom done on the elderly. In other words, no one knows what millions of these older people actually die from. [31] [Emphasis added.]

Dr. Robert Mendelsohn also admitted that "Doctors do not report drug deaths." [32] This suppression of the truth is destroying America's health. It is high time it stopped and poisonous drugs exposed for just what they are—poisons. Ladies and gentlemen of the jury, all drugs are poisons, whose exact mode of operation is not always known and they possess side effects, the extent of which is also not always known. All drugs are poisons; Dr. Andrew Weil admitted this fact in 1983 when he wrote in *Health and Healing*;

Because I have made a special study of drugs in the course of my professional career, I have a lot to say about them.

Pharmacology is the science of drugs. That word [pharmacology] also comes from Greek, derived from an ancient term for poison. The first point I must emphasize is that the only difference between a drug and a poison is dose ... Toxicity (poisoning) from drugs is their great drawback, and allopathic medicine now produces a tremendous amount of it. Adverse drug reactions account for the lion's share of iatrogenic (doctor caused) illness. [33]

Eli Lilly admits that "a drug without a toxic effect is no drug." [34] The

Physician's Desk Reference, the bible for drug medicine, made this admission about the mysterious action of drugs, "Nalfon is a non-steroidal, anti-inflammatory, anti-arthritic drug that also possesses analgesic and antipyretic activities. *Its exact mode of action is unknown,* but it is thought that prostaglandin synthesis inhibition is involved." [Emphasis added] [35] Dr. Robert Mendelsohn also admitted that physicians do not always know how drugs work. [36] Producing effects is not the same as understanding the mechanism involved and equally unknown is the mechanisms which provide the expected and unknowable side effects.

Even if the drug companies have greater knowledge on *how* their drugs work in the body, they do not always correctly predict their side effects or even anticipate some of them. Dr. Douglass admitted:

> With alarming frequency, drugs cause serious and often fatal side effects that the drug makers and the FDA were unable to identify before the drug was approved. This was the conclusion of a report from the General Accounting Office of your government. [37]

So can we trust FDA approved drugs for safety? Definitely not, was the admission of Dr. Brian Strom.

> People have this very important misconception that drugs are safe when they are FDA approved. [38]

What percentage of drugs have serious adverse side effects? And how many people are to the point of needing hospitalization? The answer will alarm you.

> According to Dr. Brian Strom, a leading specialist in pharmaco-epidemiology, 20 percent of all drug therapies cause adverse side effects ranging from nausea to fatal ailments. Side effects put an estimated 1.6 million people in the hospital yearly. Up to 160,000 of these patients die. Hospital costs from these disasters amount to $20 billion yearly. [39]

The regulatory bodies ignore this epidemic of death and disease caused by the non-emergency use of poisonous drugs, yet they will excoriate the nutritionist physician who may never have harmed a patient in all the years of his practice. Is this a double standard? You be the judge.

Pharmaceutical medicine is indeed costly, both in money and health. Another area of damage in the use of drugs is drug interactions that cause mysterious illness and often death. What is worse the doctor may think the effects of drug interactions are just more symptoms to be treated by yet more drugs! This was precisely the situation with the use of the deadly mercuric drugs of the last century. Has pharmaceutical medicine advance at all beyond this cycle of entrapment? Many experts do not think so.

Many doctors don't pay enough attention to drug interactions. They go on happily prescribing more drugs for what they see as more illnesses. The circle is complete; the patient is trapped. [40]

One feels hopeless before the ominous words: "The circle is complete; the patient is trapped."

Ladies and gentlemen of the jury, the testimony by unbiased researchers have admitted that drug-based medicine is ineffective in curing chronic degenerative diseases and often makes the condition worse, even precipitating the death of the patient.

Consider the testimony of Dr. Robert S. Mendelsohn. For many years he was a professor at the University of Illinois Medical School, Director of Chicago's Michael Reese Hospital, Director of Project Head Start, and chairman of the Medical Licensure Committee for the state of Illinois, before he became "The People's Doctor" in his nationally syndicated column which ran for many years. In his eye-opening book, *Confessions of a Medical Heretic*, he made the following admission about the inefficacy of modern medicines, particularly in the treatment of chronic degenerative diseases:

I believe that modern medicine's treatments for diseases are seldom effective, *and that they are often more dangerous than the diseases they are designed to treat.* [41] [Emphasis added.]

Amazing admission coming from a professor of a prestigious medical school! Reflecting the opinion of many physicians through the decades, including Supreme Court justice Oliver Wendell Holmes, Dr. Mendelsohn further admitted:

I believe that more than 90% of modern medicine could disappear from the face of the earth—doctors, hospitals, drugs, and equipment—and the effect on our health would be immediate and beneficial. [42]

This statement was made by the late justice Oliver Wendell Holmes, so it cannot be assigned to ignorance or to hysterical bias. Justice Holmes was willing to indict medicine to a far greater extent that this trial undertakes to do. If you, the jury, were to hand down a finding of indictment against the medical cartel in this trial, you could rest assured you would be in the company of one of America's finest jurists. What is more striking is that this opinion or prophecy was fulfilled in the medical history of three countries. In Columbia, Israel and California deaths from doctor-induced illness fell when there was a doctors' strike in those countries! Dr. Mendelsohn reported:

In 1976 in Bogota, Colombia, there was a fifty-two-day period in which doctors disappeared altogether except for emergency care. The "National Catholic Reporter" described "a string of unusual side effects" from the strike. The death rate went down thirty-five percent. A spokesman for the National Mortifications Association said, "it might be a coincidence but it is a fact." [43]

Lest one think this is a phenomenon of third-world medicine, a similar occurrence happened in Los Angeles, California.

An eighteen percent drop in the death rate occurred in Los Angeles County in 1976 when doctors there went on strike to protest soaring malpractice insurance premiums. Dr. Milton Roemer, Professor of Health Care Administration at UCLA, surveyed seventeen major hospitals and found that sixty percent fewer operations were performed. When the strike ended and the medical machine machines started grinding again, the death rate went right back up to where it had been before the strike. [44]

A more pronounced drop in death rates occurred in Israel in 1953 and 1973 as a result of doctor strikes. Commenting on the 1973 doctors' strike in Israel, Dr. Mendelsohn admitted:

The strike lasted a month. According to the Jerusalem Burial Society, the Israeli death rate dropped fifty percent during that month. There had not been such a profound decrease in mortality since the last doctors' strike twenty years before. [45]

We tend to think that doctors are the ministers of life and health. But the sad fact is that their capitulation to the pharmaceutical industry has transformed them into ministers of mayhem and death in too many instances. They no longer dispense health; they merely *manage* chronic diseases, being careful not to cure the patient lest business dries up. Consider this admission by Dr. Mendelsohn:

> Modern medicine does not address itself to health, for it does not believe a person can do anything about staying healthy. [46]

Dr. Andrew Weil, in *Natural Health, Natural Medicine*, also admitted that Allopathic drug-oriented medicine is ineffective in treating chronic degenerative diseases. In 1995 he admitted:

> In short, allopathic medicine is very good at managing trauma, acute bacterial infections, medical and surgical emergencies, and other crises. It is very bad at managing viral infections, chronic degenerative diseases, allergy and auto-immunity, many of the serious kinds of cancer, mental illness, etc [47]

Dr. Mendelsohn agreed. He made these two startling admissions about the deadly effects of applying Allopathic drug-based medicine:

> The doctor, once the agent of cure, has become the agent of disease. By going too far and diffusing the power of the extreme on the mean, modern medicine has weakened and corrupted even the management of extreme cases. The miracle I and other doctors were once proud to take part in has become a miracle of mayhem. [48]

> Doctor prescribed drugs kill more people than street drugs. [49]

Ladies and gentlemen of the jury, when was the last time you heard such a statement from the FDA ? Perhaps never. You will never hear these devastating admissions about Allopathic medicine in the media. They are part of the program to perpetuate the pharmaceutical monopoly of medicine.

Drugs have proven to be dangerous and even lethal, when drugs are used whose symptoms are the same as the disease. Dr. Mendelsohn advised us to beware of these class of drugs. One cannot tell which symptoms are genuine, requiring treatment, and which are the side effects of the drug! Again the patient is trapped. And who wins? Certainly not the patient! The drug companies do. This is the height of insanity. As the symptoms increase due to the drug side effects, more drugs are administered. [50] This is no longer the practice of medicine. Is there a profit motive? You be the judge.

Section 5

ADMISSION: THE WAR ON CANCER IS A "BLOODY ROUT"

We are not only losing the war against cancer, it's a bloody rout.

Michael Colgan, Ph. D.

Ladies and gentlemen of the jury, unbiased investigation reveals that radiation therapy not only fails to prevent cancer, it creates cancer, and is one of the causes of the epidemic of breast and prostate cancer today.

Does radiation therapy help cancer victims? Allow Dr. Irwin Bross to answer this question.

> There is very little factual evidence that there are any benefits to cancer patients from the role of radiologists in the medical management of cancer. Rather the importance of radiologists in cancer or cancer research is largely based on medical mythology—on the deadliest myth and any number of collateral myths about the value of radiology. [1]

Dr. Irwin Bross stated that the myth that low level radiation is harmless got a flying start at Crossroads and became the deadliest scientific myth in human history. [2] Then he made this serious admission in *Fifty Years of Folly and Fraud in the Name of Science*:

> The NCI payoff to radiologists and oncologists for supporting the myth resulted in a series of new cancer epidemics. [3]

How did radiation therapy cause an epidemic of new cancer deaths? Dr. Bross stated that the biggest payoff to the radiologists was the mass screening by mammography (the historic *Breast Cancer Detection Demonstration Project)* despite warnings that the radiation would increase cancer among the women screened. The evidence showed that the project did indeed identify cancer—at an alarming rate for it was the causative agent in much of the breast cancer it was detecting! [4]

Dr. Bross noted that the National Cancer Institute refused to do follow-up studies on women exposed to mammography to determine if it was effective. But the Canadians did. A randomized Canadian study showed that screening by mammography did nothing to reduce the deaths from breast cancer. What the statistical results reported in the *Lancet*, a leading British medical journal, showed was that there were actually significantly *more* deaths from breast cancer in the Canadian women under fifty-five who had been screened! [5] While the original study was designed to show how great mammography was, it actually demonstrated significantly more deaths from iatrogenic devices such a radiation and chemotherapy. [6]

Dr. Bross had predicted in several scientific journals that the NCI program would cause an epidemic in breast cancer. Because of the long latent period of cancer growth it was not until 1992 that his prediction was verified by studies yielding solid scientific proof. [7] The facts revealed that treatment of breast cancer was *worse than the disease*, for it actually speeded up the disease process. [8] Research showed that mutagenic treatment can convert latent cancer into metastatic cancer; and this is how the NCI programs in the 1970s caused an epidemic of cancer and cancer deaths Dr. Bross observed. [9]

Dr. Robert Mendelsohn also admitted that x-rays have been linked to diabetes, cardiovascular disease, stroke, high blood pressure, cataracts, cancers, and tumors of the central nervous system. [10] He also admitted that childhood leukemia was linked to prenatal radiation, [11] and that mammography would cause more breast cancer than it will detect because of the latent period for cancer growth. [12]

Dr. Bross explained why there is a lag between radiation treatment and the discovery of the deadly harvest of new cancers caused by it. Since cancer is mutagenic, low levels of radiation or chemotherapy are not harmless, but cause cancer. [13] But a cancer cell needs thirty-two doublings before it can be detected. Thus the cancer mass is first seen only after sixteen years. Ten to twenty years, depending on the rate of doublings in each individual. [14]

Ladies and gentlemen of the jury, unbiased investigation has revealed that chemotherapy frequently activates the cancer it is supposed to kill and is 100% *ineffective against metastatic cancer.*

In the 1960s chemotherapy had as its goal killing every last tumor cell. [15] This brute force approach meant that the dosage was raised until the patient was on the brink of death in order to kill every last tumor cell. Dr. Bross admitted that this goal was not achieved for studies showed that the drug would kill the patient long before the last tumor cell was killed, and so the patient was often pushed to the brink of death and even death. [16] But even at the death of the patient the reason assigned for failure was insufficient dosages were given ! [17]

Dr. Bross admitted that clinical studies clearly showed that the higher doses were counterproductive; but as is almost inevitable in medical establishments, he continued, mere statistical facts were never a deterrent to folly when this folly happened to be highly profitable to the establishment. [18] Dr. Bross sadly lamented that despite its inherent absurdity, *heroic chemotherapy* quickly became the dominant U. S. Doctrine for cancer therapy in the cancer establishment. [19]

As the nation's ranking epidemiologist, Dr. Irwin Bross was thickly enmeshed in cancer research, so he was in a position to know and assess the facts. He admitted that although there were numerous claims of success for the chemotherapy of major solid tumors at the time of the first *Adjuvant Study* (1960s) that he led out in, *none of them were valid claims.* Neither chemotherapy nor radiation had shown much value for the major solid cancers. [20] Rather, Dr. Bross admitted, the NCI's policies transformed the benign cancers into malignant forms by their radiation and chemotherapy. [21]

> Treatment does not benefit those with latent or benign cancer and is not necessary. Treatment does not benefit metastasized cancer [and it is equally unnecessary.] [22]

The survival rate for metastasized cancer is three years. Numerous studies show that it makes no difference for their survival if metastatic patients receive orthodox treatment, alternative treatment or no treatment at all. [23]

Ladies and gentlemen of the jury, unbiased investigation has revealed that surgery not only fails to cure cancer, it often promotes the spread of cancer, at best it removes only the symptom of cancer, the visible mass, but does nothing to reverse the underlying cause, the metabolic and immune dysfunction of the organism.

Dr. Raymond Brown observed that cancer has traditionally been considered an uncontrolled tissue growth which originates in a single cell and spreads to overwhelm the body with its parasitic overgrowths. This conception of a malign autonomous process has dominated medical thinking so that classic therapy has been largely surgical, seeking early recognition and complete extirpation of the tumor before its roots have penetrated and its tendrils have spread. In the United States, this philosophy has been the basis for the popularity among surgeons of radical mastectomy for breast cancer despite the physical and psychic mutilation of the patient. [24]

Ladies and gentlemen of the jury, Dr. Irwin Bross admitted that at the turn of the twentieth century, modified mastectomy was shown to give equally good results as radical mastectomy, but physicians preferred to continue with radical surgery for professional pride and economic reasons. [25] Thus from 1900 to 1960 radical mastectomy remained the treatment of choice for breast cancer until the *Adjuvant Study* showed its uselessness and it was virtually abandoned. But Dr. Bross admitted that what replaced it, surgery and radiation in combination, was worse. [26]

Dr. George Moon discovered that surgery can spread cancer. But he then advocated chemotherapy to kill these dispersing cancer cells. But Dr. Bross admitted that this only worked where the cancer had not yet spread. [27] While improved radiation technology made possible the selective destruction of cancer cells, radiation doses still had to be limited by damage to adjacent tissue. [28] However Dr. Brown admitted that the therapeutic benefit of surgery, radiation and chemotherapy has been counterbalanced by their toxic and often delayed side effects. Use of these modalities had obscured the evidence that cancer is essentially a chronic disease. [29]

Consider the opinion of Dr. Max Gerson, who first began to investigate nutritional cures to cancer after a London doctor suggested to him that surgery might contribute to the growth of cancer rather than eradicate it. After a period of investigation and experimentation, he discovered that cancer was a disease of the whole body and that nutrition helped the whole body to fight it. Many patients came to him terminally ill after receiving no help from the orthodox methods, and he cured many of them.

In some cases their former doctors destroyed their records so that these could not be used to independently corroborate Dr. Gerson's successes. [30]

Dr. Michael Feldman and colleagues at the Weizmann Institute in Israel corroborated earlier findings in America regarding the risks of cancer surgery. They also discovered that surgery can spread cancer and spur the growth of deadly metastatic cells which are actually inhibited by the tumor itself. [31] Deep surgery was also thought to entail massive shock which upset the natural immune system which could overcome the disorder in many cases. [32]

Ladies and gentlemen of the jury, the National Cancer Society's War against Cancer has not only failed, it has produced cancer epidemics according to their own statistics and records.

Dr. Irwin Bross admitted that the NCI's own statistics show that there has been little or no actual advance in the treatment of the major solid cancers since the 1970s. [33] When the incidence of cancer in 1973 (the date the NCI's war on cancer began), is compared with the incidence of cancer for the year 1986 (allowing for fourteen years of mutagenic incubation), the NCI statics revealed that all the five solid cancers examined had significant increases, except for colon cancer which increased at a slower rate [34].

Type of Cancer	1973	1986	% Increase
All cancers	318.60	365.30	15
Lung (female)	17.90	37.00	107
Prostate	62.40	87.70	41
Breast	83.80	107.30	28
Lung (male)	72.50	80.30	11
Colon Rectum	46.80	50.30	7

Dr. Bross drew the following conclusion from these statistics:

Thus, NCI's own statistics show that the cancer problem today
is far worse than it was when the NCI's "Conquest of Cancer"
program began in the 1970s. NCI's "prevention programs have
been worse than a total fiasco." [35]

Specifically addressing the significant increase in breast and prostate cancers since 1973, Dr. Irwin Bross admitted that they may reflect doctor
induced (iatrogenic) cancer. This was particularly true for routine radiation screening for breast cancer. The radiation itself induced an epidemic
of new cancer cases in women. Dr. Bross observed:

The other two [breast and prostate] may reflect iatrogenic
epidemics caused by mutagenic medical modalities promoted in
NCI's "Conquest of Cancer" programs. In sum: NCI's prevention
programs have not only failed to prevent cancer, they may have
caused tens of thousands of excess new cases of cancer every year.
[36]

Dr. Bross further admitted that progress in cancer prevention was virtually halted in the 1970s after the "Conquest of Cancer" program began
because the NCI stopped funding any study that found positive radiological effects on the incidence of cancer. Before that date, the NCI actively
encouraged and funded studies of the health effects of low-level ionizing
radiation and from medical diagnostic x-rays. [37]

The first major investigation of cancer cures ever done in the U.S. was
performed by Robert Houston and Gary Hull. The study is known as the
Houston-Hull Analysis, and it was performed in 1978–1979. Their research
led them to conclude that Nixon's War against cancer was a hopeless failure. They were puzzled by this finding considering the billions that were
spent on the program. They speculated that the reason for the lack of
progress on finding a cure for cancer was that:

A solution to cancer would mean the termination of research
programs, the obsolescence of skills, the end of dreams of personal
glory; triumph over cancer would dry up contributions to self-
perpetuating charities and cut off funding from Congress, it would
mortally threaten the present clinical establishment by rendering

obsolete the expensive surgical, radiological and chemotherapeutic treatments in which so much money, training and equipment is invested. [38]

Of course almost every important newspaper refused to run the results of the analysis. The *Houston-Hull Analysis* uncovered that the "war on cancer" was a screen for the real war against alternative cancer treatments by the medical establishment in league with governmental agencies.

The American Cancer Society, as the medical church of the current Dark Age of cancer, has managed to blacklist the most innovative and promising lines of cancer research. The FDA, obedient to policy positions of the AMA and ACS, has added muscle to the witch hunt, harassing and prosecuting proponents of alternative therapies, and road-blocking all reasonable attempts at fair testing. The truth eventually must be confronted that the real enemy is not cancer—a natural phenomenon—but the cancer establishment itself, which consistently moves to destroy whatever is hopeful against the disease, and to enlarge its predatory position as a parasite on human suffering. [39]

Ladies and gentlemen of the jury, support for their conclusions came from an unlikely source, the archives of the NCI itself! Dr. Dean Burk, Head of Cytochemistry Section of the National Cancer Institute, made several revealing admissions in a 1973 letter to Dr. Frank Rauscher, then Director of the National Cancer Institute.

I would submit that no less than six, at the very least, of the ACS's 'Unproven Methods' would be worthy of immediate scientific investigation by the NCI on a basis of non-toxic but potential efficacy. [40]

FDA approved anti-cancer drugs are toxic, immunosuppressive and carcinogenic [41]

Virtually all the conventional anti-cancer drugs had been found to cause cancer in NCI's own studies. [42]

Dr. Dean Burk was not a whistle blower. He was a loyal member of the NCI but an honest and impartial medical scientist. If he was correct that the NCI's anti-cancer drugs were themselves causing cancer, it was not surprising that the cancer treatments were a failure. Ladies and gentlemen of the jury, consider well the final appeal that Houston and Hull made to the American public.

> Right now, our generals in the battle against cancer are inept. The guns of the medical petrochemical complex are pointed in the wrong direction—straight at us. We must demand our most inalienable right, the right to life—and, therefore, to health. [43]

Dr. Irwin Bross admitted that the war on cancer itself may constitute medical fraud.

> Most of the hundreds of billions now spent for cancer care are going for treatments that are at best worthless and often constitute medical fraud. [44]

Ladies and gentlemen, Dr. Irwin Bross asked a very sobering rhetorical question to provoke us to serious thought—if there is scientific evidence about the dismal failure of the vast majority of the current cancer treatments, why do doctors continue to give these treatments and why do patients continue to accept them? Bross answered his own question for us. He stated that the answer is that patients put their faith in the prestige of the institutions behind the "war on cancer" programs.

> These [cancer] treatments are supported by official government agencies such as the NCI and by pillars of the cancer establishment, such as the American Cancer Society and by the American College of Radiologists and by the mass media. [45]

Dr. Bross charged that although it has been scientifically demonstrated over the last thirty-five years that radiological and chemical mutagens cause cancer, the National Cancer Institute has done nothing effective to protect the public. On the contrary, he pointed out, the NCI has played a key role in the cover-up of the health hazards of their treatment protocols since 1957. To make matters worse, the NCI has taken lines of action that make the public health problem more severe. [46]

Dr. Brown observed that the overuse and misuse of chemotherapy and radiation in cancer are comparable to the overuse and misuse of antibiotics in medicine. Someday, he prophesized, these barbaric methods will be viewed as we now view the treatment of war wounds before Ambroise Pare (the fifteenth-century French surgeon whose humane treatment of injuries abolished the use of boiling oil that had previously been standard therapy) or the late eighteenth-century practice of bleeding and purging terminally ill patients, such as was done to President George Washington. [47]

Ladies and gentlemen of the jury, the testimony throughout this trial has revealed that some of the best minds in medical science have advocated a return to the nutritional modalities practiced by Hippocrates and other medical geniuses though the centuries. But the testimony is also abundantly clear that some of the best minds within the cancer establishment have admitted the failure of the so-called proven, but hopelessly inefficacious methods advocated by conventional medicine. Consider the testimony of Dr. James Watson, another Nobel Prize winner. Criticizing the War on cancer James Watson, Director of Cold Spring Harbor Laboratory, admitted at a symposium in 1975 at MIT, that "The American public is being sold a nasty bill of goods about cancer." [48]

Hans Ruesch observed that despite the recognition that the majority of cancers are linked to nutritional causes less than 1% of the NCI budge is devoted to nutritional studies; and even that small amount had to be force upon the NCI by the special amendment to the National Cancer Act in 1974. [49] He also accused the medical establishment of closing their doors to nutritional cures:

> The directed research practices and other activities of the National Cancer institute and of the American Cancer Society have been scandalously counterproductive in the conquest of cancer, in spite of the billions of dollars expended. The cancer establishment is closed to new approaches and ideas, thus creating a self-perpetuating system with no clear objective even remotely insight. [50]

If cancer treatments are useless or counterproductive—why is it that some cancer patients *seem* to do well and others poorly? Ladies and gentlemen of the jury, this is a very important issue. You must consider carefully the testimony of Dr. Irvin Bross on this critical issue for it exposes many of the false claims for "cures" by the cancer establishment.

> Doctors fail to distinguish between tumors that have not yet metastasized (which cannot kill you) and those that have already metastasized. [51]

Bross argued that the *two-disease model for* cancer can explain a lot of the confusion over claims for cancer cures. The thing to grasp is that there are two kinds of breast cancer—one highly malignant and the other virtually benign. Both look similar to a pathologist. However *more than half* of the tumors diagnosed as *early breast cancers* were really cancers of the benign form. It is the same with prostate cancer for men. Dr. Bross stated that this type of benign cancer needed no treatment, and he backed it up with some very impressive evidence. [52] In 1992 a Swedish study reported in the *Journal of the American Medical Association* revealed that the ten-year survival rate for male prostate cancer is 86.8%. The reason: About 80% of prostate cancer is latent, un-metastasized tumors with a certain risk of local growth but no metastatic potential. [53] In the U.S. the NCI reported survival rate of 76% for breast and 74% for prostate cancers. Dr. Bross contends that what is being detected is latent un-metastasized cancer which does not need treatment. [54]

Dr. Bross further argued that treatment does not benefit those with latent cancer and is not necessary. Treatment does not benefit metastasized cancer and it is equally unnecessary. [55] Dr. Bross warned that the NCI's policies transformed the benign cancers to the malignant forms by their radiation and chemotherapy. [56]

Ladies and gentlemen of the jury, medical experts admit that the treatment of Chronic Degenerative Diseases with pharmaceutical drugs, does not cure the disease, is often ineffective, often aggravates the problem, and is often worse than the disease.

Dr. Bross admitted that the medical administration pedals false hope by their symptomatic treatment of chronic diseases:

> The basic fact of life that the U.S. healthcare system and most Americans have refused to face is this: for the vast majority of cancer patients there is no good treatment. This grim situation is not unique for cancer. For a number of the major chronic disease,

there is no good treatment. The medical [establishment] covers this simple truth by peddling false hope. [57]

Dr. Robert Mendelsohn also admitted that "Modern medicine neutralizes the effect of preventive action by ignoring the true causes of disease." [58] And often the remedy exacerbates the problem. For example the December 23/24, 1978, issue of the *International Heralds Tribune* reported on a study in Germany of the cholesterol lowering drug Atromid S which revealed that users did not have fewer fatal heart attacks than comparable non-users. Rather, the finding was *Atromid S users in the study had a sharply higher rate of deaths from cancer and other diseases*—principally of the liver, gall bladder and intestines. [59] It has now become known that Urethane used to cure leukemia causes cancer of the liver, lungs and bone marrow. [60]

Cyclo-phosphamide, another drug used to fight cancer, provokes widespread necrosis which starts in the liver and the lungs and usually kills the patient much sooner than the cancer would. [61] In light of these and similar facts, Bross commented that the enormous waste of money in cancer research and treatment is largely responsible for the present healthcare crisis. One-third of the money spent on healthcare goes for cancer and other chronic diseases where there is currently on good treatment. [62] If insurance payments were made only for treatments that provided benefits, this waste would stop. [63] Our healthcare budget has now exceeded the $2 trillion mark annually.

Dr. Robert Brown observed that in 1969 there was much perplexity when Dr. Hardin Jones, a reputable statistician at the University of California, reported that *statistically the life expectancy of cancer patients is greater without treatment.* [64] He contended that this remarkable conclusion is probably explained by the depression of our reticulo-endothelial systems from well meant but imperceptive use of therapeutic technology; we have used meat cleavers instead of dissection knives. It may be that Ivan Illich's thesis of the illness-producing capacity of modern medicine is best illustrated in the cancer field.

While Dr. Hardin Jones was a professor of Medical Physics and Physiology at Berkeley, California, he performed his famous twenty-five-year study of cancer onset and treatment. He reported to the *Science Writer's Seminar* sponsored by the ACS in 1969, that,

> Untreated cancer patients do not die sooner than patients getting the full conventional cut-burn-poison treatment *approved* by the medical establishment, rather in many case they live longer. [65] [Emphasis added.]

Ladies and gentlemen of the jury, this is a very important piece of testimony. It is not an aberrant isolated study. The study has been confirmed by three other studies. [66] Unbelievably, Dr. Jones and others report that the survival in breast cancer is four times longer without conventional treatment.

> People who refused treatment lived for an average of 12.5 years. Those who accepted surgery and other kinds of treatment lived an average of only 3 years. Beyond the shadow of a doubt, radical surgery on cancer patients does more harm than good. [67]

Ladies and gentlemen, you will not hear this sobering admission from the medical establishment. You will not hear it from the elite media who get their large and obscene advertizing revenues from the pharmaceutical industries. You will not hear it from governmental agencies who are promoting the pharmaceutical monopoly in medicine and who have long ceased to protect you. It rest with you to make this testimony known to your sisters, wives, mothers and daughters. Their lives may very well depend on it.

Section 6

ADMISSION: NUTRITIONAL MEDICINE IS ADVOCATED BY MEDICAL GENIUSES

Ladies and gentlemen of the jury, members of the medical establishment have admitted that empirical and nutritional medicine is advocated by some of the best minds and even medical geniuses in medicine.

Although the controversy between pharmaceutical and nutritional medicine began with Hippocrates, the concerted attack on nutritional medicine began in earnest in 1847 after the minority of doctors practicing pharmaceutical medicine formed the American Medical Association, a closed-knit union of Allopathic doctors whose goal was to eliminate the completion and create a medical monopoly for pharmaceutical medicine. They succeed in this endeavor when they formed an alliance with the emerging petro-chemical industry at the beginning of the twentieth century. The Allopathic doctors first began their attack against Homoeopathy which was the dominant type of medicine practiced in the mid to late nineteenth century. It was a turf war between two completely opposite philosophies about disease and healthcare.

But amid this war of words and yellow journalism, many Allopathic doctors admitted that their enemy was in many cases superior to them in learning and ability. Hence we find in the mid nineteenth century an Allopathic physician admitting the high learning of the Homoeopathic physicians.

So far as my knowledge of them extends, they are the flower of the profession. Men of talents and worth. Men, too, who have been well educated in the profession and had acquired a good reputation in the practice of medicine according to old school orthodoxy—but who were driven to a change of views and practice by the observation of facts. [1]

This admission not only extols the practitioners of alternative medicine, but unintentionally indicts Allopathy as unscientific, due to its disregard of the facts, the very backbone of good scientific medicine. No less a figure than Sir John Forbes recognized the revolutionary genius of Hahnemann and the scientific system of medicine that he devised. Sir John Forbes admitted that Hahnemann was:

A man of genius ... a very extraordinary man ... founder of an original system of medicine ... destined probably to be the remote, if not the immediate, cause of more important fundamental changes in the practice of the healing art that have resulted from any promulgated since the days of Galen himself. In the history of medicine his name will appear in the same list with those of the greatest systematists and theorists. [2]

In 1911 Dr. J. N. McCormack, the leader of the AMA's drive to absorb Homoeopathy, admitted in very unambiguous language, the economic motive for the war against alternative medicine.

We must admit that we have never fought the homoeopaths on matters of principle; we fought him because he came into the community and got the business. [3]

Harris Coulter quoted a number of nineteenth-century physicians who recognized the serious threat of Homoeopathy to Allopathic medicine.

... a revolution in science is to follow their reception, and a new system is to be based upon their assumptions. [4]

If Hahnemann be true, then all the past recorded experience of physicians from time immemorial is to be thrown away with all past theories. [5]

This admission is over-broad. What is overthrown is centuries of drug-based medicine; and what is affirmed is centuries of nutrition-based medicine which has followed in the foot-steps of Hippocrates. The next admission, taken from the *Boston Medical and Surgical Journal,* recognized that the real issue was which of the two medical models was truly scientific and hence true medical practice? Both could not be true. With Allopathy clearly admitting that it does not take *all* of the symptoms into consideration in deriving its therapeutics, the decision is not hard to make: *only that medical model which follows Sir Francis Bacon's emphasis on building theories on all the facts of experience is truly scientific medicine.* The *Journal* admitted:

> If we establish the truth of either, the utter fallacy of the other is equally proven. They are wide asunder as the poles, and the *middle ground* would prove as impracticable and untenable as a farm in Symmes' Hole. [6]

Ladies and gentlemen of the jury, although the NCI, ACS and FDA would have us believe that alternative cancer cures come from unqualified charlatans, *a study showed that fully* 80% *of these nutritional experts were physicians, biochemists and biologists of the first rank,* many of them like Dr. Morvyth McQueen-Williams and Dr. Max Gerson, acclaimed medical geniuses by their peers. [7] Partial lists of the medical geniuses who have embraced nutritional medicine after Hippocrates are as follows:

Foremost among these nutritional physicians was the great Paracelsus (1493–1541) who is now recognized as the Father of modern medicine.

The Dutch physician Hermann Boerhaave (1668–1738) was without peer in his day. You may recall that he once received a letter from China hailing him as the most famous physician in Europe. [8]

Thomas Sydenham (1624–1689) in England who advocated a return to the scientific empiricism of Hippocrates in medicine must also be added to the list of medical geniuses. Giorgio Baglivi (1668–1707) modeled his medical science after Sydenham, and he called him the "profoundest observer after Hippocrates." [9]

Another medical genius who abandoned chemical-based medicine for the pure Hippocratic medicine was German Professor of Medicine, Georg Ernst Stahl (1660–1734). Referring to Stahl's attempts to cleanse medical practice of the harmful influence of the chemical drug-based model of medicine, Theophile Bordeu stated this was the, "dream of Stahl ... the dream of one of the greatest geniuses medicine has ever known." [10]

Finally a biochemist of the highest rank who has received belated recognition is Dr. Antoine Bechamp (1816–1908), physician, scientist and
biologist. He discovered the pleomorphic nature of antigens. His work
discredited the theory that the germ or antigen caused the disease. He
demonstrated that it was the metabolic dysfunction of the organism
resulting in abnormal blood acidity that transforms benign organisms into
pathogens. Pharmaceutical medicine dares not acknowledge his revolutionary findings for it will utterly discredit their regime of treating only
the external symptoms of chronic degenerative diseases.

We must not overlook Dr. Linus Pauling (1901–1994), who received
Ph. Ds in physical chemistry and mathematical physicists *Summa Cum
Laude* in 1925. Among the many awards and prizes for his work in physics
and chemistry and medicine he twice received the Nobel peace prize for
his work in chemistry and medicine. Dr. Pauling was recognized as the
Father of Molecular Biology and the Founder of Quantum Chemistry.
When the British Magazine *New Scientist* drew up their list of the twenty
greatest scientists of all time, they chose Albert Einstein and Dr. Linus
Pauling to represent the twentieth century. Dr. Pauling was a strong advocate of nutritional medicine. Although the American medical establishment may have despised his work in nutritional medicine, the two Nobel
peace prizes and numerous other prizes he was awarded are a more prestigious endorsement of his worth and integrity.

Section 7

ADMISSION: THE PETRO-CHEMICAL INDUSTRY CONTROLS MEDICINE

Ladies and gentlemen of the jury, the modern medical establishment and their Cartel partners admit that medicine is under the control and direction of the Petro-chemical Industry.

Several decades ago Duncan Roads remarked in the *Nexus New Times* that "The Rockefellers own more than half of the pharmaceutical industry in America." [1] Eustace Mullins, in *Murder by Injection*, exposed the funding of medical schools by the owners of pharmaceutical companies in order to influence the direction and content of medical education.

Rockefeller's General Education Board has spent more than $100 million to gain control of the nation's medical schools and turn our physicians into physicians of the allopathic school, dedicated to surgery and the heavy use of drugs. [2]

Eustace Mullins went on to sum up the monopolistic control that Rockefeller interests have achieved over cancer research and treatment. To our knowledge this assertion has not been denied by the Cartel and therefore stands as an admission.

In medicine, the Rockefeller influence remains entrenched in its Medical Monopoly. We have mentioned its control of the cancer industry through the Sloan Kettering Cancer center. We have listed the directors of the major drug firms, each with its director from Chase Manhattan bank, the Standard Oil Company or other

Rockefeller firms. The American College of Surgeons maintains a monopolistic control of hospitals through the powerful Hospital Survey Committee, with members Winthrop Aldrich and David McAlpine Pyle representing the Rockefeller control. [3]

Ladies and gentlemen of the jury, the critical question is, does the medical establishment admit to the control of their profession by the drug industry? Dr. John McDougall admitted that the medical profession has lost credibility because "the medical profession and the drug companies are in bed together." [4]

The problem with doctors starts with our education. The whole system is paid for by the drug industry, from education to research. The drug industry has bought the minds of the medical profession. It starts the day you enter medical school. All the way through medical school everything is supported by the drug industry. [5]

Dr. McDougall is not alone. Here are some more admissions. Dr. P. Baird made this telling admission in the *Canadian Medical Association Journal* in 2003:

Research and academic medicine merely carry out the pharmaceutical industry's bidding. This can happen because: the drug companies and not researchers may design the research, which allows the company to *rig* the study. [6] [Emphasis added.]

Dr. T. Colin Campbell, in his now famous work *The China Study*, noted several ways a drug company can get academic medicine to do its bidding. Firstly, he stated, "The researchers may have a direct financial stake in the drug company whose product they are studying." [7] In other situations he admitted, "The drug company may be responsible for collecting and collating the raw data, and then only selectively allowing researchers to view the data." [8] In other cases he noted "The drug company may hire a communications firm to write the scientific article, and then find researchers willing to attach their names as authors of the paper after it has already been written." [9] These are incredible admissions concerning the fraud behind much of medical research.

Dr. Marcia Angel, past editor of the *New England Journal of Medicine*, raised the ominous question whether academic medicine is for sale.

The tie between clinical researchers and industry include not only grant support, but also a host of other financial arrangements. Researchers serve as consultants to companies whose products they are studying, joint advisory boards and speakers bureaus, enter into patent and royalty arrangements, agree to be listed authors of articles ghostwritten by interested companies, promote drugs and devises at company-sponsored symposiums and allow themselves to be plied with expensive gifts and trips to luxurious settings. Many also have equity interests in the companies. [10]

Dr. Campbell contended that the only research permitted by the drug companies are those designed to find a pill for every problem while ignoring nutritional remedies, despite the fact that the leading killers among the chronic degenerative diseases can be prevented and ever reversed by using good nutrition. [11]

Even more dangerous than the threat of fraudulent findings is the fact that the only type of research that is funded and recognized is research on drugs. Research on the causes of disease and non-drug interventions simply doesn't occur in medical education settings. For example, academic researchers may be furiously trying to find a pill that will treat the symptoms of obesity, but not be devoting any time or money to teaching people how to live a healthier life. [12]

Dr. Vernon Coleman, a well-known British physician, admitted in 1975 that physicians have lost control of their own profession.

As it stands, the drug industry seems to be running the medical profession. Doctors are pushed around and bullied and bribed by the drug industry. They have undoubtedly lost control of their own profession and must subsequently be held responsible for all the disasters and errors which bad prescribing produces. It is not fair simply to blame the drug industry (whose sole purpose is to make a profit) for not having strong ethics. The responsibility must be laid fairly and squarely on the medical profession which, now that it is reduced to receiving instructions and accepting commandments from a trade, can hardly claim to be still described as a profession. [13]

Ladies and gentlemen of the jury, let us consider who the Medical Establishment is today and how it controls the practice of medicine.
Like the proverbial Trojan horse, the pharmaceutical industry has wheeled its way inside the medical establishment and has become part of it. Dr. Raymond Brown stated that the Medical Establishment is a loose web of Academia (schools, hospitals and research institutions), professional associations, governmental health and regulatory agencies, health foundations and the pharmaceutical industry. [14] Within the Medical Establishment, orthodoxy is maintained by control of medical education, research funding and professional publications. What is not popular is seldom funded or published. [15]
Dr. Raymond Brown further outlined how the establishment and its satellite institutions control medicine.

The National Institutes of Health (NIH), the government medical research center and the major funding agency for medical research throughout the country, is a bastion of conservatism and scientific fashion. Its guidelines, like military rules and regulations, protect the conventional while discouraging originality or independence. By its control of funding (the life blood of research), it has disseminated and perpetuated the conservatism of its advisors and consultants, who are drawn almost exclusively from teaching and research centers. [16]

Dr. Campbell stated that the U.S. National Institutes of Health (NIH) is responsible for funding at least 80% of all biomedical and nutritional-related research that is published in the scientific literature. [17] It is made up of twenty-seven institutions, including the National Cancer Institute (NCI) and the National Heart, Lung and Blood Institute. It had a budget of $29 billion in 2005. It is the center of the nation's gigantic medical research efforts, yet, unbelievably, Dr. Campbell observed, "The NIH devotes very little time or money to the role of nutrition in preventing or reversing chronic degenerative diseases." [18]

None of the twenty-seven institutes and centers at the NIH is devoted to nutrition, despite the pivotal nature of nutrition in health, and despite the public interest in the subject. One of the arguments against having a separate institute for nutrition is that the existing institutes already concern themselves with nutrition. But this does not happen …

Of the $28 billion NIH budget proposed for 20004, only about 3.66% is designed for projects that are related in some way to nutrition and 24% for projects related to prevention. That may not sound too bad. But these figures are seriously misleading.

Most of the prevention and nutrition budgets have absolutely nothing to do with prevention and nutrition. [19]

Where does the money ear-marked for nutrition and prevention go? By a strained definition of prevention, the money is allotted to developing drugs that *inhibit* malignancy and otherwise promote preventative measures! [20] Dr. Bross also admitted that the role of the scientific and medical establishments in health issues has usually been to support the most powerful governmental agencies irrespective of the scientific or medical merits of the matter. [21]

The inadequacies of the NIH have been most evident in cancer research. Dr. Raymond Brown stated that when the NIH was founded in the 1940s its major interest was the role of nutrition in cancer, but this line of research, he admitted, "was totally discarded as chemotherapy and virology permeated and dominated research thinking. Money, talent and time were expended over three decades in a search for cancer's viral cause and chemical cure." [22]

Section 8

ADMISSION: THE FDA PROTECTS THE DRUG-BASED MEDICAL MONOPOLY

Ladies and gentlemen of the jury, the evidence is now overwhelming that the Food and Drug Administration (FDA) has been diverted from an honest broker in the protection of America's health to an ally of the medical establishment and chemical and food industry.

In 1970 Dr. Herbert Ley, former head of the FDA, made the following incredible admission:

> The thing that bugs me is that the people think the FDA is protecting them. It isn't. What the FDA is doing and what the public thinks it's doing are as different as night and day. [1]

Whose interests then, is the FDA sponsoring? On August 3, 1970, FDA Commissioner, Dr. Charles C. Edwards, admited that it was "not our policy to jeopardize the financial interests of the pharmaceutical companies." [2] Congressman Craig Hosmer soundly criticized the FDA for its war against the nutrition and vitamin industry while winking at the enormous harm that drugs produce. Omar Garrison, in his book *The Dictocrats*, quoted Congressman Hosmer:

> I have been informed that there never has been an accidental death due to vitamin overdose, but it is said one person dies every three days from taking lethal doses of aspirin ... But, despite the fact that Americans buy twenty-million pounds of aspirin a year, the FDA has never publically considered any kind of regulation or warning

in labels. Instead, the agency has spent its time and millions of the taxpayer's dollars establishing arbitrary daily dosages for harmless vitamins and minerals. [3]

The double standard is quite evident. The policy is also quite dangerous to the American population: *overlook the epidemic of drug deaths and strain at finding the least miniscule harm a vitamin may do.* It is clear that science is not at work here. At work is a malignant profit motive and a heartless quest for power and monopoly.

Senator William Proxmire threw light on the true role of the FDA when he stated in his 1973 campaign to pass the *Food Supplements Amendment Act*, that it was the goal of the FDA to drive the natural health food industry out business.

The FDA and much, but not all, of the orthodox medical profession are actively hostile against the manufacture, sale and distribution of vitamins and minerals as food or food supplements. They are out to get the health food industry and to drive the health food stores out of business. And they are trying to do this out of active hostility and prejudice. [4]

Senator Proxmire did not name the beneficiaries of the FDA's policy of driving the health foods out of business, but the answer is obvious. The processed food industry and the pharmaceutical industry are the real beneficiaries of the FDA's policy. The winners and losers are clear from this next quote from Martin Walker's book, *Dirty Medicine.*

It [the FDA] is heavy against vegetarianism and in favor of the meat industry. Most pointedly, in terms of powerful vested interests, the FDA has always supported the international sugar industry, while launching frequent assaults on honey and anyone who makes health claims for it. [5]

The FDA's unsuccessful drive in 1975 to limit the availability of vitamins, minerals, and other nutritional supplements to the general public was part of a larger establishment drive against nutritional and naturopathic therapies. Where cancer is concerned, Dr. Raymond Brown admitted that the FDA has been more effective than the AMA or the American Cancer Society in curtailing the use of alternative cancer therapies. [6]

Ladies and gentlemen of the jury, the evidence shows that the FDA emerged from obscurity within the Agriculture Department in 1938 when Congress passed the Food, Drug and Cosmetic Act in response to more than one hundred deaths which resulted from faultily manufactured Sulfanilamide. This legislation required that new drugs must pass *safety tests* and that relevant data be submitted to the government for clearance prior to licensing. [7] The power of the FDA was further augmented in 1975 when it acquired the power to control all aspects of medical devices and equipment on the basis of *effectiveness* as well as *safety*. [8]

But Dr. Raymond Brown contended that the FDA soon strayed from its original purpose.

The FDA, probably the most powerful and essential institution of the Medical Establishment, has probably been the most demoralized, inept, and excoriated of any regulatory agency within the government.

Founded for the purpose of achieving purity and safety in our food and medicines, the FDA has never achieved its goals ... Functioning virtually as a National Department of Medicine, its current role far exceeds the original intent of Congress. [9]

Another admission from Dr. Raymond Brown explains why the FDA winks at the weaknesses in the part of the industries it is supposed to regulate: FDA offices go to work for the agencies they are responsible for regulating.

The agency's close ties to industry, from which FDA officials are frequently drawn, and to which they return following government service, have produced FDA leniency toward safety standards for many industry products. [10]

Thus the FDA has turned 180 degrees away from its original purpose: To protect the health and well-being of Americans by prohibiting unsafe practices in medicine and food manufacture. Dr. William Campbell Douglass, also indicted the FDA in *Bad Medicine*. He admitted that the FDA protects the drug industry, in order to protect their job opportunities after leaving the agency.

What about the FDA—the supposed watchdog of the drug industry? FDA bureaucrats are part of the problem, not the solution. Do they protect the public or just protect their jobs?

The incestuous relationship between drug companies and the FDA is legendary. The level of corruption and collusion is unparalleled. The FDA protects the interests of the major drug companies. That has always been paramount to well-paid FDA officials because they are well taken care of by the drug boys after they finish their "tour" at FDA. [11]

Ladies and gentlemen of the jury, the evidence is becoming clear that because of the ineffectiveness of the FDA and its partiality toward the drug industry, America is being endangered.

Year in and year out, drug companies parade an endless line of new drugs before the FDA; year in and year out the FDA approves these drugs—ignoring the negative test data—while the agency officials end up on the payroll of the very drug companies they are supposed to be monitoring. [12]

Every year a new scandal about FDA neglect and corrupt consortium with the drug companies seem to burst upon us like comets darting across the sky, leaving only their fiery fleeting emblems to remind us of the event. On June 4, 2007 Evelyn Pringle reported in *CounterPounch* magazine that a study published by the *New England Journal of Medicine* on May 21, 2007, revealed that GlaxoSmithKline's diabetes drug Avandia was associated with a 43% increase in heart attacks and possibly a 64% increase in cardiovascular death. Millions of Americans with Type II diabetes have taken it to control their blood sugar. What is truly scandalous, the article went on to say, is that documents dating back 7 years reveal that the FDA knew about the risks associated with Avandia and did nothing to protect consumers.

On June 6, 2007, the US House of representatives Committee on Oversight and Government Reform held a meeting to assess the FDA's role in the evaluation of the safety of Avandia. As usual there was much talk and no action. Meanwhile over in the Senate Senator Chuck Grassley opined: "We need to know if this is another Vioxx where the FDA sat on its hands and endangered lives." Senator Max Baucus chimmed in: "What we are hearing about the handling of Avandia by both GlaxoSmithKline and the FDA is appalling and unacceptable." Not to be out done a representative of the medical establishment added: "The FDA is going to have an extremely tough time wriggling out from under the rug of blame for this regulatory failure." Meanwhile American taxpayers have spent millions of dollars on this drug to protect them from exactly what the drug delivers: heart failure. Not surprisingly Avandia is the top selling drug for diabetes, with sales of over $2.2 billion in 2006. Was there a profit motive for suppressing the deadly evidence? You the jury must decide this question.

America is also being malnourished by the failure of the FDA to see that wholesome foods are put on the market. Martin Walker, in *Dirty Medicine,* observed that *food production in the modern world has nothing to do with nutrition.* Processed foods have become another channel through which the chemical companies reap big dividends by the process of *enriching* foods with chemicals:

In processed foods, and especially in "luxury entertainments," such as sweets, cakes, chocolates and soft drinks, a great array of chemicals are added to make items more palatable and to extend their shelf life. It becomes increasingly difficult to understand what we are eating and the effect it will ultimately have on our bodies and minds.

Food production and consumption in the modern world have nothing to do with nutrition or health. Like all capitalist production, food production aims for the highest number of manufactured units at the lowest cost and the maximum profit. We have radically departed from the path of simple nutritious food and strayed into a world where we take into our systems, as if in a dream, a wide range of toxic substances which play no part in constructing a healthy body.

The chemical companies, the pharmaceutical companies, agribusiness, the processed food industry, the water supply companies and the health care sectors represent a global market for chemicals.

Firms which are part of this market tend to have the same marketing strategies, the same friends—and the same enemies. [13]

The 1971 FDA's Fact Sheet on *Nutritional Nonsense—and Sense* shows their bias towards the processed food industry in making the following blatantly untrue statements:

In general, there is little difference between fresh and processed foods. Modern processing methods retain most vitamin and mineral values ...

Nutrition Research has shown that a diet containing white bread made with enriched flour has nearly the same value as one containing whole grain bread ...

Chemical fertilizers are not poisoning our soil. Modern fertilizers are needed to produce enough food for our population ...

Vitamins are specific chemical compounds, and the human body can use them equally well whether they are synthesized by a chemist or by nature. [14]

Ladies and gentlemen of the jury, the evidence is also overwhelming that, protected by the government agencies, the modern medical establishment promotes the pharmaceutical management of chronic degenerative disease and wages war against alternative medicine for the sake of profits.

Dr. Colin Campbell made the revealing admission that the medical system responsible for caring for the health of Americans is failing us because it is putting profits before health.

When was the last time that you went to the doctor and he or she told you what to eat or what not to eat? You've probably never had that experience. But the vast majority of Americans fall prey to one of the chronic diseases of affluence discussed ... and as you have seen, there is a wealth of published research that suggests these diseases are a result of poor nutrition, not poor genes or bad luck. So why doesn't the medical system take nutrition seriously?

Four words: money, ego, power and control. While it is unfair to generalize about individual doctors, it is safe to say that the system they work in, the system that currently takes responsibility for promoting the health of Americans, is failing us. [15] [Emphasis added.]

On September 7, 1979, the *Philadelphia Inquirer* carried this commentary on the cancer industry:

It's a terrible thing to say, but the fact remains that conventional cancer therapy is a multimillion-dollar industry. It does not cure cancer ... But naturopathic (using all resources, including doctors, chiropractors and diet) therapy is very inexpensive. And if naturopathy was made legal in the United States as far as cancer is concerned, a lot of people would lose a lot of money. [16]

On June 30, 1975, the Albuquerque *Tribune* revealed that the AMA has been engaged in a relentless campaign against its *economic* competitors. [17] Commenting on this assault on our medical freedom by the AMA and compliant governmental agencies, P. Joseph Lisa revealed the economic motivation of the antagonists.

For the past thirty years, the American Medical Association and its allies in and out of government have waged a war against their economic competitors in alternative medicine. They have not been above using covert operations, dirty tricks, *fixing* government studies, adversely influencing government policy and insurance company coverage, and much, much, more. [18] [Emphasis added.]

Dr. Sidney Wolfe testified before the Congressional subcommittee in 1977 and made the following admission, "prevention cuts into the profit margin of existing industries which have thus far been able to escape the costs of the cancer they cause." [19] Regrettably, the goal of the medical establishment today is not to protect the people's health but their own profit. [20]

CLOSING STATEMENT:

A Call for Accountability

REDEFINING MEDICAL MALPRACTICE

Ladies and Gentlemen of the jury, the responsibility has fallen upon your shoulders to bring conventional pharmaceutical medicine to the bar of justice for putting the health of America at risk by routinely treating, in non-emergency cases, chronic degenerative diseases by the use of poisonous drugs without seriously attempting to cure the underlying diseases. In order for you to fulfill your duty we need a new definition of what constitutes medical malpractice, particularly in the treatment of chronic degenerative diseases. Presently the standard for medical malpractice is weighed in the favor of conventional medicine and is designed to shield it from the atrocious consequences of its often reckless and unscientific practices.

In the courts of law the conduct of a physician will amount to malpractice *only when the doctor's actions or omissions constitute a departure from the acceptable medical standards to be expected from a specialist or practitioner similarly situated.* [1] The problem with this standard is that conventional pharmaceutical medicine determines what acceptable medical practice is! But the evidence clearly demonstrates that it is based on a false conception of science. If the science is false, then the therapeutics based on that medical science is false. The medical community is thus able to give its stamp of approval to their so-called *proven* methods of treatment, while condemning as heretical all other approaches, despite clear and convincing evidence that these so-called proven and acceptable methods are maiming and killing literally thousands (perhaps millions, if the whole truth were known) of patients every year. [2] No one in the medical club dare call it medical malpractice or the whole spurious fabrication by which they earn a living will collapse. They fear the storming of their medical *Bastille* by the angry mob of aroused patients.

Likewise the standard in product liability cases for determining when a pharmaceutical company should be held liable for the harm done by its poisonous drugs designed for treating chronic degenerative diseases is weighted in favor of the manufacturers. The Third Restatement of the Law of Torts section 6 states in part:

> c. A prescription drug or medical device is not reasonably safe due to defective design if the foreseeable risks of harm posed by the drug or medical device are sufficiently great in relations to its foreseeable therapeutic benefits that *reasonable healthcare providers,* knowing of such foreseeable risks and therapeutics benefits, would not prescribe the drug or medical device for any class of patients. [3] [Emphasis added.]

The problem with this definition is that the "reasonable healthcare providers" who are to determine whether the risks of harm done by the drug out weight the benefits, exclude, by convention, nutritional doctors. Their opinions do not count in this risk/benefit analysis. So of course pharmaceutical doctors who have a vested interest in profiting by the continuation of pharmaceutical medicine will not be too ready to pass judgment on the drugs they use in their therapeutics. Again this standard must be changed to include nutritional doctors who practice in the tradition of Hippocrates. Drugs may have a place in emergency situations. It is the non-emergency and routine use of drugs in chronic degenerative diseases to the exclusion of nutritional modalities that is in question in this trial.

Another unfair design in the Law of Torts is the refusal to apply section 2 subsection (b) of the Restatement of Torts (which states that a product is defective if there was a reasonable alternative design) to drug manufacturers in section 6 of the Restatement. The standard for determining whether a product is defective is defined by section 2 of the Restatement Third of Torts as follows:

> A product is defective when, at the time of sale or distribution, it contains a manufacturing defect, is defective in design, or is defective because of inadequate instructions or warnings. A product:

> a) Contains a manufacturing defect when the product departs from its intended design even though all possible care was exercised in the preparation and marketing of the product;

INDICTED!   419

b) Is defective in design when the foreseeable risks of harm posed by the product could have been reduced or avoided by the *adoption of a reasonable alternative design* by the seller or other distributor, or a predecessor in the commercial chain of distribution, and the omission of the alternative design renders the product not reasonably safe;

c) is defective because of inadequate instructions or warnings when the foreseeable risks of harm posed by the product could have been reduced or avoided by the provision of reasonable instructions or warnings by the seller or other distributor, or a predecessor in the commercial chain of distribution, and the omission of the instructions or warnings renders the product not reasonably safe. [4]

Notice that while all these subsections generally apply to any kind of product, in the case of drugs, subsection (b) is deleted when this section is adopted by section 6 of the Restatement which defines safe and unsafe drugs. This is a crucial deletion; for the adoption of an *alternative reasonable design* is precisely what alternative nutritional medicine provides medical therapeutics. Nutritional medicine is deliberately excluded by the Law of Torts so as to shield pharmaceutical drugs from a risk/benefit analysis that takes into consideration the alternative harmless approach of nutritional modalities as advocated by Hippocrates and other nutritional physicians. This loophole in the law has to be changed. It is a change that will revolutionize the practice of medicine and enhance the safety and health of patients throughout the land.

Ladies and gentlemen, the standards for medical malpractice and product liability must be taken out of the hands of the medical fraternity and placed in the hands of the public acting through an accountable legislature, one not beholden to the Cartel of big business in league with the medical and pharmaceutical establishments. We need a commonsense objective standard for medical malpractice and pharmaceutical negligence that conforms to *empirical scientific criteria*. The standard must be *empirical* because *rationalistic* science and medicine, which are the foundations of present medical practice, are based on false theories and result in harmful therapeutics.

Dr. Andrew Weil cited an example of the disconnect between empirical science and medical therapeutics. He observed that the foundation upon which pharmaceutical medicine is based is faulty and unscientific and hence the therapeutics will be faulty, unscientific and harmful. Recognizing that most of our drugs (as much as 70%) are obtained from plants, [5] he observed that pharmaceutical medicine is based on the erroneous concept that drug plants owe their effects to single *active* compounds and the *inactive* ingredients can be discarded and ignored. [6] In *Health and Healing*, America's foremost herbal and nutritional doctor stated:

In their enthusiasm at isolating the active principles of drug plants, researchers of the last century made a serious mistake. They came to believe that all of a plant's desirable properties could be accounted for by a single compound, that it would always be better to conduct research and treat disease with the purified compound than with the whole plant. In this belief, they forgot the plants once they had the active principles out of them, called all the other principles "inactive" and advanced the notion that prescribing refined white powders was more *scientific* and up to date than using crude green plants.

The idea that plants owe their effects to single compounds is simply untrue. Drug plants are always complex mixtures of chemicals, all of which contribute to the effect of the whole ...

The erroneous idea that plants and isolated active principles are equivalent has become fixed dogma in pharmacology and medicine today. [7] [Emphasis added.]

Drugs in their phyto-chemical matrix would present a *reasonable alternative design* of present therapeutic remedies, and this would be in keeping with nutritional medicine, for nutritional medicine generally recognizes the benefits of herbal medicine. The issue is whether the so-called active ingredient of the plant or herb should be isolated and used as a drug in medical therapeutics or whether the whole herb should be used. This is the line that divides pharmaceutical medicine from nutritional medicine. The drug used in non-emergency situations has greater risks than benefits.

The herb, though slower acting, has fewer risks if any at all, and all the benefits.

Dr. Weil could not have summed up *rationalistic* medicine more succinctly. In the area of pharmacology, it exalts expert opinion *above* the facts of nature. It commits the cardinal scientific sin which Sir Francis Bacon labored to expel at the birth of modern science: *it is the error of basing a scientific hypothesis or axiom upon too few facts.* [8] Bacon argued that these erroneous axioms are held on to even when contradicted by the facts of experience.

> The axioms in use are derived from a scanty handful, as it were, of experience and a few particulars of frequent occurrence ... and if any neglected or unknown instance occurs the axiom is saved by some frivolous distinctions, when it would be more consistent with truth to amend it. [9]

Today, as in the Dark Age of Scholastic science, the goal is not truth but political correctness. Rationalist physicians and scientists today do not amend their erroneous ideas when they are confronted with additional facts. Dr. Weil stated that they often label the facts *anecdotal;* thus justifying their decision to ignore them, and to hold on to their cherished but erroneous ideas. Referencing a testimonial about the benefits of the herb Ginkgo, Dr. Weil stated:

> This letter is a classic example of a testimonial to a health product. As such it would be likely be dismissed by most medical scientists, who tend to drop all testimonials into wastebaskets labeled Anecdotal Evidence. In medical usage, "anecdotal evidence" means "of no scientific value or importance." I take a different view of this material, and I am interested in why so many doctors have a hard time with it.

> I suppose the simplest answer is that doctors and scientists do not like to be made to look like fools, and they sense danger in endorsing products or techniques whose claimed effects may turn out to be false or unprovable by controlled experiments. But it is equally foolish to ignore testimonial evidence, because it may

suggest directions for experimental inquiry as well as provide clues to the nature of healing. [10]

Ladies and gentlemen of the jury, this is the crux of the problem with the present standard for medical practice: *a false rationalistic science is determining what acceptable medical practice* is. As such, physicians and pharmaceutical companies can commit atrocities and still not be found liable for the death and disability and suffering they are causing in society today, for their actions and medications are determined to be politically acceptable and legally correct. It has become accepted public policy to enforce the false and erroneous *rationalistic science* of the chemical and drug industries. The Cartel owns the legislatures and Congress.

Ladies and gentlemen of the jury, the problem is that we have silently and imperceptibly retreated into the metaphysical and Scholastic pseudo-science of the Dark Ages and have abandoned Baconian and Newtonian science in which all theories are strictly held accountable to the facts. Dr. Weil reminded us what good science is—it is taking *all of the facts* into account and not dismissing awkward facts because they do not support a preconceived concept.

Many scientists reject testimonials out of hand on the assumption that the information is false, that people are either deluded or have simply made up the stories for one reason or another.

The essence of good science is open-minded inquiry, so would it not make sense to try, at least, to verify the stories? ...

Science is the orderly gathering of knowledge by methodical inquiry and experiment, but where do you get ideas to inquire about or experiment with except through your experience of the world around you? Experimenting blindly, without starting from reasonable hypotheses suggested by experience, often wastes time, money, and effort. [11] [Emphasis added.]

Dr. Weil succinctly summed up the essence of the dispute between nutritional physicians and conventional medicine that is steeped in the use of poisonous drugs. Medical science has been corrupted by big business and by the drive by the chemical and oil industries to made outrageous profits.

Government agencies like the FDA serve as handmaids to this politically correct medical monopoly. Only time and eternity will expose the untold suffering caused by erroneous conclusions drawn from faulty science. Dr. Weil observed that rejecting herbal medicine out of hand can lead to harm through toxic drugs.

> It is useful to know how drugs differ from pure compounds derived from them, because the differences have great practical import.

> In general, isolated and refined drugs are much more toxic than their botanical sources. They also tend to produce effects of more rapid onset, greater intensity, and shorter duration. [12]

Dr. Weil is not alone in *indicting* the faulty science of the medical and pharmaceutical establishment. Harris Coulter and others testified emphatically that the rationalist or Allopathic, drug-based medicine of today is *not* science and it should not be favored over other medical theories. [13] Why do modern medical scientists adhere to the harmful pharmaceutical practice of treating chronic degenerative diseases with chemical *silver-bullets* and not employ natural means of healing? Dr. Weil provided one answer. Whereas his approach to medical therapeutics is built on the foundation that "the body can heal itself," that it can do so because it has a healing mechanism [14], rationalistic medical scientists put little faith on natural healing processes and pursue man-made silver-bullets to either strike down the microbe or manage the disease by manipulating the chemical balance of the body.

> The possibility that secondary compounds of medical plants may be valuable in their own right or may modify the effects of dominant compounds in good ways seems unremarkable to me. Nevertheless, I find I have to explain it to allopathic physicians and pharmacologists with great patience. I notice that I make many of these people uneasy when I impute any "wisdom" to nature; they seem to resent the suggestion that natural substances may be better then man-made ones.

> All I can say is that, empirically, I find such a difference, at least in the case of medical plants versus isolated drugs. [15]

On the use of herbs to promote the natural healing ability of the body, Ellen White wrote,

> This is God's method. The herbs that grow for benefit of man, and the little handful of herbs kept and steeped and used for sudden ailments have served tenfold, yes, one hundred fold better purposes than all the drugs hidden under mysterious names and dealt out to the sick. [16]

But philosophical differences over the ability of nature to heal diseases, is not the only reason driving the medical and pharmaceutical establishment to use drugs. The reason is as sordid as it is callous: *profits.* Yes, raw, filthy profits. Dr. Weil gave an instance of this. Whereas many drugs were derived from plants, today the synthetic drug market is thriving. Dr. Weil stated that it is incorrect to think that pharmaceutical companies create drugs to cure or manage a *specific* disease. [17] To do this may give the process a semblance of scientific credibility. But the very opposite of medical science is often at work here. The reverse happens: they invent drugs and then go looking for a disease condition that the drug might help! [18].

> People who do not know the ways of pharmaceutical companies imagine that they study diseases and try to invent drugs to fill medical needs. Such is not the case. More often, the companies hire chemists specializing in particular classes of molecules, and those chemists try to come up with new patentable molecules. A patentable molecule is one different enough from a molecule some other company already markets to merit a patent of its own. When a company obtains a patent on a molecule variant of an existing drug, the job then is to find a way to sell it. That is, the company attempts to fit a disease to its chemical. [19]

Ladies and gentlemen of the jury, this is an astonishing bit of information. Mark this well, because the plant molecules existing in nature are not patentable, the drug company has little interest in marketing a natural remedy. There is no money in it. So man-made drugs are feverishly sought after. Dr. Andrew Weil related a story in which, as a young man, he was hired by a doctor to study the effects of a new molecule that had psychotic effects. They selected a number of psychiatric patients and administered the drug to see what effect it would have upon them and hence determine what illness it might be of benefit to. After the drug had killed one patient and injured many others, he wrote up a detailed report noting the dangerous side effects of the drug. Because of his report, the drug company decided not to market it. [20] But eight years later, when he was interning at a hospital in San Francisco, he came across the same drug, listing all of the side effects he had written up, but passed off now as a pre-anesthetic medication! He stated that the drug company had invested so much money in the new molecule that they had to get their money's worth out of it. [21] And they dare call this scientific medicine?

Ladies and gentlemen of the jury, I appeal to you in all earnestness, the standard for medical malpractice must be based on *commonsense*. If a practice or procedure results in death and more suffering than the disease, it must be condemned outright, regardless of the support of the conventional medical community for this harmful practice. In addition the opinions of the alternative physicians who base their practice on sound empirical principles, should be admitted as competence evidence on the conduct or practice being called into question.

Ladies and gentlemen, the core issue here is the *method* by which a *scientific* truth is verified. True empirical science and medicine subjects all truth, theories or practices to the acid test of *conformity to the observed facts*. Of vital importance to the public is that these empirical facts are within the knowledge and province of the layman possessing common sense and the faculty of reason. This concept is dreaded by the handful of elitist mercenaries who control the medical Cartel. False rationalistic science and medicine gives more weight to the agreement of its theories with its religious (non-creationist) and metaphysical worldview. These rationalists believe that knowledge can be obtained by *a priori* reasoning and not through observing the facts of nature and experience. Modern medical science has sunk to the low level that facts must not overrule theory. This is why the theories of conventional medicine, which are clearly out of touch with reality, are tenaciously clung to despite the colossal harm perpetrated by them.

Philipp Frank stated that the difference between ancient science (the metaphysical science of Pythagoras, Plato and Aristotle) and modern science (the empirical science that grew out of the biblical worldview of the Reformation) was the criteria, by which a discovered principle was recognized to be valid.

The method of "verification" is different now; more weight is given to the agreement of the results with observed facts than to the agreement of the principles with a world picture that has been accepted for what we called ... "philosophical" reasons. [22]

Ladies and gentlemen of the jury, we have *lost* this perspective which gave birth to modern empirical science and have reverted to Dark Age Scholastic pseudo-science. Using true scientific criteria for validating all theories and medical practices by the objective facts of experience, the common man will have then a standard to judge the efficacy of a medical theory or practice. Does it do harm? Does experience demonstrate that the *treatment* is *worse* that the disease? Does it suppress symptoms while aggravating the underlying chronic degenerative disease? Do nutritional modalities on the other hand go to the core of the problem and thus remove, not only the symptoms, but the cause of the disease? If these things are true, then conventional medicine must be brought to the bar of accountability. Conventional medicine must re-adopt the injunction of Hippocrates to all physicians, *first do no harm.*

THE VERDICT

REQUEST FOR AN INDICTMENT

Ladies and gentlemen of the jury, utilizing the commonsense criteria of empirical science, which incorporates the objective standard for validating all theories and medical practices by the objective facts of experience, I urge you to find that it *should* be medical malpractice to exclude nutritional modalities and treat cancer (excepting emergency cases), only by surgery, radiation, and chemotherapy, as these treat only the *symptoms of a metabolic disease* and in the case of the two latter approaches, result in the near total destruction of the patient's immune system, and often result in the generation of more cancer cells. [1]

It should be malpractice to treat high blood pressure by drugs such as diuretics, when it has been clearly shown that high blood pressure medication does positive harm, aggravates the cause of the disease and increases the mortality rate. [2]

It should be medical malpractice to shun dietary remedies and treat Type II diabetics with insulin only, when aggressive treatment with insulin causes progressive damage to the retina, often leading to total blindness. [3] The use of drugs or insulin to treat Type II individuals is a classic case of symptom management. High blood sugar is the symptom of a deeper metabolic problem that leads to some very serious medical complications, including heart disease, blindness and death. Treating the symptoms of high blood sugar does nothing to stop the relentless progress of these life impairing diseases that diabetics are prone to.

Ladies and gentlemen of the jury, it should be medical malpractice to encourage the victim of osteoporosis to drink more milk to replenish calcium stores in the body when study after study, including epidemiological evidence, show that the excessive protein in milk and animal products cause a negative calcium balance in people using these products. [4]

It should be medical malpractice to treat arthritis with drugs that suppress only the symptoms of the disease. Indicted are drugs such as

Indomethacin when the side effects are severe headaches, dizziness, rashes, and depression. [5] It should be medical malpractice to treat arthritis with the hormone cortisone, when the side effects are worse than the disease, causing damage to the nerves, blood, bones and other vital organs of the body, peptic ulcers, osteoporosis with spontaneous fractures, mental disturbances, psychosis, neuropathy or degeneration of the nerves, posterior subcapsular cataracts, diabetes, hypertension, disturbances in the metabolism and utilization of protein and fats, acne, and excessive hair growth in women. [6]

It should be medical malpractice to treat heart disease with cholesterol-lowering drugs such as Niacin and Lovastatin, in light of the fact that diet can completely control cholesterol levels, and the side effects of these drugs are liver damage, glucose intolerance, gout, headaches, itching, skin flushing, and cataracts. [7]

Ladies and gentlemen, what should drive this need to redefine medical malpractice is not only the gruesome toll of patient suffering and death, but the rising cost of healthcare in America. This cost was estimated to reach $1.6 trillion by the year 2000 and to consume 28% of the GNP by the year 2010 if allowed to continue at present trends. [8] The cost of healthcare is now over $2 trillion annually. The vast majority of these healthcare dollars are unnecessarily spent on treating the symptoms of disease that are largely or completely prevented or cured by lifestyle and dietary changes.

In *Your Body's many Cries for Water*, Dr. Batmanghelidj demonstrated the folly of treating the symptoms of thirst by medication, when the simple remedy is to drink more water! [9] Hence, ladies and gentlemen of the jury, it should be medical malpractice to treat dyspeptic pain with antacids and histamine-blocking agents, when the simple remedy is drinking more water! [10] In light of his clinical work, it should also be medical malpractice to treat high blood pressure with diuretics when simply exercising more and drinking more water is the solution to the problem. Dr. Batmanghelidj stated that high blood pressure is simply the result of an adaptive process to a gross body water deficiency. [11] Accordingly he criticized the pharmaceutical approach to treating high blood pressure.

The present way of treating hypertension is wrong to the point of *scientific absurdity*. The body is trying to retain its water volume, and we say to the designer of nature in us: "No, you do not understand—you must take diuretics and get rid of water!" [12]

Ladies and gentlemen, it should be medical malpractice to treat asthma with antihistamines, when the simple remedy according to Dr. Batmanghelidj is drinking more water [13], and also avoidance of excessive sugar [14], and dairy products [25]

The list of the medical and scientific absurdities of pharmaceutical medicine can go on and on *ad infinitum* and *ad nauseam*. The bottom line is that we must not abandon our commonsense because the medical community tells us we must subject ourselves to their endless round of drug-induced death and suffering. To do so would be to yield our medical freedom to a profit making Cartel that is callous of human suffering.

In summary, ladies and gentlemen of the jury, it *should* be medical malpractice and medical fraud to treat the symptoms of a disease with pharmaceutical remedies which only *suppress* the symptoms, while making the underlying disease worse and more expensive to treat and more life-threatening to the patient. On the other hand, medical science should emphasize *nutritional remedies, including exercise, adequate water intake and lifestyle changes,* that the evidence has demonstrated in this trial, to be highly efficacious in not only preventing but in reversing chronic degenerative diseases.

Ladies and gentlemen my last efforts in this trial will be to appeal to you to make a difference in America today.

AMERICA AT A CROSSROADS

STANDING UP FOR MEDICAL FREEDOM

Is life so dear, or peace so sweet

As to be purchased at the price of chains and slavery?

Forbid it, Almighty God!

I know not what course others may take,

But as for me,

Give me liberty, or give me death!

Patrick Henry. March 23, 1775

Ladies and gentlemen of the jury, in closing, it is crystal clear from the evidence we have presented to you that the chronic degenerative diseases now epidemic in America, are due primarily to our lifestyle choices in eating, drinking and pleasure seeking, and secondarily by the poisonous drugs we ingest. By our lifestyle we are violating the natural laws that were designed by our Creator to keep our bodies in health. It is lifestyle that is killing us. The proper treatment for diseases that flow from the violation of natural law is to adopt a lifestyle and eating pattern that conforms to natural law. When we do this the body heals itself. This was the ancient teaching of Hippocrates, the Father of both ancient and modern medicine, and it was also the teaching of Moses, the lawgiver for our Western civilization. Ellen G. White, the most prolific woman writer in American history, also wrote extensively in this area. Her highly acclaimed books, *Ministry of Healing*, *Temperance*, and *Counsel on Diet and Foods*, teach us how to reclaim our health by living in compliance with the principles of natural law.

Of equal or greater concern is the fact that this epidemic of chronic degenerative disease is to a great extent iatrogenic; that is, physician induced. [1] Physicians are contributing to this epidemic of chronic diseases by their disdain for nutritional medicine, while relying on pharmaceutical drugs that treat only symptoms, while leaving intact and in some cases even aggravating, the underlying degenerative disease. I will remind you of the testimony of Harris Coulter, author of the massive four-volume *Divided Legacy.*

> The major drug diseases, as will be shown below, are coextensive with the principal chronic diseases afflicting the populations of the twentieth-century industrialized societies: allergic hypertension, hypertension, ulcers, deafness, asthma, heart disease, mental illness, cancer, diabetes, congenital defects, neurologic disorders, and arteriosclerosis. To what extent, therefore, does drug use contribute to chronic disease? Or, in other words, how much chronic disease is really drug disease? [2]

Ladies and gentlemen of the jury, you have seen how Harris Coulter then proceeded to present devastating evidence of the link between pharmaceutical medicine and a variety of chronic diseases. Coulter is not the only voice crying in the wilderness, travailing to be heard on the link between the free and abandoned use of pharmaceutical medicine to cure chronic degenerative diseases and the rising epidemic of these same diseases. In 1863 Ellen White wrote:

> I was shown that more deaths have been caused by drug taking than from all other causes combined. If there was in the land one physician in the place of thousands, a vast amount of premature mortality would be prevented. Multitudes of physicians, and multitudes of drugs, have cursed the inhabitants of the earth, and have carried thousands and tens of thousands to untimely graves. [3]

Ellen White was consistent and constant in her warning about the harmfulness of pharmaceutical drugs in the care of the sick. Thirty years later, in 1895, even after the more deadly drugs such as Calomel, mercury compounds and Nux Vomica were discarded for more scientifically created drugs, Ellen White wrote:

Many of the physicians in our world are of no benefit to the human family. The drug science has been exalted, but if every bottle that comes from every such institution was done away with, there would be fewer invalids in the world today. Drug medication should never have been introduced into our institutions. [4]

Helen White advocated in the place of harmful pharmaceutical drugs, the use of the herbs themselves from which most of these drugs are extracted:

The true method of healing the sick is to tell them of the herbs that grow for the benefit of man. Scientists have attached large names to these simplest preparations, but true education will lead us to teach the sick that they need not call in a doctor any more than they would call in a lawyer. They themselves administer the simple herbs if necessary. To educate the human family that the doctor alone knows all the ills of infants and persons of every age is false teaching, and the sooner we as a people stand on the principles of health reform, the greater will be the blessing that will come to those who would do true medical missionary work.

There is a work to be done in treating the sick with water, and teaching them to make the most of the sunshine and physical exercise. Thus in simple language we may teach the people how to preserve health, how to avoid sickness. This is the work our sanitariums are called upon to do. This is true science. [5]

Ellen White is not alone. Just before the turn of the twentieth century, Oliver Wendell Holmes—a contemporary of Ellen White who became one of our most eminent Justices—gave his opinion of the value of pharmaceutical medicine.

I firmly believe that if the whole materia medica as now used could be sunk to the bottom of the sea, it would be all the better for mankind and all the worse for the fishes. [6]

One of the most eminent herbal healers today, and a prominent pioneer in nutritional medicine, is Dr. Andrew Weil. He has eloquently warned

America time and again about the dangers stemming from the promiscu-
ous use of pharmaceutical drugs.

The average patient in a hospital today is placed on half a dozen
drugs simultaneously. How some of these chemicals react with
each other is anybody's guess. Moreover, a significant percentage
of drug doses in hospitals involve errors: the wrong drug, the
wrong patient, the wrong dosage, and the wrong time. As I wrote
earlier, adverse drug reactions are the leading variety of iatrogenic
(doctor induced) illnesses.

The kinds of drugs Allopaths chose to give favor these reactions.
They also account for a high proportion of soaring medical
costs, often fail to improve health, and frequently make patients
dependent on pharmacies and pills. [7]

Dr. Weil stated in his 1995 best seller, *Spontaneous Healing*, that when he
graduated from Harvard Medical School in 1969, he made a conscious
decision *not* to practice the medicine he had just learned. [8] Why?

The logical reason was that most of the treatments I had learned
in four years at Harvard Medical School and one of internship
*do not get to the root of disease processes and promote healing but
rather suppressed theses processes or merely counteracted the visible
symptoms of disease.* I had learned almost nothing about health and
its maintenance, about how to prevent illness—a great omission,
because I have always believed that the primary function of doctors
should be to teach people how not to get sick in the first place.
The word *doctor* comes from the Latin word *teacher.* Teaching
preventions should be primary; treatment of existing disease,
secondary. [9] [Emphasis added.]

Dr. Weil's explanation of why he decided to reserve drug medicine for only
serious emergency cases highlights the theme of this trial: pharmaceutical
drugs have dangerous side effects and can even exacerbate the disease they
are trying to cure.

I have no objections to use of these treatments on a short-term
basis for the management of very serious conditions. But I came to

realize, early in my hospital days, that if you rely on such measures as the main strategy for treating illness, you create two kinds of problems.

First, you expose patients to risk, because, by their nature, pharmaceutical weapons are strong and toxic. Their desired effects are too often offset by side effects, by toxicity. Adverse reactions to the counteractive drugs of conventional medicine are a great black mark against the system, and I saw more than enough of them in my clinical training to know that there had to be a better way.

The second problem, less visible but more worrisome, is the chance that over time suppressive treatments may actually strengthen disease processes instead of resolving them. [10]

What type of medicine did Dr. Andrew Weil turn to?

Botanical medicine appealed to me because it offered the possibility of finding safe, natural alternatives to the drugs I had been taught to use. [11]

As a physician with botanical training, I recommend herbal treatments for a wide range of diseases. Unfortunately, few allopathic physicians have the knowledge or experience to do this … Herbal medicines tend to be milder than chemical drugs and produce their effects more slowly; they are also much less likely to cause toxicity, because they are dilute forms of drugs rather than concentrated ones. [12]

Ladies and gentlemen, Harris Coulter stated that the true extent of drug-induced chronic diseases will remain concealed from the public so long as Allopathic medicine controls public debate. [13] There is no sustained effort to record the true grim statistics of those injured from drugs or by drug induced chronic diseases. Dr. Leighton Cuff stated in *Controversies in Therapeutics* in 1908 that the true cause of death is *not* always recorded, National Health statistics do not reflect the magnitude of the problem of drug-induced diseases. A death certificate may indicate that a person died of renal failure, but it may not state that the disease was caused by a drug. [14]

Ladies and gentlemen of the jury, the health and safety of the public demand an accounting by the medical profession. For too long a *false* rationalistic medicine has been passed off as *scientific* medicine. [15] This fallacy must be exposed. Once the public understands that rationalistic drug-based medicine is *not* science but an ancient moribund religious and metaphysical fallacy taught by Pythagoras, Plato and Aristotle, which now masquerades as science, it will throw of the yoke of bondage it has so patiently borne. This metaphysical tradition held that matter is evil and therefore nature cannot provide reliable knowledge, and that true knowledge can only be obtained from the unseen or occult world, the abode of the gods, which was accessible only to the elite. This Greek religious tradition not only undermined true science [16], but it set the stage for reducing mankind to bondage by making knowledge inaccessible to the common man. In *The Origin of Science and the Science of its Origin*, professor Stanley Jaki stated that "Aristotle killed Greek science and postponed its rise for 2,000 years." [17] The belief that nature cannot provide reliable knowledge influenced rise of the pseudo rationalistic science which exalts opinion over the facts of nature in formulating its theories. We have seen how this rationalistic science of the Dark Ages, at one time overthrown by the empirical, fact-based science of Sir Francis Bacon, was resurrected by Rene Descartes and it came to dominate modern science and medicine.

Opposed to this dogmatic and tyrannical tradition is the biblical perspective of the ancient Hebrews and the Sixteenth Century Reformation. This worldview holds that the heavens and earth declare the Glory of God who provided every man with commonsense and the faculty of reason, by which he can access the knowledge God placed in his creation (Psalms 19; Romans 1). It was this understanding that gave rise to true empirical science. [18] And because knowledge is power, this biblical tradition opens the door to liberty in all spheres, not just political and religious, but medical. The layman *can* understand the natural laws that govern his body in health and healing. Thus he need no longer be the pawn and victim of the physician claiming a false superior knowledge inaccessible to the common man.

Both Hippocratic and Mosaic medicine *alone* stand in the tradition of true empirical science. Empirical science is good science because it conforms to natural law. Whenever medicine has followed in the path of empirical science it has brought health and healing to mankind. On the other hand rationalistic science is a false science that has always confounded medical science. Its worldview warps the thinking of the physician. Conventional rationalistic medicine advocates only man-made solutions that not only trample upon natural laws, but invariably bring death and disease where there should be healing. This is the lesson of the history of medical science as traced in the author's next book, *The Whisper of the Serpent*. The evidence is overwhelming that medicine which does not conform to the empirical facts of natural law is the harbinger of death. The issue is not the sufficiency of the scientific evidence—it is rebellion. A rebellion from the laws of our Creator who beckons us to return:

Then I saw another angel flying in the midst of heaven, having the everlasting gospel to preach to those who dwell on the earth—to every nation, tribe, tongue, and people—saying with a loud voice, "Fear God and give glory to Him, for the hour off His judgement has come; and worship Him who made heaven and earth, the sea and springs of water."

Revelation 14: 6,7

When ever mankind asserts his autonomy and rejects the wisdom and advice of his Creator, he takes yet another step nearer to the grave. Solomon recognized this when he stated that there is a way that seems right unto a man, but the way thereof is the path to death. Proverbs 14:12. He was right. Both ancient and modern rationalistic medicine demonstrate this. Conventional medicine seeks to help mankind avoid the immediate *consequences* of violating the health laws that regulate his being, while encouraging him, perhaps inadvertently, to continue to violate those natural laws, obedience to which, is health and life. But it fails to do even this. It only manages to *suppress* the symptoms of the diseases we bring upon ourselves, while the disease rages on beneath the surface.

Ladies and gentlemen, modern pharmaceutical medicine is substantially destructive to our health, especially in its attempts to treat chronic degenerative diseases by means of poisonous drugs. It is a betrayal of our trust. It teaches us to live as we please, yet be sure to buy its *magic-bullet* remedies. But alas, these magic *silver-bullet* remedies are often more destructive than the disease, and at best they compound the disease. It is high time that the public woke up to the fraud and abuse that is being perpetrated upon them. It is time that they brought conventional medicine to the bar of justice.

Of course, I speak not of medicine in its empirically scientific sense. Empirical medicine along with empirical science has given us the best acute care system in the world. Let us preserve it. I speak of the false rationalistic medicine that presumes to treat chronic degenerative disease with pharmaceutical weapons that shoot down not only the microbe, but the host—the unsuspecting patient. Pharmaceutical medicine, based on the false rationalistic science that was spawned by the false theories about the nature of man and the nature of the natural world, has drunk deep from the *Whispered lies* of that old Serpent, the enemy of mankind.

The public must shake off the metaphysical and pseudo-scientific shackles by which the modern Medical Deity keeps them in bondage and in exploitation. It is time that we educate ourselves and assume responsibility for our own health and happiness. We have nothing to lose but our medical chains. We have a world of health to gain. Is not life a precious gift to hold fast?

Ladies and gentlemen of the jury, I end this closing statement, with a warning and a prayer. The warning is the prophetic words of Dr. Benjamin Rush, signer of the Declaration of Independence and a member of the Continental Congress. This warning is repeated because it was a prophecy that sadly came to pass. In it he foretold the loss of medical freedom in America.

Unless we put medical freedom into the Constitution, the time will come when medicine will organize into an undercover dictatorship ... To restrict the art of healing to one class of men and deny equal privileges to others will constitute the Bastille of medical science. All such laws are un-American and despotic ... and have no place in a republic ... The Constitution of this republic should make special provision for medical freedom as well as religious freedom. [19]

Dr. Benjamin Rush's prediction has come to pass. We lost medical freedom in a century—1850 to 1950. Ironically it was Rush's Allopathic school of medicine that has established this medical dictatorship. We have been under medical bondage for all of the twentieth century. Ladies and gentlemen of the jury, if you hesitate to believe this, let me remind you of the graphic assessment of medical freedom in our day by Dr. J. W. Hodge, a physician in Niagara Falls, New York.

> The medical monopoly or medical trust, euphemistically called the American Medical Association, is not merely the meanest monopoly ever organized, but the most arrogant, dangerous and despotic organization which ever managed a free people in this or any other age. Any and all methods of healing the sick by means of safe, simple and natural remedies are sure to be assailed and denounced by the arrogant leaders of the AMA doctors' trust as "fakes, frauds and humbugs." Every practitioner of the healing art who does not ally himself with the medical trust is denounced as a "dangerous quack" and imposter by the predatory trust doctors. Every sanitarian who attempts to restore the sick to a state of health by natural means without resort to the knife or poisonous drugs, disease imparting serums, deadly toxins or vaccine, is at once pounded upon by these medical tyrants and fanatics, bitterly denounced, vilified and persecuted to the fullest extent. [20]

The Dark Ages lasted over ten centuries because the organs of the government, the Church, the Scholastic academies and the professions perpetuated the false rationalistic science of Pythagoras, Plato and Aristotle. Today we have thrown off the empirical science of Sir Francis Bacon and have bought into this false rationalistic science that dominated the Dark Ages. Consequently, we have lost medical freedom. And with it our rationality.

If the past throws any light on the future, we may never regain our medical freedom for another ten centuries unless each one of us stands up to be counted.

Ladies and gentlemen of the jury, are you willing to stand and be counted? Are you willing to tell the medical and pharmaceutical High Priests who now rule over us, enough is enough?

Will you, the jury, stand up for truth? If not you, who? If not now, when? Will you help Americans reclaim their God-given freedom? William Penn once warned,

> Those people who are not governed by God will be ruled by tyrants.

America now stands at this crossroads. Wither America?

I rest my case on your shoulders; bear this responsibility with virtue and courage, and you too will live free.

End Notes for Indicted!

Preface:

1. The Hippocratic Oath.
2. Hippocrates, On Ancient Medicine, translated By Francis Adams, part 3: Classics.mit. edu/Hippocrates/ancimed.3.3
3. Hippocrates, On Ancient Medicine, ibid, 20.20
4. Hippocrates, On Ancient Medicine, ibid, 14.14
5. Kevin Trudeau, Natural Cures "They" Don't Want You to Know About, 2004, p. 38
6. Garden of Praise.com/ibdhipp.htm.

THE INDICTMENT

Count 1: Profiteering with our Health.

1. T. Colin Campbell, and Thomas M. Campbell, The *China Study*, 2006, p. 315.
2. Ellen G. White Selected Messages, volume 2, p. 289
3. Ellen G. White, Medical Ministry, p. 281.
4. Campbell, *The China Study*, ibid, p. 340.
5. Campbell, *The China Study*, ibid, p. 353.
6. Campbell, *The China Study*, ibid, pp. 340, 348.
7. Campbell, *The China Study*, ibid, p. 340.
8. Campbell, *The China Study*, ibid, p. 340
9. Campbell, *The China Study*, ibid, p. 340
10. Campbell, *The China Study*, ibid, p. 340
11. Campbell, *The China Study*, ibid, p. 327
12. Jeffrey Novick, Effects of a Nutrition Education Program on the Related Knowledge and Behaviors of Family Practice Residents, 2001, www.beyondveg.com/ novick-j/nutrition-education/physicians-1.shtml

Count 2: Reaping a Harvest of Chronic Degenerative Diseases

1. Andrew Weil, Health and Healing, 1983, p. 21, note.
2. Harris Coulter Divided Legacy, A History of the Schism in Medical Thought, Vol. 4: Twentieth Century Medicine: The Biological Era, 1994, p. 570.
3. Coulter, *Divided Legacy, A History of the Schism*, ibid, p. 571.
4. Coulter, *Divided Legacy, A History of the Schism*, ibid, p. 571.

5. Coulter, *Divided Legacy, A History of the Schism*, ibid, p. 572.
6. Coulter, *Divided Legacy, A History of the Schism*, ibid, p. 572.
7. Harris Coulter, *Divided Legacy: Twentieth- Century Medicine, vol.* 4, *ibid,* p. 502.
8. Coulter, *Divided Legacy: vol.* 4. Ibid, p. 564, 565.
9. Julian Whitaker, *Whitaker's Guide to Natural Healing,* p. 3.
10. John McDougall, *The McDougall Program for a Health Heart,* p. 5.
11. Dean Ornish, *Reversing Heart Disease,* pp. 11, 56
12. McDougall, *The McDougall Program for a Health Heart,* p. 213.
13. Whitaker, *Whitaker's Guide to Natural Healing,* p. 222.
14. James Balch, *Prescription for Nutritional Healing,* p. 229.
15. John McDougall, *McDougall Program for Maximum Weight Loss,* p. 8.
16. Jason Theodosakis & Brenda Adderly, Ph.D., *The Arthritis Cure,* pp. 3, 19.
17. Whitaker, *Whitaker's Guide to Natural Healing,* p. 315.
18. T. Colin Campbell and Thomas M. Campbell, *The China Study,* 2006, p. 16.
19. Campbell, *China Study,* ibid, p. 16.
20. Andrew Weil, *Health and Healing,* 1983, p. 21.

Count 3: A New Dark Age:

1. Campbell, *The China Study,* ibid, p. 341 Emphasis added.
2. Francis Schaefer, *Escape From Reason,* p. 34.
3. Coulter, *Divided Legacy, vol.* 4, *ibid,* pp. xvii, 684.

Count 4: Turning the Wheel of Knowledge Backwards.

1. Henry Morris, *Men of Science, Men of God,* 1982, p. 9.
2. Stanley Jaki, *The Origin of Science and the Science of its Origin,* 1978, p. 93.
3. Stanley Jaki, *The Origin of Science,* ibid, p.69.
4. Stanley Jaki, *The Origin of Science,* ibid, p. 70.
5. Stanley Jaki, *The Origin of Science,* ibid, pp. 9, 105
6. Stanley Jaki, *The Origin of Science,* ibid, pp. 21, 73, 85
7. Dan Graves, *Scientists of Faith,* 1996, p. 8.
8. Morris, *Men of Science,* ibid, p. 1.
9. Stanley Jaki, *The Origin of Science,* ibid, p. 12

Count 5: The Plot: Suppressing Symptoms While Refusing to Cure the Disease

1. Max Gerson, *A Cancer Therapy, The Powerful Nutritional Therapy that has Healed Thousands,* 1958, p. 133
2. Patrick Quillin, *Beating Cancer by Nutrition,* 1994, pp. 29, 30.
3. Gerson, *A Cancer Therapy,* ibid, p. 45
4. Gerson, *A Cancer Therapy,* ibid, p. 42.
5. Gerson, A cancer Therapy, ibid, pp. 38, 39.
6. Julian Whitaker, *Reversing Diabetes,* 1987, pp. 108, 109.
7. Campbell, *The China Study,* Ibid, pp.151, 152.

8. John McDougall, *A Challenging Second Opinion,* 1985, pp. 74, 75.
9. McDougall, *A Challenging Second Opinion,* ibid, p. 67.
10. McDougall, *A Challenging Second Opinion,* ibid, p. 75.
11. Jason Theodosakis & Brenda Adderly, *The Arthritis Cure,* 1997, p. 4.
12. Paavo Airola, *There is a Cure for Arthritis,* p. 37.
13. Campbell, *The China Study,* ibid, p. 124.
14. Campbell, *The China Study,* ibid, pp. 126, 127,130.
15. Campbell, *The China Study,* ibid, p. 123.
16. F. Batmanghelidj, Water, ibid, page 2.
17. F. Batmanghelidj, Water, ibid, page 71.
18. F. Batmanghelidj, Water, ibid, page 75.
19. Campbell, *The China Study,* ibid, pp. 22, 23.

OPENING STATEMENT: An Overview of the Field of Conflict.

Section 1: The War on Nutrition

1. Whitaker, *Reversing Heart Disease,* ibid, p. xxi.
2. Julian Whitaker, *Reversing Heart Disease,* ibid, p. xv.
3. Whitaker, *Whitaker's Guide,* ibid, p. xiii
4. John Robbins, *Reclaiming our Health,* p. 6.
5. The Bob Livingston Letter.
6. Whitaker, *Whitaker's Guide,* ibid, p. 4.
7. Whitaker, *Whitaker's Guide,* ibid, pp. 110,111.
8. Harvey Bigelsen, Robert E. Smith, Ph.D., Phronda Keala Smith, *Your Cure for Cancer,* pp. 65, 66.
9. Harvey Bigelsen, *Your Cure for Cancer,* ibid, p. 73.
10. Louise Tenney, *The Immune System, A Nutritional Approach,* p. 3.
11. Elinor Levy, Ph.D. and Tom Monte, *The Ten Best Tools to Boost Your Immune System,* p. 5.
12. Levy, *The Ten Best Tools,* ibid, p. 5.
13. Weil, *Spontaneous Healing* ibid, p. 53.
14. Whitaker, *Whitaker's Guide,* ibid, p. 113.
15. Whitaker, *Whitaker's Guide,* ibid, p. 114.
16. John McDougall, *The McDougall Program for Maximum Weight Loss,* p. 5.
17. McDougall, *The McDougall Program,* ibid, p. 5.
18. McDougall, *The McDougall Program,* ibid, p. 5.
19. T. Collin Campbell, Wellnessnow.us/discoveries/ A China Study, 2007.
20. McDougall, *The McDougall Program,* ibid, p. 5.
21. 21. U C Davis Medicine, Fall 2007, p. 28.
22. Max Gerson, *A Cancer Therapy,* p, 89.
23. Gerson, Ibid, p. 93.
24. Gerson, Ibid, p, 163.
25. Gerson, Ibid, p. 163.

26. Gerson, Ibid, p, 130

27. Michael Colgan, *Prevent Caner Now,* pp. 30, 40, 45.

28. Michael Colgan, *Prevent Caner Now,* p. 48.

29. Michael Colgan, *Prevent Caner Now,* p. 49.

30. Michael Colgan, *Prevent Caner Now,* p. 50.

31. Michael Colgan, *Prevent Caner Now,* p. 50.

32. Michael Colgan, *Prevent Caner Now,* p. 49.

33. Michael Colgan, *Prevent Caner Now,* p. 50.

34. T. Colin Campbell, The China Study, pp. 5, 50.

35. T. Colin Campbell, The China Study, p. 81.

36. T. Colin Campbell, The China Study, p. 242

37. T. Colin Campbell, The China Study, p. 242.

38. Nancy Appleton, *Lick The Sugar Habit*, pp. 12, 13

39. Nancy Appleton, *Lick The Sugar Habit*, p. 20.

40. Nancy Appleton, *Lick The Sugar Habit*, p. 28.

41. Nancy Appleton, *Lick The Sugar Habit*, p. 31.

42. Nancy Appleton, *Lick The Sugar Habit*, p. 40.

43. Nancy Appleton, *Lick The Sugar Habit*, p. 40.

44. Nancy Appleton, *Lick The Sugar Habit*, p. 13.

45. Nancy Appleton, *Lick The Sugar Habit*, p. 13.

46. Nancy Appleton, *Lick The Sugar Habit*, p. 28.

47. Nancy Appleton, *Lick The Sugar Habit*, p. 28.

48. Nancy Appleton, *Lick The Sugar Habit*, p. 28.

Section 2: The Causes of Chronic Degenerative Diseases

1. John McDougall, *The McDougall Plan*, ibid, pp. 3, 4, 5.

2. Mike Colgan, *Optimum Sports Nutrition*, p. 95.

3. McDougall, *The McDougall Program*, ibid, p. 8.

4. McDougall, *The McDougall Program*, ibid, p. 8.

5. Whitaker, *Reversing Health Risks*, ibid, p. 85.

6. Whitaker, *Reversing Health Risks*, p ibid, p. 53.

7. Whitaker, *Reversing Health Risks*, ibid, pp. 53, 54.

8. Whitaker, *Reversing Health Risks*, ibid, p. 54.

9 Nancy Appleton, *Lick the Sugar Habit*, p. 42.

10. Appleton, *Lick the Sugar Habit*, ibid, p. 13.

11. Appleton, *Lick the Sugar Habit*, ibid, p. 12.

12. Appleton, *Lick the Sugar Habit*, ibid, pp. 12, 19.

13. Appleton, *Lick the Sugar Habit*, ibid, p. 13

14. Appleton, *Lick the Sugar Habit*, ibid, p. 37.

15. McDougall, *The McDougall Plan*, ibid, p. 14.

16. McDougall, *The McDougall Plan*, ibid, p. 19.

17. McDougall, *The McDougall Plan*, ibid, p. 19.

18. McDougall, *The McDougall Plan*, ibid, p. 19.

19. McDougall, *The McDougall Plan*, ibid, p. 5.

20. McDougall, *The McDougall Plan*, ibid, p. 16.

21. McDougall, *The McDougall Plan*, ibid, p. 16.

22. McDougall, *The McDougall Plan*, ibid, pp. 16, 17.

23. McDougall, *The McDougall Plan*, ibid, p. 17.

24. Robbins, *Diet for a New America*, ibid, p., 176.

25. John Robbins, *Diet for a New America*, ibid, p. 176.

26. Genesis chapters 4 thru 11

27. Robbins, *Diet for a New America*, ibid, p. 178.

28. McDougall, *The McDougall Plan*, ibid, p. 97.

29. McDougall, *The McDougall Plan*, ibid, p. 5.

30. Robbins, *Diet for a New America*, ibid, p. 175.

31. Leslie van Romer, Lifedynamic.com/articles/nutrition/meat_and_protein, 2007.

32. McDougall, *The McDougall Plan*, ibid, pp. 5, 38.

33. Whitaker, *Reversing Heart Disease*, ibid, p. 79.

34. Julian Whitaker, *Reversing Diabetes*, ibid, p. 46.

35. McDougall, *The McDougall Plan*, ibid, p. 5.

36. McDougall, *The McDougall Plan*, ibid, pp. 5, 6, 49.

37. McDougall, *The McDougall Plan*, ibid, pp. 5, 6, 49.

38. Whitaker, *Reversing Diabetes*, ibid, pp. 55, 56.

39. Whitaker, *Reversing Diabetes*, ibid, pp. 51–56.

40. Whitaker, *Reversing Diabetes*, ibid, pp. 51–56.

41. Robbins, *Diet For a New America*, ibid, p. xv.

Section 3: The Nutritional Experts and Medical Geniuses.

1. McDougall, *The McDougall Program*, ibid, p. 9.

Section 4: Foods That Heal: One Woman's Journey into Health

1. Appleton, *Lick the Sugar Habit*, ibid, p. 61.

2. Richard Schulze, AAm Evening with Dr. Schulze" DVD Series.

3. Whitaker, *Reversing Heart Disease*, ibid, p. 88.

4. Dharma Singh Khalsa, *Brain Longevity*, ibid, p. 205.

5. Khalsa, *Brain Longevity*, ibid, pp. 9, 10.

6. Khalsa, *Brain Longevity*, ibid, pp. 205, 206.

7. Khalsa, *Brain Longevity*, ibid, p. 347.

8. Khalsa, *Brain Longevity*, ibid, p. 348.

9. Khalsa, *Brain Longevity*, ibid, p. 348.

10. Khalsa, *Brain Longevity*, ibid, p. 348.

11. Gary Null, *The Vegetarian Handbook*, ibid, p. 7.

Section 5: Recapturing our Medical Freedom

1. See the companion book by the same author, *The Whisper of the Serpent, Part Two: How we Lost Medical Freedom*.

2. Patrick Quillin, *Beating Cancer with Nutrition*, ibid, p. 13.
3. G. Edward Griffin, *World without Cancer*, ibid, pp. 357, 358.
4. Coulter, *Divided Legacy, A History of the Schism*, ibid, p. 685.
5. Campbell, *The China Study*, ibid, p. 345.

THE EVIDENCE

Arthritis: Section 1: Why Africans Don't Get Arthritis.

1. Paavo O. Airola, N.D., *There is a Cure for Arthritis*, p. xii.
2. Jason Theodosakis & Brenda Adderly Ph.D., *The Arthritis Cure*, p. 2.
3. John McDougall, A Challenging Second Opinion, p. 232.
4. McDougall, *A Challenging Second Opinion*, ibid, p. 231.
5. Paavo O. Airola, *There is a Cure for Arthritis*, ibid, p. xi.
6. Theodosakis & Adderly, *The Arthritis Cure*, ibid, p. 3, 19
7. McDougall, *A Challenging Second Opinion*, ibid, p. 231.
8. McDougall, *A Challenging Second Opinion*, ibid, p. 234.
9. Theodosakis & Adderly, *The Arthritis Cure*, ibid, p. 4.
10. John McDougall, *A Challenging Second Opinion*, ibid, p. 239
11. John McDougall, *A Challenging Second Opinion*, ibid, p. 239.
12. John McDougall, *A Challenging Second Opinion*, ibid, p. 234.
13. John McDougall, *A Challenging Second Opinion*, ibid, p. 234.
14. John McDougall, A Challenging Second Opinion, ibid, p. 234.
15. John McDougall, *A Challenging Second* Opinion, ibid, p. 236.
16. Jason Theodosakis & Brenda Adderly, *The Arthritis Cure*, ibid, p. 3.
17. John McDougall, *A Challenging Second Opinion*, ibid, p. 237.
18. Jason Theodosakis & Brenda Adderly, ibid, p. 8.
19. John McDougall, *A Challenging Second Opinion*, ibid, p. 238.
20. Theodosakis & Adderly, *The Arthritis Cure*, ibid, pp. 22,23.
21. Theodosakis & Adderly, *The Arthritis Cure*, ibid, pp. 22, 23.
22. Theodosakis & Adderly, *The Arthritis Cure*, ibid, p 23.
23. McDougall, *A Challenging Second Opinion*, ibid, p. 239.
24. McDougall, *A Challenging Second Opinion*, ibid, p. 239.
25. Theodosakis & Brenda Adderly, *The Arthritis Cure*, ibid, p. 13.
26. Theodosakis & Adderly, *The Arthritis Cure*, ibid, p. 15.
27. Theodosakis & Adderly, *The Arthritis Cure*, ibid, p. 15.
28. Theodosakis & Adderly, *The Arthritis Cure*, ibid, p. 16.
29. Theodosakis & Adderly, *The Arthritis Cure*, ibid, pp. 16, 17.
30. McDougall, *A Challenging Second Opinion*, ibid, p. 240.
31. Theodosakis & Adderly, ibid, p. 19.
32. McDougall, *A Challenging Second Opinion*, ibid, p. 240.
33. McDougall, *A Challenging Second Opinion*, ibid, p. 240.

34. McDougall, *A Challenging Second Opinion*, ibid, p. 241.

35. McDougall, *A Challenging Second Opinion*, ibid, p. 242.

36. McDougall, A Challenging Second Opinion, ibid, p. 243.

37. McDougall, *A Challenging Second Opinion*, ibid, p. 243.

38. Appleton, *Lick the Sugar Habit*, ibid, p. 23,50.

39. McDougall, *A Challenging Second Opinion*, ibid, p. 246.

40. McDougall, *A Challenging Second Opinion*, ibid, p. 247.

41. McDougall, *A Challenging Second Opinion*, ibid, p. 247.

42. McDougall, *A Challenging Second Opinion*, ibid, p. 246.

43. McDougall, *A Challenging Second Opinion*, ibid, p. 248

Arthritis Section 2: Drug Therapy: A False Hope For The Arthritic

1. Paavo O. Airola, N.D., *There is a Cure for Arthritis*, p. 33.

2. Airola, *There is a Cure for Arthritis* ibid, p. 33.

3. Jason Theodosakis. & Dr. Brenda Adderly, *The Arthritis Cure*, p. 4.

4. John McDougall, *A Challenging Second Opinion*, ibid, p. 232.

5. John McDougall, *A Challenging Second Opinion*, ibid, p. 236.

6. John McDougall, *A Challenging Second Opinion*, ibid, p. 237.

7. Jason Dr. Theodosakis. & Dr. Brenda Adderly, *The Arthritis Cure*, ibid, p. 106.

8. Airola, *There is a Cure for Arthritis* ibid, p. 35.

9. Journal of the American Medical Association, *Acetylsalicylic Acid Poisoning*, Nov. 15, 1947, in Airola, p. 35.

10. Airola, *There is a Cure for Arthritis*, ibid, p. 35. .

11. Airola, *There is a Cure for Arthritis*, ibid, p. 36.

12. Airola, *There is a Cure for Arthritis*, ibid, p. 35.

13. Airola, *There is a Cure for Arthritis*, ibid, p. 35.

14. Airola, *There is a Cure for Arthritis*, ibid, pp. 35, 36.

15. Theodosakis. & Adderly, *The Arthritis Cure*, ibid, p. 103, 104.

16. Theodosakis. & Adderly, *The Arthritis Cure*, ibid, p. 104.

17. Theodosakis. & Brenda Adderly, *The Arthritis Cure*, ibid, p. 104.

18. Theodosakis. & Adderly, *The Arthritis Cure*, ibid, p. 105.

19. Theodosakis. & Adderly, *The Arthritis Cure*, ibid, p. 106.

20. Theodosakis. & Adderly, *The Arthritis Cure*, ibid, pp. 106, 107.

21. Airola, *There is a Cure for Arthritis*, ibid, p. 36.

22. Airola, *There is a Cure for Arthritis*, ibid, p. 37.

23. Airola, *There is a Cure for Arthritis*, ibid, p. 37.

25. Airola, *There is a Cure for Arthritis*, ibid, p. 38.

26. Airola, *There is a Cure for Arthritis*, ibid, pp. 37, 38.

27. Theodosakis. & Adderly, *The Arthritis Cure*, ibid, p. ibid, p. 155.

28. Airola, *There is a Cure for Arthritis*, ibid, p. 37.

29. McDougall, *A Challenging Second Opinion*, ibid, p. 242.

30. McDougall, *A Challenging Second Opinion*, ibid, p. 243.
31. Airola, *There is a Cure for Arthritis*, ibid, p. 39.
32. Airola, *There is a Cure for Arthritis*, ibid, p. 39.
33. McDougall, *A Challenging Second Opinion*, ibid, p. 248.

Arthritis section 3: Reversing Arthritis By Nutrition

1. John McDougall, *A Challenging Second Opinion*, p. 235.
2. McDougall, *A Challenging Second Opinion*, ibid, p. 235.
3. McDougall, *A Challenging Second Opinion*, ibid, p. 235.
4. McDougall, *A Challenging Second Opinion*, ibid, p. 235.
5. McDougall, *A Challenging Second Opinion*, ibid, p. 236.
6. McDougall, *A Challenging Second Opinion*, ibid, p. 237.
7. McDougall, *A Challenging Second Opinion*, ibid, p. 239.
8. McDougall, *A Challenging Second Opinion*, ibid, p. 239.
9. McDougall, *A Challenging Second Opinion*, ibid, p. 243.
10. McDougall, *A Challenging Second Opinion*, ibid, p. 243.
11. McDougall, *A Challenging Second Opinion*, ibid, pp. 245, 246.
12. McDougall, *A Challenging Second Opinion*, ibid, p. 247.
13. McDougall, *A Challenging Second Opinion*, ibid, p. 246.
14. McDougall, *A Challenging Second Opinion*, ibid, p. 246.
15. McDougall, *A Challenging Second Opinion*, ibid, p. 246.
16. McDougall, *A Challenging Second Opinion*, ibid, p. 244.
17. McDougall, *A Challenging Second Opinion*, ibid, p. 246.
18. Prevention *Joints Feel the Weight*. 41:10, February 1989.
19. Theodosakis. & Adderly, ibid, p. 15.
20. Theodosakis. & Adderly, *The Arthritis Cure*, ibid, p. 65.
21. Theodosakis. & Adderly, *The Arthritis Cure*, ibid, p. 65.
22. Theodosakis. & Adderly, ibid, p. 148.
23. Theodosakis. & Adderly, *The Arthritis Cure*, ibid, p. 65.
24. Theodosakis. & Adderly, *The Arthritis Cure*, ibid, p. 151.
25. Theodosakis. & Adderly, *The Arthritis Cure*, ibid, p. 151.
26. Theodosakis. & Adderly, *The Arthritis Cure*, ibid, p. 152.
27. Theodosakis. & Adderly, *The Arthritis Cure*, ibid, p. 152.
28. Theodosakis. & Adderly, *The Arthritis Cure*, ibid, p. 153.
29. Theodosakis. & Adderly, *The Arthritis Cure*, ibid, p. 115.
30. Theodosakis. & Adderly, *The Arthritis Cure*, ibid, p. 117.
31. Theodosakis. & Adderly, *The Arthritis Cure*, ibid, pp. 14, 116
32. Theodosakis. & Adderly, *The Arthritis Cure*, ibid, p. 117.
33. Theodosakis. & Adderly, *The Arthritis Cure*, ibid, p. 116.

Cancer Section 1: A Profile of a Killer Epidemic.

1. Patrick Quillin, *Beating Cancer With Nutrition*, 1994, p. xv.

2. Scott Gottlieb, Deputy Commissioner for Medical and Scientific Affairs, FDA, 3/07/06. www.fda.gov/oc/speceches/2006/cancerprogress0307.html.

3. Quillin, *Beating Cancer, ibid,* p. xv.

4. Quillin, *Beating Cancer, ibid,* p. xv.

5. Quillin, *Beating Cancer, ibid,* p. 25.

6. Quillin, *Beating Cancer, ibid,* pp. 25, 30.

7. James W. Anderson, Maury M. Breecher, Dr. Anderson's Antioxidant, Antiaging Health Program, 1996, p. 55.

8. Michael Colgan, *Prevent Cancer Now,* 1990, p.1, 2, 6.

9. John Robbins, *Diet For a New America,* 1987, page 248.

10. John Robbins, *Diet, ibid,* p. 250.

11. John Robbins, *Diet, ibid,* p. 251.

12. Quillin, *Beating Cancer, ibid,* p. xiv.

13. Donald McAlvany, *The McAlvany Intelligence Advisor,* Nov. 1997, p. 6.

14. McAlvany, ibid, Nov. 1997, p. 6

15. Neal Barnard, *The Power of your Plate,* 1990, p. 52.

16. Quillin, *Beating Cancer, ibid,* p. 27.

17. McAlvany, ibid, Nov. 1997, p. 5.

18. Andrew Weil, *Spontaneous Healing,* 1995, p. 274.

19. Max Gerson, *A Cancer Therapy,* 1958, p. 12.

20 Andrew Weil, *Health and Healing,* 1983, p. 74

21. Anne E. Frahm with David J. Frahm, *A Cancer Battle Plan,* 1992, p. 30.

22. Weil, *Spontaneous Healing,* p. 267.

23. John McDougall, *A Challenging Second Opinion,* 1985, p. 30.

24. McDougall, *A Challenging Second Opinion,* p. 30.

25. Colgan, *Prevent Cancer Now,* p. 4.

26. Weil, *Spontaneous Healing,* p. 268.

27. Gerson, *A Cancer Therapy, ibid,* p. 6.

28. Gerson, *A Cancer Therapy, ibid,* p. 45.

29. Andrew Weil, *Natural Health, Natural Medicine,* p. 174.

30. James Anderson, *Dr. Anderson's Antioxidant, ibid,* p. 58.

31. Ellen White, *Health, or How to Live,* cited into Selected Messages, Bk. 2, p. 449.

32. Ellen White, *The Ministry of Healing,* p. 313.

33. Anderson *Dr. Anderson's Antioxidant, ibid,* p. 58.

34. Anderson *Dr. Anderson's Antioxidant, ibid,* p. 57.

35. Anderson *Dr. Anderson's Antioxidant, ibid,* p. 58.

36. Anderson *Dr. Anderson's Antioxidant, ibid,* p. 59.

37. Griffin, *World Without Cancer,* 1997, p. 74.

38. Griffin, *World Without Cancer,* ibid, pp. 75, 83.

39. Griffin, *World Without Cancer, ibid,* pp. 75, 83.

40. Griffin, *World Without Cancer, ibid,* p. 76.

41. Griffin, *World Without Cancer, ibid,* p. 77.

42. Griffin, *World Without Cancer, ibid,* p. 77.

43. Griffin, *World Without Cancer, ibid,* p. 78.

44. Griffin, *World Without Cancer, ibid,* p. 84

45. Griffin, *World Without Cancer, ibid,* p. 79.

46. Gerson, *A Cancer Therapy, ibid,* p. 20.

47. Griffin, *World Without Cancer, ibid,* p. 84.

48. Gerson, *A Cancer Therapy, ibid,* p. 61.

49. Gerson, *A Cancer Therapy, ibid,* p. 40.

50. Neil Barnard, *ibid,* p. 55.

51. Tortora & Anagnostakos, *Principles of Anatomy & Physiology,* 2nd. ed., 1975, p. 578.

52. Tortora & Anagnostakos, *ibid,* p. 578.

53. Gerson, *A Cancer Therapy, ibid,* p. 25.

54. Tortora & Anagnostakos, *ibid,* p. 578.

55. Gerson, *A Cancer Therapy, ibid,* pp. 27,28.

56. Tortora & Anagnostakos, *ibid,* p. 578.

57. Gerson, *A Cancer Therapy, ibid,* p. 24.

58. Gerson, *A Cancer Therapy, ibid,* p. 25.

59. Quillin, *Beating Cancer, ibid,* p. 16.

60. Gerson, *A Cancer Therapy, ibid,* p. 24.

61. Gerson, *A Cancer Therapy, ibid,* p. 24.

62. Gerson, *A Cancer Therapy, ibid,* p. 25.

63. Gerson, *A Cancer Therapy, ibid,* p. 25.

64. Gerson, *A Cancer Therapy, ibid,* p. 26.

65. Gerson, *A Cancer Therapy, ibid,* p. 163.

66. Quillin, *Beating Cancer, ibid,* pp. 16, 17.

67. Quillin, *Beating Cancer, ibid,* pp. 16, 17.

68. Nancy Appleton, *Lick the Sugar Habit,* 1988, p. 54.

69. Appleton, *ibid,* p. 54.

70. Julian Whitaker, Dr. Whitaker's Guide to Natural Healing, p. 40.

71. Appleton, *ibid,* pp. 54, 55.

72. Gerson, *A Cancer Therapy, ibid,* p. 7.

73. Gerson, *A Cancer Therapy, ibid,* p. 67.

74. Gerson, *A Cancer Therapy, ibid,* p. 125.

75. Quillin, *Beating Cancer, ibid,* p. 53.

76. Quillin, *Beating Cancer, ibid,* p. 39.

77. Appleton, *ibid,* p. 55.

78. McDougall, *A Challenging Second Opinion,* pp. 20, 21.

79. Appleton, *Lick the Sugar Habit, ibid,* p. 56.

80. McDougall, *A Challenging Second Opinion,* p. 23.

81. McDougall, *A Challenging Second Opinion,* p. 20.

82. Weil, *Natural Health Natural Medicine,* p. 172.

83. Weil, *Natural Health, Natural Medicine,* p. 175.

84. McDougall, *A Challenging Second Opinion,* p. 43.

85. McDougall, *A Challenging Second Opinion,* p. 20.

86. Weil, *Natural Health, Natural Medicine,* p.172.

87. McDougall, A Challenging Second Opinion, p.21.

88. McDougall, A Challenging Second Opinion, p.21.

89. McDougall, *A Challenging Second Opinion,* p. 45.

90. Quillin, *Beating Cancer, ibid*, p. 112.
91. McDougall, *A Challenging Second Opinion, ibid*, p. 21.
92. McDougall, A Challenging Second Opinion, pp. 21, 22.
93. McDougall, A Challenging Second Opinion, p. 22.
94. Barnard, *The Power of your Plate, ibid*, p. 56.
95. Barnard, *The Power of your Plate, ibid*, p. 56.
96. McDougall, *A Challenging Second Opinion*, p. 22.
97. McDougall, *A Challenging Second Opinion*, p. 22.
98. Barnard, *The Power of Your plate*, p. 60.
99. Quillin, *Beating Cancer, ibid*, p. 46.
100. McDougall, *A Challenging Second Opinion*, p. 48.
101. Whitaker, *Dr. Whitaker's Guide, ibid*, p. 56.
102. Whitaker, *Dr. Whitaker's Guide, ibid*, p. 49.
103. Whitaker, *Dr. Whitaker's Guide, ibid*, p. 49.
104. Neal Barnard, *Eat Right Live Longer*, p. 121.
105. Barnard, *Eat Right Live Longer*, p. 121.
106. Barnard, *Eat Right Live Longer*, p. 122..
107. Quillin, *Beating Cancer*, 64,.
108. Weil, *Natural Health, Natural Medicine*, p.171.
109. Gerson, *A Cancer Therapy, ibid*, p. 80.
110. Barnard, *The Power of Your Plate*, p. 62.
111. Barnard, *The Power of Your Plate*, p. 62.
112. Gerson, *A Cancer Therapy, ibid*, p. 146.
113. Colin Campbell & Thomas Campbell, *The China Study*, 2006, pp. 48, 49.
114. Campbell i*bid, China Study*, p.50.
115. Campbell i*bid, The China Study,*, p. 50.
116. Campbell i*bid, The China Study*, pp. 52, 53.
117. Campbell i*bid, The China Study,*, p. 54.
118. Campbell i*bid, The China Study,*, p. 57.
119. Campbell i*bid, The China Study,*, p. 58.
120. Campbell i*bid, The China Study,*, p. 57.
121. Campbell i*bid, The China Study,*, p. 61.
122. Campbell i*bid, The China Study,*, p. 60.
123. Campbell i*bid, The China Study,*, p. 72, 73.
124. Campbell i*bid, The China Study*, p. 78.
125. Campbell i*bid, The China Study,*, pp. 78, 79.
126. Campbell i*bid, The China Study,*, pp. 80, 81.
127. Campbell i*bid, The China Study*, p. 92.
128. Campbell i*bid, China Study*, p.92.
129. Campbell i*bid, China Study*, p.94.
130. Campbell i*bid, China Study*, p.87.
131. Campbell i*bid, China Study*, p.104.
132. Weil, *Natural Health, Natural Medicine*, p. 30.
133. Barnard, *The Power of Your Plate*, p. 63.
134. Weil, *Natural Health, Natural Medicine*, p. 16.

135. Quillin, *Beating Cancer, ibid,* p.
136. Quillin, *Beating Cancer, ibid,* p. 124.
137. Weil, Natural Health , Natural Medicine, p. 175.
138. Weil, *Natural Health, Natural Medicine,* p. 178.
139. Weil, *Natural Health, Natural Medicine,* p. 180.
140. Weil, *Natural Health, Natural Medicine,* p. 180.
141. Weil, Natural Health, Natural Medicine, p. 181.
142. Weil, *Natural Health, Natural Medicine,* pp. 182, 183.
143. Whitaker, *Dr. Whitaker' Guide, ibid,* p. 29.
144. Barnard, *The Power of Your Plate,* p. 107.
145. Weil, *Natural Health, Natural Medicine,* p. 184.
146. Gerson, *A Cancer Therapy, ibid,* p. 64.
147. Gerson, *A Cancer Therapy, ibid,* p. 64.
148. Gerson, *A Cancer Therapy, ibid,* p. 64.
149. Gerson, *A Cancer Therapy, ibid,* p. 64.
150. Gerson, *A Cancer Therapy, ibid,* pp. 64, 65.
151. Gerson, *A Cancer Therapy, ibid,* pp. 68, 69.
152. Gerson, *A Cancer Therapy,* page 65.
153. Gerson, *A Cancer Therapy, ibid,* p. 66.
154. Gerson, *A Cancer Therapy, ibid,* p. 66.
155. Gerson, *A Cancer Therapy, ibid,* p. 67.
156. Gerson, *A Cancer Therapy, ibid,* p. 68.
157. Gerson, *A Cancer Therapy, ibid,* p. 69.
158. Gerson, *A Cancer Therapy, ibid,* p. 68.
159. John Robbins, *Diet for a New America,* p. 252.
160. John Robbins, *Diet for a New America,* p. 252.
161. John Robbins, *Diet for a New America,* p. 251.
162. Max Gerson, *A Cancer Therapy, ibid,* p. 146.
163. Max Gerson, *A Cancer Therapy, ibid,* pp. 141, 142.
164. Robbins, *Diet for a New America,* p. 253.
165. Robbins, *Diet for a New America,* p. 254.
166. Robbins, *Diet for a New America,* pp. 254, 260.
167. Whitaker, *Reversing Heart Disease,* 1985, p. 63.
168. Robbins, *Diet for a New America,* p. 256.
169. Campbell *ibid, China Study,* p. 89.
170. Campbell *ibid, China Study,* p. 89.
171. Colgan, *Prevent Cancer Now,* p. 40.
172. Robbins, *Diet for a New America,* p. 256.
173. Robbins, *Diet for a New America,* p. 258.
174. Robbins, *Diet for a New America,* p. 258.
175. Robbins, *Diet for a New America,* p. 260.
176. Robbins, Diet for a New America, p. 262.
177. Ellen White, *Testimonies to the Church,* vol. 9, p.156.
178. Harvey Bigelsen, Robert E. Smith, Phronda Keala Smith, *Your Cancer,* p. 99.
179. Bigelsen, *Cancer, ibid,* p. 63.

180. Bigelsen, *Cancer, ibid,* p. 64.

181. Bigelsen, *Cancer, ibid,* p. 64.

182. Bigelsen, *Cancer, ibid,* p. 64.

183. Bigelsen, *Cancer,* ibid, pp. 65, 66.

184. Bigelsen, *Cancer, ibid,* p. 66.

185. Bigelsen, *Cancer, ibid,* p. 67.

186. Bigelsen, *Cancer, ibid,* pp. 68, 69.

187. Bigelsen, *Cancer,* ibid, p. 69, 70.

188. Bigelsen, *Cancer, ibid,* p. 70.

189. Bigelsen, *Cancer, ibid,* p. 70.

190. Bigelsen, *Cancer, ibid,* p. 69.

191. Bigelsen, *Cancer, ibid,* p. 74.

192. Bigelsen, *Cancer, ibid,* p. 74.

193. Bigelsen, *Cancer, ibid,* pp. 75, 99.

194. Bigelsen, *Cancer,* page 75.

195. Bigelsen, *Cancer, ibid,* p. 79.

196. Bigelsen, *Cancer, ibid,* p. 80.

197. Bigelsen, *Cancer, ibid,* p. 85.

198. Julian Whitaker, Are you and your doctor making these COMMON MISTAKES with your health? Special Medical Alert, July 1999, p.27.

199. Whitaker, Are you and your doctor making these COMMON MISTAKES, *ibid,* p. 27.

200. Quillin, *Beating Cancer, ibid,* p. 13.

Cancer Section: 2 Cut Burn & Poison: The Politics of Death

1. G. Edward Griffin, *World Without Cancer, ibid,* p. 22.

2. John McDougall, *A Challenging Second Opinion,* p. 40.

3. Max Gerson, *A Cancer Therapy, ibid,* pp 13, 14.

4. Patrick Quillin, *Beating Cancer, ibid,* p. 10.

5. Donald McAlvany, *ibid,* p. Nov. 1997, page 5

6. McDougall, A Challenging Second Opinion, pp. 30, 31, 33.

7. Gerson, *A Cancer Therapy, ibid,* pp 16,17.

8. Gerson, *A Cancer Therapy,* pages 11, 119.

9. Gerson, *A Cancer Therapy, ibid,* p. 35.

10. Gerson, *A Cancer Therapy, ibid,* p. 66.

11. Gerson, *A Cancer Therapy, ibid,* p. 47.

12. Quillin, *Beating Cancer, ibid,* p. 4.

13. Gerson, *A Cancer Therapy, ibid,* p. 18.

14. Griffin, *World Without Cancer, ibid,* p. 138.

15. Griffin, *World Without Cancer, ibid,* p. 138.

16. Griffin, *World Without Cancer, ibid,* p. 141.

17. McDougall, *A Challenging Second Opinion,* p. 34.

18. Quillin, *Beating Cancer, ibid,* p. 32.

19. Quillin, *Beating Cancer, ibid,* p. 12.

20. Quillin, *ibid,* p. 58.

21. Donald McAlvany, *ibid,* p. Nov. 1997 p. 9.

22. Quillin, *Beating Cancer, ibid,* p. 14.

23. McDougall, *A challenging second Opinion,* p. 28.

24. Quillin, *ibid,* p. 10.

25. McDougall, *ibid,* p. 28.

26. McDougall, *A challenging second Opinion,* p. 29.

27. McDougall, *A challenging second Opinion,* p. 29.

28. Andrew Weil, *Health and Healing,* p. 87.

29. McDougall, *A Challenging Second Opinion,* p. 36.

30. McDougall, *A challenging Second Opinion,* p. 30.

31. McDougall, *A Challenging Second Opinion,* p. 31.

32. McDougall, *A Challenging Second Opinion,* p. 33.

33. McDougall, *A Challenging Second Opinion,* p. 30.

34. Quillin, *Beating Cancer, ibid,* p. 24.

35. Quillin, *Beating Cancer, ibid,* p. 24.

36. Quillin, *Beating Cancer, ibid,* p. xv.

37. Quillin, *Beating Cancer, ibid,* p. 25.

38. Quillin, *Beating Cancer, ibid,* p. 34.

39. Quillin, *Beating Cancer, ibid,* p. 33.

40. Quillin, *Beating Cancer, ibid,* p. 10.

41. Griffin, *World Without Cancer, ibid,* p. 139.

42. Griffin, *World Without Cancer, ibid,* p. 139.

43. Griffin, *World Without Cancer, ibid,* p. 139.

44. Griffin, *World Without Cancer, ibid,* p. 139.

45. Griffin, *World Without Cancer, ibid,* p. 141.

46. Griffin, *World Without Cancer, ibid,* p. 411.

47. Quillin, *Beating Cancer, ibid,* p. 30.

48. Gary Null and Carolyn Dean, *Death by Medicine,* 2003, p. 19.

49. Kenny Ausubel, *When Healing Becomes a Crime: The Amazing Story of the Hoxsey Clinics and the Return of Alternative Therapies,* 2000, p. 268.

50. Griffin, *World Without Cancer, ibid,* p. 142.

51. Griffin, *World Without Cancer, ibid,* p. 142.

52. McDougall, *A Challenging Second Opinion,* p. 36.

53. Quillin, *Beating Cancer, ibid,* p. 31.

54. Griffin, *World Without Cancer, ibid,* p. 144.

55. McDougall, *A Challenging Second Opinion,* p. 37.

56. McDougall, *A Challenging Second Opinion,* p. 37

57. McDougall, *A Challenging Second Opinion,* p. 37.

58. Griffin, *World Without Cancer, ibid,* p. 144.

59. Griffin, *World Without Cancer, ibid,* p. 145.

60. Quillin, *ibid,* p. 30.

61. Griffin, *World Without Cancer, ibid,* p. 143.

62. Griffin, *World Without Cancer, ibid,* p. 147.

63. Griffin, *World Without Cancer, ibid,* p. 145.
64. Quillin, *Beating Cancer, ibid,* p. 9.
65. Quillin, *Beating Cancer, ibid,* p. 9.
66. Quillin, *Beating Cancer, ibid,* p. 29.
67. Quillin, *Beating Cancer, ibid,* p. 29.
68. Quillin, *Beating Cancer, ibid,* p. 29.
69. Quillin, *Beating Cancer, ibid,* p. 30.
70. Quillin, *Beating Cancer, ibid,* p. 30.
71. Quillin, *Beating Cancer, ibid,* p. 32.
72. Griffin, *World Without Cancer, ibid,* p. 152.
73. Quillin, Quillin, *Beating Cancer, ibid,* p. 42.
74. Griffin, *World Without Cancer, ibid,* p. 152.
75. McDougall, *A Challenging Second Opinion,* p. 41.
76. McDougall, *A Challenging Second Opinion,* p. 41.
77. Griffin, *ibid,* p. 153. Open letter to Interested Doctors, Nov. 1972.
78. Griffin, *World Without Cancer, ibid,* p. 154.
79. Griffin, *World Without Cancer, ibid,* p. 155..
80. Griffin, *World Without Cancer, ibid,* p. 155..
81. Griffin, *World Without Cancer, ibid,* p. 156..
82. Griffin, *World Without Cancer, ibid,* p. 156..
>83. Griffin, *World Without Cancer, ibid,* p 146.9.
84. Griffin, *World Without Cancer, ibid,* p. 146.
85. Griffin, *World Without Cancer, ibid,* p. 146.
86. Griffin, *World Without Cancer, ibid,* p. 147.

Cancer: Section 3 Nutritional Remedies

1. Patrick Quillin, *Beating Cancer With Nutrition,* p. 12.
2. Griffin, *World Without Cancer,* ibid, p. 155.
3. I. William Lane, Linda Comac, *Sharks Don't get Cancer,* p. 87.
4. Quillin, *Beating Cancer,* ibid, p. 13.
5. Griffin, *World Without Cancer,* ibid, p. 155..
6. Griffin, *World Without Cancer,* ibid, p. 157.
7. Griffin, *World Without Cancer,* ibid, p. 157, 168.
8. Griffin, *World Without Cancer,* ibid, p. 169.
9. Griffin, *World Without Cancer,* ibid, p. 80.
10. Griffin, *World Without Cancer,* ibid, p. 81.
11. Griffin, *World Without Cancer,* ibid, p. 81.
12. Griffin, *World Without Cancer,* ibid, p. 82.
13. Griffin, *World Without Cancer,* ibid, p. 88.
14. Griffin, *World Without Cancer,* ibid, pp. 88, 89.
15. Griffin, *World Without Cancer,* ibid, p., 89.
16. Griffin, *World Without Cancer,* ibid, p. 91.
17. Griffin, *World Without Cancer,* ibid, p. 115.
18. G. Edward Griffin, *World Without Cancer,* ibid, p. 115.

19. Griffin, *World Without Cancer*, page 115.
20. Griffin, *World Without Cancer*, ibid, p. 127.
21. Griffin, *World Without Cancer*, ibid, p. 117.
22. Griffin, *World Without Cancer*, ibid, pp. 127.
23. Griffin, *World Without Cancer*, ibid, pp. 127.
24. Griffin, *World Without Cancer*, ibid, p. 128.
25. Griffin, *World Without Cancer*, ibid, p. 92.
26. Griffin, *World Without Cancer*, ibid, p. 83.
27. Gerson, *A Cancer Therapy*, ibid, pp. 35, 36.
28. Gerson, *A Cancer Therapy*, p. 37.
29. Gerson, *A Cancer Therapy*, ibid, p. 37.
30. Gerson, *A Cancer Therapy*, ibid, p. 133.
31. Gerson, *A Cancer Therapy*, ibid, p. 35.
32. Gerson, *A Cancer Therapy*, ibid, pp. 37, 125.
33. Gerson, *A Cancer Therapy*, ibid, pp. 37, 125.
34. Gerson, *A Cancer Therapy*, ibid, p. 37.
35. Gerson, *A Cancer Therapy*, ibid, p. 56.
36. Gerson, *A Cancer Therapy*, ibid, pp. 61, 62.
37. Gerson, *A Cancer Therapy*, ibid, p. 40.
38. Gerson, *A Cancer Therapy*, ibid, pp. 98,99.
39. Gerson, *A Cancer Therapy*, ibid, p. 40.
40. Gerson, *A Cancer Therapy*, ibid, p. 67.
41. Gerson, *A Cancer Therapy*, ibid, p. 66.
42. Gerson, *A Cancer Therapy*, ibid, p. 63.
43. Gerson, *A Cancer Therapy*, ibid, pp. 63. 64.
44. Gerson, *A Cancer Therapy*, ibid, pp. 130, 131.
45. Gerson, *A Cancer Therapy*, ibid, p. 131.
46. Gerson, *A Cancer Therapy*, ibid, p. 132.
47. Gerson, *A Cancer Therapy*, ibid, p. 80.
48. Gerson, *A Cancer Therapy*, ibid, p. 80.
49. Gerson, *A Cancer Therapy*, ibid, p. 80.
50. Gerson, *A Cancer Therapy*, ibid, p. 80.
51. Gerson, *A Cancer Therapy*, ibid, p. 132.
52. Gerson, *A Cancer Therapy*, ibid, p. 25.
53. Gerson, *A Cancer Therapy*, ibid, p. 91.
54. Gerson, *A Cancer Therapy*, ibid, p. 89, 90, 91.
55. Gerson, *A Cancer Therapy*, ibid, p. 165.
56. Gerson, *A Cancer Therapy*, ibid, p. 164.
57. Gerson, *A Cancer Therapy*, ibid, p. 97.
58. Gerson, *A Cancer Therapy*, ibid, p. 164.
59. Gerson, *A Cancer Therapy*, ibid, p. 164.
60. Gerson, *A Cancer Therapy*, ibid, p. 165.
61. Gerson, *A Cancer Therapy*, ibid, pp. 96, 97.
62. Gerson, *A Cancer Therapy*, ibid, p. 130.
63. Gerson, *A Cancer Therapy*, ibid, p. 82.

64. Gerson, *A Cancer Therapy*, ibid, p. 83.
65. Gerson, *A Cancer Therapy*, ibid, p. 81.
66. Gerson, *A Cancer Therapy*, ibid, p. 142.
67. Gerson, *A Cancer Therapy*, ibid, pp. 3,4.
68. I. William Lane, *Sharks Don't Get Cancer*, 1993, p. 142.
69. I. William Lane, *Sharks*, ibid, p. 143.
70. I. William Lane, *Sharks*, ibid, pp. 144, 145.
71. I. William Lane, *Sharks*, ibid, p. 40.
72. I. William Lane, *Sharks*, ibid, p. 38.
73. I. William Lane, *Sharks*, ibid, p. 41.
74. I. William Lane, *Sharks*, ibid, p. 41.
75. I. William Lane, *Sharks*, ibid, p. 41.
76. I. William Lane, *Sharks*, ibid, p. 43.
77. I. William Lane, *Sharks*, ibid, p. 44.
78. I. William Lane, *Sharks*, ibid, p. 45.
79. I. William Lane, *Sharks*, ibid, p. 48.
80. I. William Lane, *Sharks*, ibid, p. 49.
81. I. William Lane, *Sharks*, ibid, p. 50.
82. I. William Lane, *Sharks*, ibid, p. 54.
83. I. William Lane, *Sharks*, ibid, pp. 50, 51.
84. I. William Lane, *Sharks*, ibid, p. 66.
85. I. William Lane, *Sharks*, ibid, p. 68.
86, I. William Lane, *Sharks*, ibid, p. 69.
87. I. William Lane, *Sharks*, ibid, pp. 69, 70.
88. I. William Lane, *Sharks*, ibid, p. 88.
89. I. William Lane, *Sharks*, ibid, p. 99.
90. I. William Lane, *Sharks*, ibid, p. 99.
91. I. William Lane, *Sharks*, ibid, p. 101.
92. I. William Lane, *Sharks*, ibid, p. 101.
93. I. William Lane, *Sharks*, ibid, p. 102.
94. I. William Lane, *Sharks*, ibid, p. 144.
95. I. William Lane, *Sharks*, ibid, p. 144.
96. Richard Passwater, *Cancer Prevention and Nutritional Therapies*, p. 111.
97. Richard Passwater, *Cancer Prevention* ibid, p. 4.
98. Richard Passwater, *Cancer Prevention* ibid, p. 5.
99. Richard Passwater, *Cancer Prevention* ibid, pp. 4,5.
100. Richard Passwater, *Cancer Prevention* ibid, p. 5.
101. Richard Passwater, *Cancer Prevention* ibid, p. 13.
102. Richard Passwater, *Cancer Prevention* ibid, p. 16.
103. Richard Passwater, *Cancer Prevention* ibid, p. 6.
104. Richard Passwater, *Cancer Prevention* ibid, p. 31.
105. Richard Passwater, *Cancer Prevention* ibid, p. 31.
106. Richard Passwater, *Cancer Prevention* ibid, p. 31,32.
107. Richard Passwater, *Cancer Prevention* ibid, p. 30.
108. Richard Passwater, *Cancer Prevention* ibid, p. 31.

109. Richard Passwater, *Cancer Prevention* ibid, p. 31.
110. Passwater, *Cancer Prevention* ibid, p. 35.
111. Passwater, *Cancer Prevention* ibid, p. 35.
112. Richard Passwater, *Cancer Prevention* ibid, p. 36.
113. Richard Passwater, *Cancer Prevention* ibid, pp. 36, 37.
114. Richard Passwater, *Cancer Prevention* ibid, p. 36.
115. Richard Passwater, *Cancer Prevention* ibid, p. 36.
116. Richard Passwater, ibid, p. 38.
117. Passwater, *Cancer Prevention* ibid, pp. 38, 39.
118. Passwater, *Cancer Prevention* ibid, p. 39.
119. Richard Passwater, *Cancer Prevention* ibid, p. 40.
120. Richard Passwater, *Cancer Prevention* ibid, p. 40.
121. Loraine Day, A*Diseases Just Don't Happen*, video tape series.
122. Passwater, *Cancer Prevention* ibid, p. 42.
123. Passwater, *Cancer Prevention* ibid, pp. 43.44, citing Gladys Block.
124. Passwater, *Cancer Prevention* ibid, p. 44, citing Harish Padh.
125. Richard Passwater, *Cancer Prevention* ibid, pp. 44, 45.
126. Richard Passwater, *Cancer Prevention* ibid, p. 45.
127. Richard Passwater, *Cancer Prevention* ibid, p. 46.
128. Richard Passwater, *Cancer Prevention* ibid, p. 46.
129. Richard Passwater, *Cancer Prevention* ibid, p. 47.
130. Richard Passwater, *Cancer Prevention* ibid, p. 51.
131. Richard Passwater, *Cancer Prevention* ibid, p. 51.
132. Richard Passwater, *Cancer Prevention* ibid, p. 54.
133. Richard Passwater, *Cancer Prevention* ibid, p. 52.
134. Richard Passwater, *Cancer Prevention* ibid, p. 51.
135. Passwater, *Cancer Prevention* ibid, p. 52.
136. Passwater, *Cancer Prevention* ibid, p. 53.
137. Richard Passwater, *Cancer Prevention* ibid, p. 54.
138. Richard Passwater, *Cancer Prevention* ibid, p. 55.
139. Richard Passwater, *Cancer Prevention* ibid, p. 56.
140. Richard Passwater, *Cancer Prevention* ibid, p. 56.
141. Patrick Quillin, *Beating Cancer,* ibid, p. x.
142. Patrick Quillin, *Beating Cancer,* ibid, p. xi.
143. Patrick Quillin, *Beating Cancer,* ibid, p. 23.
144. James Duke, *The Green Pharmacy*, p. 110.
145. Michael Colgan, *Prevent Cancer Now,* p. 8.
146. Michael Colgan, *Prevent Cancer* ibid, p. 9.
147. Michael Colgan, *Prevent Cancer* ibid, p. 51.
148. Michael Colgan, *Prevent Cancer* ibid, p. 49.
149. Michael Colgan, *Prevent Cancer* ibid, pp. 49, 50.
150. Michael Colgan, *Prevent Cancer* ibid, p. 50.
151. Colgan, *Prevent Cancer* ibid, p. 50.
152. Michael Colgan, *Prevent Cancer* ibid, p. page 51.
153. Michael Colgan, *Prevent Cancer* ibid, pp. 53–73.

154. Michael Colgan, *Prevent Cancer* ibid, p. 57.

155. Michael Colgan, *Prevent Cancer* ibid, p. 58.

156. Michael Colgan, *Prevent Cancer* ibid, p. 58.

157. Michael Colgan, *Prevent Cancer* ibid, p. 81.

158. Michael Colgan, *Prevent Cancer* ibid, pp. 115, 116.

159. Michael Colgan, *Prevent Cancer* ibid, p. 124, 125.

160. Neal Barnard, *Eat Right Live Longer*, p. 208.

161. Neal Barnard, *Eat Right, ibid,* p. 208.

162. Neal Barnard, *Eat Right ,ibid,* p. 208.

163. Neal Barnard, *Eat Right ibid,* p. 208.

164. Neal Barnard, *Eat Right ,ibid,* p. 208.

165. Neal Barnard, *Eat Right ,ibid,* p. 209.

165. Neal Barnard, *Eat Right ,ibid,* p. 209.

166. Neal Barnard, *Eat Right ,ibid,* p. 209.

167. Neal Barnard, *Eat Right ,ibid,* p. 209.

168. Harvey Bigelsen, Robert E. Smith, Phronda Keala Smith, *Your Cure for Cancer*, p. 204.

169. Harvey Bigelsen, Cancer, ibid, ibid, p. 62.

171. Harvey Bigelsen, Cancer, ibid, p. 65.

172. Harvey Bigelsen, Cancer, ibid, p. 81.

173. Harvey Bigelsen, Cancer, ibid, p. 99.

174. Harvey Bigelsen, Cancer, ibid, pp. 118, 119.

175. Harvey Bigelsen, Cancer, ibid, pp. 114, 120, 121.

176. Harvey Bigelsen, Cancer, ibid, p. 120.

177. Harvey Bigelsen, Cancer, ibid, pp. 75, 77.

178. Harvey Bigelsen, Cancer, ibid, p. 216.

179. Harvey Bigelsen, Cancer, ibid, p. 207.

180. Campbell i*bid, China Study,* ibid, p.75.

181. Campbell i*bid, China Study, ,ibid,* p.104.

182. Campbell i*bid, China Study, ibid,* pp. 52, 53.

183. Campbell i*bid, China Study,* ibid, p. 54.

184. Campbell i*bid, China Study bid,* p. 61.

185. Campbell i*bid, China Study, ibid ,* p. 57.

186. Campbell i*bid, China Study, ibid* p.50.

187. Campbell i*bid, China Study, ibid,* p. 50.

188. Campbell i*bid, China Study,,* ibid, p. 60.

189. Campbell i*bid, China Study,* p. 78.

190. Campbell i*bid, China Study, ibid,* pp. 80, 81.

191. Campbell i*bid, China Study, ibid,* pp. 78, 79.

192. Campbell i*bid, China Study, ibid,* p.92.

193. Campbell i*bid, China Study,* ibid, p.94.

194. Campbell i*bid, China Study,* ibid, p.87.

195. Johanna Budwig www.positivehealth.com/permit/Articles/Nutrition/tumer60.htm.

196. Budwig ibid.

197. Budwig, ibid.

198. Budwig, ibid.

Diabetes: Section 1: Fat and a Cluster of Villains.

1. James A. Duke, Ph.D., *The Green Pharmacy*, page 161.
2. James A. Duke, *Green Pharmacy, ibid*, p. 161.
3. Julian Whitaker, *Reversing Diabetes*, p. xxi.
4. Julian Whitaker, *Whitaker's Guide to Natural Healing*, p. 222.
5. James Balch, *Prescription for Nutritional Healing*, p. 229.
6. Whitaker, *Reversing Diabetes*, p. xxi.
7. Julian Whitaker, *Whitaker's Guide, ibid*, p. 222.
8. Whitaker, *Reversing Diabetes*, p. 5.
9. Julian Whitaker, *Whitaker, Guide, ibid*, pp. 222, 226.
10. Whitaker, *Whitaker's Guide, ibid*, p. 223.
11. Whitaker, *Reversing Diabetes*, p. 4.
12. Agatha & Calvin Thrash, *Diabetes & The Hypoglycemic Syndrome*, p. 164.
13. Andrew Weil, *Natural Healing Natural Medicine*, p. 281.
14. Whitaker, *Whitaker's Guide, ibid*, p. 222.
15. Thrash, *Diabetes, ibid*, p. 81.
16. Whitaker, *Whitaker's Guide, ibid*, p. 222.
17. Thrash, *Diabetes, ibid*, p. 27.
18. Thrash, *Diabetes, ibid*, pp. 27, 28.
19. Weil, *Natural Health Natural Medicine*, p.281.
20. Whitaker, Whitaker, *Reversing Diabetes*, p. 65.
21. Whitaker, *Whitaker's Guide, ibid*, p. 223.
22. Whitaker, *Reversing Diabetes*, p. 31.
23. John McDougall, A *Challenging Second Opinion*, p. 213.
24. Whitaker, *Reversing Diabetes*, p. 27.
25. McDougall, A *Challenging Second Opinion*, p.212.
26. McDougall, *A Challenging Second Opinion*, p. 218.
27. McDougall, *A Challenging Second Opinion*, p. 222.
28. Whitaker, *Whitaker's Guide, ibid*, p. 227.
29. Nancy Appleton, *Lick the Sugar Habit*, p. 44.
30. Appleton, *Lick the Sugar Habit, ibid*, p. 45.
31. Appleton, *Lick the Sugar Habit, ibid*, p. 45.
32. Appleton, *Lick the Sugar Habit, ibid*, p. 45.
33. McDougall, *A Challenging Second Opinion*, pp. 212, 215.
34. Whitaker, *Whitaker's Guide, ibid*, pp. 222, 226.
35. Whitaker, *Reversing Diabetes*, pp. 31, 32.
36. Dean Ornish, *Stress, Diet. & Your Heart*, p.8.
37. Ornish, *Stress, ibid*, p. 48.
38. Whitaker, *Reversing Diabetes*, p. 46.
39. Whitaker, *Reversing Diabetes*, p.51.
40. Whitaker, *Reversing Diabetes*, p.51.
41. Whitaker, *Reversing Diabetes*, pp. 51, 52.
42. Whitaker, *Reversing Diabetes*, pp. 52, 53.
43. Whitaker, *Reversing Diabetes*, p. 53.

44. Whitaker, *Reversing Diabetes*, p. 54.

45. Campbell, *The China Study*, ibid, p. 58.

46. McDougall, *A Challenging Second Opinion*, pp. 214, 215.

47. McDougall, *A Challenging Second Opinion*, pp. 215, 216.

48. Thrash, *Stress, ibid*, p. 164:

49. Thrash, *Stress, ibid*, p. 80.

50. Thrash, *Diabetes, ibid*, p. 81.

51. Thrash, *Diabetes, ibid*, p. 80.

52. Thrash, *Diabetes, ibid*, p. 74.

53. Thrash, *Diabetes, ibid*, p. 81.

54. Thrash, *Diabetes, ibid*, p. 81.

55. Thrash, *Diabetes*, 82.

56. F. Batmanghelidj, *Your Body Many Cries For Water*, p. 124.

57. Batmanghelidj, *Water, ibid*, p. 125.

58. Batmanghelidj, *Water, ibid*, p. 126.

59. Batmanghelidj, *Water, ibid*, p. 128.

60. Thrash, *ibid*, p. 164.

61. Ornish, *Reversing Heart Disease*, pp. xxxiii, xxxiv.

62. Ornish, *Reversing Heart Disease*, p. xxxiv.

63. Ornish, *Reversing Heart Disease*, p. xxxiv.

64. Thrash, *Diabetes, ibid*, p. 63.

65. Thrash, *Diabetes, ibid*, p. 65.

66. Thrash, *Diabetes, ibid*, p. 64.

67. Thrash, *Diabetes, ibid*, p. 64.

68. Thrash, *Diabetes, ibid*, p. 66.

69. Thrash, *Diabetes, ibid*, p. 28.

70. Thrash, *Diabetes, ibid*, p. 28.

71. Thrash, *Diabetes, ibid*, p. 28.

72. Thrash, *Diabetes, ibid*, p. 29.

73. Thrash, *Diabetes, ibid*, pp. 29, 30.

Diabetes Section 2: The Drug Therapy Racket.

1. Julian Whitaker, *Whitaker's Guide to Natural Healing*, p. 225.

2. Julian Whitaker, *Reversing Diabetes*, p. 130.

3. Neil Nedley, *Proof Positive, How to Reliably Combat Disease and Achieve Optional Health through Nutrition and Lifestyle*, 1998, p. 177.

4. Nedley, *Proof Positive*, ibid, p. 177.

5. Nedley, *Proof Positive*, ibid, p. 177.

6. Whitaker, *Whitaker's Guide, ibid*, p. 225.

7. Whitaker, *Whitaker's Guide, ibid*, p. 225.

8. Whitaker, *Whitaker's Guide, ibid*, p. 228.

9. Whitaker, *Whitaker's Guide, ibid*, p. 228.

10. Whitaker, *Whitaker's Guide, ibid*, p. 228.

11. Whitaker, *Reversing Diabetes*, p. 101.

12. Whitaker, *Reversing Diabetes, ibid,* pp. 102, 103.

13. Whitaker, *Reversing Diabetes, ibid, pp.* 102, 103.

14. Whitaker, *Reversing Diabetes, ibid,* p. 106.

15. Whitaker, *Reversing Diabetes, ibid,* p. 106.

16. Whitaker, *Reversing Diabetes, ibid,* p. 106.

17. Whitaker, *Reversing Diabetes, ibid,* p. 106.

18. Whitaker, *Reversing Diabetes, ibid,* p. 108.

19. Whitaker, *Reversing Diabetes, ibid,* p. 109.

20. Whitaker, *Reversing Diabetes, ibid,* pp. 110, 111.

21. Whitaker, *Reversing Diabetes, ibid,* p. 112.

22. Whitaker, *Reversing Diabetes, ibid,* p. 119.

23. Whitaker, *Reversing Diabetes,, ibid,* p.

24. Whitaker, *Reversing Diabetes, ibid,* p. 119.

25. Whitaker, *Reversing Diabetes, ibid,* p. 119.

26. Whitaker, *Reversing Diabetes, ibid,* p. 119.

27. Nedley, Proof Positive, ibid, p. 177.

28. Whitaker, *Reversing Diabetes, ibid,* p. 150.

29. Whitaker, *Reversing Diabetes, ibid,* p. 150.

30. Whitaker, *Reversing Diabetes, ibid,* p. 150.

31. Whitaker, *Reversing Diabetes, ibid,* p. 150.

32. Whitaker, *Reversing Diabetes, ibid,* p. 150.

33. Whitaker, Reversing Diabetes, *ibid,* p. 149.

34. Lynn Paige Walker, Ellen Hodgson Brown, J.D. *The Alternative Pharmacy,* 1998, p. 141.

35. Whitaker, *Reversing Diabetes, ibid,* p. 149.

36. Whitaker, *Reversing Diabetes, ibid,* p. 149.

37. McDougall, A *Challenging Second Opinion,, ibid,* p. 222.

38. McDougall, A challenging Second Opinion, *ibid,* p. 222.

39. Whitaker, *Reversing Diabetes, ibid,* p. 153.

40. Walker, *The Alternative Pharmacy,* ibid, pp. 142- 145.

41. McDougall, *A Challenging Second Opinion, ibid,* p. 222.

Diabetes Section 3: Preventing & Curing Diabetes by Nutrition

1. James A. Duke, Ph. D. *The Green Pharmacy,* p. 162.

2. Agatha and Calvin Thrash, *Diabetes & The Hypoglycemic Syndrome,* p. 151.

3. Dean Ornish, *Reversing Heart Disease,* p. xxxiv.

4. Julian Whitaker, *Whitaker's Guide to Natural Healing,* p. 227.

5. Julian Whitaker, *Reversing Diabetes,* p. 31.

6. Whitaker, *Whitaker's Guide, ibid,* p. 22.

7. John A. McDougall, *A Challenging Second Opinion, ibid,* p. 219.

8. Whitaker, *Whitaker's Guide, ibid,* p. 227.

9. Whitaker, *Whitaker's Guide, ibid,* p. 228.

10. T. Colin Campbell, The China Study, p. 152.

11. McDougall, *A Challenging Second Opinion,* ibid, p. 219.

12. McDougall, *A Challenging Second Opinion*, ibid, pp. 219, 220.
13. McDougall, *A Challenging Second Opinion*, ibid, p. 214.
14. McDougall, *A Challenging Second Opinion*, ibid, p. 215.
15. McDougall, *A Challenging Second Opinion*, ibid, p. 215.
16. McDougall, *A Challenging Second Opinion*, ibid, p. 215.
17. McDougall, *A Challenging Second Opinion*, ibid, p. 215.
18. McDougall, *A Challenging Second Opinion*, ibid, p. 216.
19. McDougall, *A Challenging Second Opinion*, ibid, p. 216
20. Whitaker, Reversing Heart Disease, p. 63.
21. John Robins, Diet for a New America, p. 256.
22. McDougall, *A Challenging Second Opinion*, ibid, pp. 215, 218.
23. McDougall, *A Challenging Second Opinion*, ibid, p. 220.
24. McDougall, *A Challenging Second Opinion*, ibid, p. 220.
25. McDougall, *A Challenging Second Opinion*, ibid, p. 221.
26. Campbell, The China Study, ibid, p. 152.
27. Andrew Weil, *Natural Health, Natural Medicine*, p. 282.
28. Neil Nedley, Proof Positive, p. 178.
29. Whitaker, *Reversing Diabetes*, ibid, p. 62.
30. Whitaker, *Reversing Diabetes*, ibid, p. 62.
31. Whitaker, *Reversing Diabetes*, ibid, p. 63.
32. Whitaker, *Reversing Diabetes*, ibid, p. 64.
33. Whitaker, *Reversing Diabetes*, ibid, p. 65.
34. Whitaker, *Reversing Diabetes*, ibid, p. 65.
35. Whitaker, *Reversing Diabetes*, ibid, p. 67.
36. Weil, *Natural Health Natural Medicine*, ibid, p. 282.
37. Whitaker, *Reversing Diabetes*, ibid, p. 68.
38. Whitaker, *Reversing Diabetes*, ibid, p. 69, 70.
39. Whitaker, *Whitaker's Guide to Natural Healing,* ibid, p. 231.
40. Duke, *Green Pharmacy*, ibid, p. 167.
41. Whitaker, *Whitaker's Guide,* ibid, p. 231.
42. Whitaker, *Reversing Diabetes*, ibid, p. 92.
43. Duke, *Green Pharmacy*, ibid, p. 163.
44. Lynne Paige Walker, *The Alternative Pharmacy*, ibid, p. 144.
45. Walker, *Alternative Pharmacy*, ibid, p. 144
46. Walker, *Alternative Pharmacy*, ibid, pp. 144, 145
47. Duke, *Green Pharmacy*, ibid, pp. 163, 165.
48. Duke, *Green Pharmacy*, ibid, pp. 163, 165. .
49. Duke, *Green Pharmacy*, ibid, p. 164.
50. Duke, *Green Pharmacy*, ibid, p. 164.
51. Duke, *Green Pharmacy*, ibid, p. 165.
52. James Marti, *The Alternative Health Medicine Encyclopedia*, p. 87.
53. Duke, *Green Pharmacy*, ibid, p. 161.
54. Whitaker, *Whitaker's Guide,* ibid, p. 232.
55. Duke, *Green Pharmacy*, ibid, p. . 163.
56. Whitaker, *Whitaker's Guide,* ibid, p. 233.

57. Whitaker, *Whitaker's Guide,* ibid, p. 41.

58. Whitaker, *Whitaker's Guide,* ibid, p. 41.

59. Whitaker, *Whitaker's Guide,,* ibid, pp. 42, 43.

60. Whitaker, *Whitaker's Guide,* ibid, p. 42.

61. Whitaker, *Whitaker's Guide,* ibid, p. 42.

62. Whitaker, *Whitaker's Guide,* ibid, p. 232.

63. Whitaker, *Whitaker's Guide,* ibid, p. 43.

64. Whitaker, *Whitaker's Guide,* ibid, p. 43.

65. Whitaker, *Whitaker's Guide,* ibid, p. 44.

66. Whitaker, *Whitaker's Guide,* ibid, p. 44.

67. Whitaker, *Whitaker's Guide,* ibid, p. 232.

68. Whitaker, *Whitaker's Guide,* ibid, p. 233.

68. Whitaker, *Whitaker's Guide,* ibid, p. 233.

70. Medicine in the Public Interest, *Learning to live with Diabetes*, p. 54.

71. Whitaker, *Reversing Diabetes*, ibid, p. 90.

72. Whitaker, *Reversing Diabetes*, ibid, p. 90.

73. Walker, *Alternative Pharmacy*, ibid, p. . 143.

74. Whitaker, *Reversing Diabetes*, ibid, p. 90.

75. Whitaker, *Whitaker's Guide,* ibid, p. 46.

76. Whitaker, *Reversing Diabetes*, ibid, p. 91.

77. Whitaker, *Reversing Diabetes*, ibid, p. 90.

78. Whitaker, *Reversing Diabetes*, ibid, p. 91.

79. Whitaker, Whitaker's Guide, ibid, p. 44.

80. Whitaker, *Whitaker's Guide,* ibid, p. 44.

81. Whitaker, *Whitaker's Guide,* ibid, p. 45.

82. Whitaker, *Whitaker's Guide,* ibid, p. 46.

83. Whitaker, *Reversing Diabetes*, ibid, p. 91.

84. Whitaker, *Whitaker's Guide,* ibid, p. 46.

85. Whitaker, *Whitaker's Guide,* ibid, p. 46.

86. Whitaker, *Whitaker's Guide,* ibid, p. 46.

87. Whitaker, *Whitaker's Guide,* ibid, p. 46.

88. Whitaker, *Whitaker's Guide,* ibid, p. 48.

89. Whitaker, *Whitaker's Guide,* ibid, p. 48.

90. Whitaker, *Whitaker's Guide,* ibid, p. 47.

91. Whitaker, *Whitaker's Guide,* ibid, p. 47.

92. Whitaker, *Whitaker's Guide,* ibid, p. 47.

93. F. Batmanghelidj, *Your Body Many Cries For Water*, p. 11.

94. Batmanghelidj, *Water*, ibid, p. 124.

95. Duke, *Green Pharmacy*, ibid, p. 163.

Heart Disease: Section 1: The Deadly Trio.

1. Dean Ornish, *Reversing Heart Disease*, p. 11.

2. Ornish, *Reversing Heart Disease*, ibid, p.11.

3. Ornish, *Reversing Heat Disease*, ibid, p 11.

4. Julian Whitaker, *Reversing Heart Disease*, p. 3.

5. Julian Whitaker, *Special Medical Alert* AAre you and your doctor making these COMMON MISTAKES with your health? p. 21.

6. Ornish, *Reversing Heart Disease*, ibid, p 56.

7. Whitaker, *Reversing Heart Disease*, ibid, p 4.

8. Ellen G. White, *Counsels on Diet and Foods*, p. 141.

9. White, *Counsels*, ibid, p. 127.

10. Whitaker, *Reversing Heart Disease*, ibid, p. xv, citing *Cardiovascular News*, Spring 1984.

11. White, *Counsels*, ibid, p. 122.

12. Ornish, *Reversing Heart Disease*, ibid, p. 50.

13. Whitaker, Reversing Heart Disease, ibid, p. 93.

14. Whitaker, *Reversing Heart Disease*, ibid, p. 159.

15. Ornish, Reversing heart disease, ibid, p. 55.

16. Whitaker, *Reversing Heart Disease*, ibid, p. 94.

17. Whitaker, *Reversing Heart Disease*, ibid, p. 96.

18. Ornish, Reversing Heart Disease, ibid, p. 262.

19. Neil Nedley, *Proof Positive*, p. 73

20. Nedley, *Proof Positive*, ibid, p. . 74

21. Nedley, *Proof Positive*, ibid, p. 74

22. Nedley, *Proof Positive*, ibid, p. . 74

23. Whitaker, *Reversing Heart Disease*, ibid, pp. 87, 88.

24. John McDougall, *The McDougall Program for a Health Heart*, ibid, p. 39.

25. Ornish, *Reversing Heart Disease*, ibid, p. 259.

26. Ornish, *Diet, Stress & your Heart*, ibid, p. 48.

27. T. Colin Campbell, *The China Study*, p. 80.

28. *Lets Live, Nutrition Insights*, page 1, Issue 4 vol. 3, April 1988.

29. Julian Whitaker, *Special Medical Alert* AAre you and your doctor making these COMMON MISTAKES with your health? p. 23.

30. Whitaker, *Reversing Heart Disease*, ibid, p. 88.

31. Whitaker, *Reversing Heart Disease*, ibid, p. 87.

32. Whitaker, *Reversing Heart Disease*, ibid, p. 87.

33. Whitaker, *Reversing Heart Disease*, ibid, p. 88.

34. Whitaker, *Reversing Heart Disease*, ibid, p. 88.

35. Whitaker, *Reversing Heart Disease*, ibid, p. 88.

36. Whitaker, *Reversing Heart Disease*, ibid, p. 88.

37. Whitaker, *Reversing Heart Disease*, ibid, p. 94.

38. Whitaker, *Reversing Heart Disease*, ibid, p. 63.

39. Ornish, *Reversing Heart Disease*, ibid, p. 66.

40. Ornish, *Reversing Heart Disease*, ibid, p. 70.

41. Ornish, *Reversing Heart Disease*, ibid, p. 70.

42. Ornish, *Diet, Stress & your Heart*, ibid, p. 52.

Heart Disease Section 2: Refined Foods

1. Nancy Appleton, *Lick the Sugar Habit*, 1996, pp.68–72.

2. American Journal of Clinical Nutrition, March 11, 2008 as cited in www.news.com.au/ story//0,23599,23349178–421,00.html.

3. Harold E. Miller et al, Antioxidant Content of Whole Grain Breakfast Cereals, Fruits and Vegetables, as cited in the Journal of American College of Nutrition, Vol. 19, No. 3, 312S-319S (200).

4. Appleton, *Sugar Habit* ibid, pp.91, 92.

5. Appleton, Sugar Habit, ibid, p. 93.

6. Appleton, *Lick the Sugar Habit,* 1988, p. 62.

7. Appleton, *Sugar Habit,* ibid, p. 64.

8. Appleton, *Sugar Habit,* ibid, p. 65.

9. Appleton, *Sugar Habit,* ibid, p. 62.

10. Appleton, Lick the *Sugar Habit,* 1996, p.25.

11. Appleton, *Lick the Sugar Habit,* 1988, p. 16.

12. Appleton, *Sugar Habit,* ibid, p. 63.

13. Appleton, *Sugar Habit,* ibid, p. 64.

14. Appleton, Lick the *Sugar Habit,* 1995, p. 89.

Heart Disease: Section 3: Surgery

1. Julian Whitaker, Special Medical Alert, AAre you and your doctor making these COMMON MISTAKES with your health?, July 1999 issue p. 24.

2. Whitaker, Special Medical Alert, ibid, p. 24.

3. Neil Nedley, *Proof Positive,* ibid, pp. 91, 92.

4. Dean Ornish, *Reversing Heart Disease,* ibid, p. 51.

5. Ornish, *Reversing Heart Disease,* ibid, p. 52.

6. Ornish, *Reversing Heart Disease,* ibid, p. 52.

7. Ornish, *Reversing Heart Disease,* ibid, p. 53.

8. Ornish, *Reversing Heart Disease,* ibid, p. 53.

9. Whitaker, Special Medical Alert, ibid, p. 24.

10. Whitaker, Special Medical Alert, ibid, p. 24, 25.

11. Julian Whitaker, *Reversing Heart Disease,* ibid, p. 33.

12. Whitaker, *Reversing Heart Disease,* ibid, p. 34.

13. Whitaker, *Reversing Heart Disease,* ibid, p. 34.

14. Whitaker, *Reversing Heart Disease,* ibid, p. 36.

15. Whitaker, *Reversing Heart Disease,* ibid, p. 37.

16. Ornish, *Reversing Heart Disease,* ibid, p. 52.

17. News Week, March 1998.

18. Ornish, *Reversing Heart Disease,* ibid, p. 53.

19. Ornish, *Reversing Heart Disease,* ibid, p. 53.

20. Ornish, *Reversing Heart Disease,* ibid, p. 54.

21. Neil Nedley, *Proof Positive,* ibid, p. 92.

22. Ornish, *Reversing Heart Disease,* ibid, p. 55.

23. John McDougall, *The McDougall Program,* ibid, p. 200.

24. McDougall, *The McDougall Program,* ibid, p. . 201.

25. McDougall, *The McDougall Program,* ibid, p. 198.

Treating Heart Disease: Section 4: Drugs

1. Julian Whitaker, *Reversing Heart Disease*, ibid, p. 67.

2. Whitaker, *Reversing Heart Disease*, ibid, p. 67.

3. Whitaker, *Reversing Heart Disease*, ibid, p. 121.

4. Dean Ornish, *Reversing Heart Disease*, ibid, p. 57.

5. Ornish, *Reversing Heart Disease*, ibid, p. 57.

6. John McDougall, *The McDougall Program*, ibid, p. . 186.

7. Ornish, *Reversing Heart Disease*, ibid, p. 57.

8. McDougall, *The McDougall Program*, ibid, p. 189.

9. Dr. Lynne Paige Walker, *The Alternative Pharmacy*, 1998, p. 128

10. McDougall, *The McDougall Program*, ibid, p. 189.

11. Walker, *Alternative Pharmacy*, ibid, p. 128.

12. McDougall, *The McDougall Program*, ibid, p. 189.

13. Lynne Paige Walker, *The Alternative Pharmacy*, p. 209.

14. Walker, *Alternative Pharmacy*, ibid, p. 210.

15. *Walker, Alternative Pharmacy*, ibid, p. 210.

16. Walker, *Alternative Pharmacy*, ibid, p. 210.

17. Whitaker, *Reversing Heart Disease*, ibid, p. 105.

18. Whitaker, *Reversing Heart Disease*, ibid, p. 105.

19. Whitaker, *Reversing Heart Disease*, ibid, p. 105.

20. Whitaker, *Reversing Heart Disease*, ibid, p. 105.

21. Whitaker, *Reversing Heart Disease*, ibid, p. 106.

22. Neil Nedley, *Proof Positive*, p. . 103.

23. Nedley, *Proof Positive*, ibid, p. 104.

24. Ornish, *Reversing Heart Disease*, ibid, p. 62.

25. Ornish, *Reversing Heart Disease*, ibid, p. 62.

26. Ornish, *Reversing Heart Disease*, ibid, p. 62.

27. Ornish, *Reversing Heart Disease*, ibid, p. 63.

28. Ornish, *Reversing Heart Disease* ibid, p. 28.

29. Whitaker, *Dr. Whitaker's Guide*, ibid, p. . 4.

30. Whitaker, *Dr. Whitaker's Guide*, ibid, p. . 40.

31. Whitaker, *Dr. Whitaker's Guide*, ibid, pp. 4, 5.

32. Whitaker, *Dr. Whitaker's Guide*, ibid, pp. 4, 5.

33. T. Colin Campbell, *The China Study*, ibid, pp. 249, 250.

34. Whitaker, *Dr. Whitaker's Guide*, ibid, p. . 5.

35. Ornish, *Reversing Heart Disease*, ibid, p. 57, 266.

36. Ray Moynihan and Alan Cassels, *Selling Sickness: How the World's Biggest Pharmaceutical Companies Are Turning us All into Patients*, 2005, pp. ix, xi

37. Moynihan and Cassels, *Selling Sickness*, ibid, pp. xii, xiii.

38. Ornish, *Reversing Heart Disease*, ibid, p. 56.

39. Ornish, Reversing Heart Disease, ibid, p. 27.

40. Ornish, Reversing Heart Disease, ibid, p. 27.

Reversing Heart Disease: Section 5: Water and Nutrition ...

1. Dean Ornish, *Reversing Heart Disease*, p. 19.
2. Ornish, *Reversing Heart Disease*, ibid, p. 18.
3. Ornish, *Reversing Heart Disease*, ibid, p. 19.
4. Ornish, *Reversing Heart Disease*, ibid, p. 20.
5. Ornish, *Reversing Heart Disease*, ibid, p. 20.
6. Ornish, *Reversing Heart Disease*, ibid, p. 25.
7. Ornish, *Reversing Heart Disease*, ibid, p. 23.
8. Ornish, *Reversing Heart Disease*, ibid, p. 17.
9. Ornish, *Reversing Heart Disease*, ibid, p. 257.
10. Ornish, *Reversing Heart Disease*, ibid, p. 256.
11. Ornish, *Reversing Heart Disease*, ibid, p. 293.
12. Neil Nedley, *Proof Positive*, p. 69.
13. Ornish, *Reversing Heart Disease*, ibid, p. 259.
14. *Let's Live Nutritional Insights*, page 6, April 1997, issue 4 vol. 3.
15. Dean Ornish, *Stress, Diet and Your Heart*, p. 48. See also Ornish, *Reversing Heart Disease*, ibid, p. 259.
16. T. Colin Campbell, *The China Study*, p. 80.
17. Ornish, *Reversing Heart Disease*, ibid, p. 259.
18. Whitaker, *Reversing Heart Disease*, ibid, p. 126.
19. Ornish, *Reversing Heart Disease*, ibid, p. 260.
20. Ornish, *Reversing Heart Disease*, ibid, p. 261.
21. McDougall, *McDougall's Program for Maximum Weight Loss*, p. 70.
22. Ornish, *Reversing Heart Disease*, ibid, p. 257.
23. Ornish, *Reversing Heart Disease*, ibid, p. 281.
24. Ornish, *Reversing Heart Disease*, ibid, p. 261.
25. Journal of the American Dietetic Association, March 1988, vol. 88, # 3, pp. 352–355.
26. Gary Null, in *The Vegetarian Handbook, Eating Right for Total Health*, 1996, p. 181.
27. Gary Null, ibid, p. . 12.
28. Let's Live Nutrition Insights, page 6, April 1998, issue 4 vol. 3.
29. Julian Whitaker, *Reversing Heart Disease*, p 117.
30. Dean Ornish, *Reversing Heart Disease*, ibid, p. 263.
31. Dean Ornish, *Reversing Heart Disease*, ibid, p. 18, 19.
32. Dean Ornish, *Reversing Heart Disease*, ibid, p. 266.
33. Dean Ornish, *Reversing Heart Disease*, ibid, p. 271.
34. Neil Nedley, *Proof Positive*, ibid, p. 77.
35. Neil Nedley, ibid, p. . 77.
36. Dean Ornish, *Reversing Heart Disease*, ibid, p. 272.
37. Dean Ornish, *Reversing Heart Disease*, ibid, p. 274.
38. Dean Ornish, *Reversing Heart Disease*, ibid, p. 278.
39. Dean Ornish, *Reversing Heart Disease*, ibid, p. 278.
40. Dean Ornish, *Reversing Heart Disease*, ibid, p. 278.
41. Neil Nedley, *Proof Positive*, ibid, p. . 135.

42. Dean Ornish, *Reversing Heart Disease*, ibid, p. 278.

43. John McDougall, McDougall's Program for a Healthy Heart, p. 77.

44. John McDougall, McDougall's Program for a Health Heart, ibid, p. 78.

45 Dean Ornish, *Reversing Heart Disease*, ibid, p. 279.

46. Dean Ornish, *Reversing Heart Disease*, ibid, p. 279.

47. Dean Ornish, *Reversing Heart Disease*, ibid, p. 279.

48. Dean Ornish, *Reversing Heart Disease*, ibid, p. 279.

49. Nedley, *Proof Positive*, ibid, p. . 121.

50. Nedley, *Proof Positive*, ibid, p. 121.

51. Nedley, *Proof Positive*, ibid, p. 122.

52. Whitaker, *Reversing Heart Disease*, ibid, pp. 145, 146.

53. Whitaker, *Reversing Heart Disease*, ibid, p. 193. .

54. Whitaker, *Reversing Heart Disease*, ibid, p. 193.

55. Whitaker, Reversing Heart Disease, ibid, p. 193.

56. Whitaker, Whitaker's Guide, ibid, p., p. 27.

57. Whitaker, Whitaker's Guide, ibid, p. 28.

58. Whitaker, Whitaker's Guide, ibid, p. 31.

59. Whitaker, Whitaker's Guide, ibid, p. 33.

60. Whitaker, Whitaker's Guide, ibid, p. 33.

61. Whitaker, Whitaker's Guide, ibid, p. 40.

62. Whitaker, Whitaker's Guide, ibid, p. 40.

63. Whitaker, Whitaker's Guide, ibid, p. 44.

64. Whitaker, Whitaker's Guide, ibid, p. 44.

65. Whitaker, Whitaker's Guide, ibid, p. 45.

66. Whitaker, Whitaker's Guide, ibid, pp. 45, 46.

67. Whitaker, Whitaker's Guide, ibid, p. 46.

68. Whitaker, Whitaker's Guide, ibid, p. 47.

69. Whitaker, Whitaker's Guide, ibid, p. 48.

70. Whitaker, Whitaker's Guide, ibid, pp. 48, 49.

71. Whitaker, Whitaker's Guide, ibid, p. 49.

72. Whitaker, Whitaker's Guide, ibid, p. 50.

73. Whitaker, Whitaker's Guide, ibid, p. 53.

74. Whitaker, Whitaker's Guide, ibid, p. 53.

75. Whitaker, Whitaker's Guide, ibid, p. 53.

76. Nedley, *Proof Positive*, ibid, p. 491.

77. Nedley, *Proof Positive*, ibid, p. 491.

78. Nedley, *Proof Positive*, ibid, p. . 38.

79. Nedley, *Proof Positive*, ibid, p. 489.

80. Nedley, *Proof Positive*, ibid, p. 37.

81. Nedley, *Proof Positive*, ibid, p. 488.

82. Whitaker, Whitaker's Guide, ibid, p. 54.

83. Whitaker, Whitaker's Guide, ibid, p. 55.

84. Whitaker, Whitaker's Guide, ibid, p. 55.

85. Whitaker, Whitaker's Guide, ibid, p. 55.

86. Whitaker, Whitaker's Guide, ibid, p. 56.

87. Whitaker, Whitaker's Guide, ibid, p. 56.

88. Whitaker, Whitaker's Guide, ibid, p. 56.

89. McDougall, McDougall's Program ibid, pp. 78, 79.

90. McDougall, McDougall's Program ibid, pp. 75.

91. F. Batmanghelidj, *Your Body's Many Cries For Water,* p. 83.

92. Batmanghelidj, *Water,* ibid, p. 83.

93. Batmanghelidj, *Water,* ibid, pp. 86, 88.

94. Batmanghelidj, *Water,* ibid, pp. 88,89.

95. Ellen G. White, Counsel on Diet and Foods, p. 419.

96. Batmanghelidj, *Water,* ibid, p. xvii.

97. White, *Counsel,* ibid, p. 419.

High Blood Pressure: Section 1: Most Medicated Illness.

1. John McDougall, *The McDougall Program for a Healthy Heart,* p. 213.

2. McDougall, *The McDougall Program,* ibid, p. 213.

3. McDougall, *The McDougall Program,* ibid, p. 232.

4. McDougall, *The McDougall Program,* ibid, p. 232.

5. Julian Whitaker, *Reversing Heart Disease,* ibid, p. 100.

6. McDougall, *The McDougall Program,* ibid, p. 213.

7. Neil Nedley, *Proof Positive,* p. 129.

8. McDougall, *The McDougall Program,* ibid, p. 216.

9. Whitaker, *Reversing Heart Disease,* ibid, p. 99.

10. Whitaker, *Reversing Heart Disease,* ibid, pp. 100–103.

11. McDougall, *The McDougall Program,* ibid, pp. 227, 238, 239.

12. Whitaker, *Reversing Heart Disease,* ibid, p. 99.

13. Whitaker, *Reversing Heart Disease,* ibid, p. 99.

14. Neil Nedley, *Proof Positive,* ibid, p. 131.

15. Neil Nedley, *Proof Positive,* ibid, p. 131.

16. John McDougall, *The McDougall Program,* ibid, p. 219.

17. John McDougall, *The McDougall Program,* ibid, p. 220.

18. Nedley, *Proof Positive,* ibid, p. 130.

19. McDougall, *The McDougall Program,* ibid, p. 220.

20. McDougall, *The McDougall Program,* ibid, p. 220.

21. T. Colin Campbell, *The China Study,* p. 80.

22. Campbell, ibid, p. 80. See also Julian Whitaker, *Reversing Heart Disease,* ibid, p.103.

23. Whitaker, *Reversing Heart Disease,* ibid, p. 103.

24. Whitaker, *Reversing Heart Disease,* ibid, p. 103.

25. *Let's Live Nutrition Insights,* May 1998, issue 5 vol. 3, p. 4.

26. Nedley, *Proof Positive,* ibid, p. 137.

27. Whitaker, *Reversing Heart Disease,* ibid, p. 100.

28. Whitaker, *Reversing Heart Disease,* ibid, p. 100.

29. Nedley, *Proof Positive,* ibid, p. 137.

30. Nedley, *Proof Positive,* ibid, p. 137.

31. McDougall, The McDougall Program, ibid, p. 218.

32. Whitaker, *Reversing Heart Disease,* ibid, p. 101, 104.

33. McDougall, The McDougall Program, ibid, p. 219.

34. Whitaker, *Reversing Heart Disease,* ibid, p. 102.

35. Whitaker, *Reversing Heart Disease,* ibid, p. 102.

36. Whitaker, *Reversing Heart Disease,* ibid, p. 103.

37. Whitaker, *Reversing Heart Disease,* ibid, p. 103.

38. Whitaker, *Reversing Heart Disease,* ibid, p. 104.

39. Thrash, *Diabetes & The Hypoglycemic Syndrome,* p. 65.

40. Thrash, *Diabetes* ,ibid, p. 64.

41. Thrash, *Diabetes* ,ibid, p. 64.

42. Thrash, *Diabetes* ,ibid, p. 64.

43. Nedley, *Proof Positive,* ibid, p.

44. McDougall, *The McDougall Program,* ibid, p. 238.

45. McDougall, *The McDougall Program,* ibid, p. 239.

46. McDougall, *The McDougall Program,* ibid, p. 239.

47. Nedley, *Proof Positive,* ibid, p. 142.

48. Nedley, *Proof Positive,* ibid, p. 142.

49. McDougall, *The McDougall Program,* ibid, p. 239.

50 Nedley, *Proof Positive,* ibid, p. 142.

51. Nedley, *Proof Positive,* ibid, p. 142.

52. McDougall, *The McDougall Program,* ibid, p. 227.

53. McDougall, *The McDougall Program,* ibid, p. 227.

54. McDougall, *The McDougall Program,* ibid, p. 228.

55. McDougall, *The McDougall Program,* ibid, p. 227.

56. F. Batmanghelidj, *Your Body's Many Cries For Water,* p. 71.

57. Batmanghelidj, *Water,* ibid, p. 73.

58. Batmanghelidj, *Water,* ibid, p. 74

59. Whitaker, *Reversing Heart Disease,* ibid, p. 105.

60. Whitaker, *Reversing Heart Disease,* ibid, p. 105.

61. McDougall, *The McDougall Program,* ibid, p. 213.

62. Nedley, *Proof Positive,* ibid, p. 131.

63. McDougall, ibid, p., ibid, p. 216.

High Blood Pressure: Section 2: Drug Medication.

1. John McDougall, *The McDougall Program for a Healthy Heart,* p. 232.

2. Julian Whitaker, *Reversing Heart Disease,* p. 05.

3. Whitaker, *Reversing Heart Disease,* ibid, p. 105.

4. Whitaker, *Reversing Heart Disease,* ibid, p. 107.

5. Lynne Paige Walker, *The Alternative Pharmacy,* p. 221

6. Walker, *Alternative Pharmacy,* ibid, p. 221.

7. Walker, *Alternative Pharmacy,* ibid, p. 221.

8. Andrew Weil, Health and Healing, p. 21.

9. McDougall, *The McDougall Program,* ibid, p. 235.

10. McDougall, *The McDougall Program*, ibid, p. 235.
11. Whitaker, *Reversing Heart Disease*, ibid, p. 105.
12. Walker, *Alternative Pharmacy*, ibid, p. 222.
13. Whitaker, *Reversing Heart Disease*, ibid, p. 105.
14. Neil Nedley, *Proof Positive*, ibid, p. 496.
15. Nedley, *Proof Positive*, ibid, p. 496.
16. Walker, *Alternative Pharmacy*, ibid, p. 222.
17. Walker, *Alternative Pharmacy*, ibid, p. 222.
18. James Marti, *Alternative Health Medicine Encyclopedia*, p. 65
19 Whitaker, *Reversing Heart Disease*, ibid, p. 105.
20. McDougall, *The McDougall Program*, ibid, p. 235.
21. Whitaker, *Reversing Heart Disease*, ibid, p. 105.
22. McDougall, *The McDougall Program*, ibid, p. 235.
23. McDougall, *The McDougall Program*, ibid, p. 235.
24. Whitaker, *Reversing Heart Disease*, ibid, p. 106.
25. Whitaker, *Reversing Heart Disease*, ibid, p. 106.
26. Nedley, *Proof Positive*, ibid, p. 135.
27. Whitaker, Reversing Heart Disease, ibid, p. 106.
28. Nedley, *Proof Positive*, ibid, p. 135.
29. Whitaker, *Reversing Heart Disease*, ibid, p. 107.
30. McDougall, *The McDougall Program*, ibid, p. 234.
31. Walker, *Alternative Pharmacy*, ibid, p. 222.
32. McDougall, *The McDougall Program*, ibid, p. 234.
33. McDougall, *The McDougall Program*, ibid, p. 234.
34. McDougall, *The McDougall Program*, ibid, p. 234.
35. Nedley, *Proof Positive*, ibid, p. 206.
36. Nedley, *Proof Positive*, ibid, p. 195.
37. Nedley, *Proof Positive*, ibid, p. 197.
38. Nedley, *Proof Positive*, ibid, p. 206.
39. McDougall, *The McDougall Program*, ibid, p. 235.
40. McDougall, *The McDougall Program*, ibid, p. 235.
41. McDougall, *The McDougall Program*, ibid, p. 235.
42. McDougall, *The McDougall Program*, ibid, p. 235.
43. McDougall, *The McDougall Program*, ibid, p. 236.
44. McDougall, *The McDougall Program*, ibid, p. 236.
45. McDougall, *The McDougall Program*, ibid, p. 236.
46. McDougall, *The McDougall Program*, ibid, p. 236.
47. Nedley, *Proof Positive*, ibid, p. 206.
48. McDougall, *The McDougall Program*, ibid, p. 236.

High Blood Pressure: Section 3: Nutritional Cures

1. John McDougall, The McDougall Program for a Healthy Heart, p. 221.
2. McDougall, The McDougall Program ibid, p. 222.
3. McDougall, The McDougall Program ibid, p. 223.

4. McDougall, The McDougall Program ibid, p. 223.
5. McDougall, The McDougall Program ibid, p. 223.
6. Neil Nedley, *Proof Positive*, p. 142.
7. Nedley, *Proof Positive*, ibid, p. 142.
8. McDougall, The McDougall Program ibid, p. 223.
9. McDougall, The McDougall Program ibid, p. 223.
10. Nedley, *Proof Positive*, ibid, p. 137.
11. Nedley, *Proof Positive*, ibid, p. 137.
12. Nedley, *Proof Positive*, ibid, p. 148.
13. Nedley, *Proof Positive*, ibid, p. 137.
14. Nedley, *Proof Positive*, ibid, p. 137.
15. Nedley, *Proof Positive*, ibid, p. 143.
16. McDougall, The McDougall Program ibid, p. 224
17. McDougall, The McDougall Program ibid, p. 224.
18. McDougall, The McDougall Program ibid, p. 224.
19. McDougall, The McDougall Program ibid, p. 224.
20. Nedley, *Proof Positive*, ibid, p. 142.
21. Nedley, *Proof Positive*, ibid, p. 142.
22. Nedley, *Proof Positive*, ibid, p. 143.
23. Nedley, *Proof Positive*, ibid, p. 143.
24. John McDougall, The McDougall Program ibid, p. 240.
25. F. Batmanghelidj, *Your Body's Many Cries For Water*, pp. 71, 74.
26. Batmanghelidj, *Water*, ibid, p. 75.
27. Batmanghelidj, *Water*, ibid, p. 76
28. . Batmanghelidj, *Water*, ibid, p. 76.
29. Batmanghelidj, *Water*, ibid, p. 75.
30. Lynne Paige Walker, *The Alternative Pharmacy*, p. 224.
31. Walker, *Alternative Pharmacy*, ibid, p. 224
32. Walker, *Alternative Pharmacy*, ibid, p. 225.
33. Walker, *Alternative Pharmacy*, ibid, p. 224.
34. James Marti, *The Alternative Health & Medicine Encyclopedia*, p. 143.
35. Walker, *Alternative Pharmacy*, ibid, p. 224.
36. Walker, *Alternative Pharmacy*, ibid, p. 224.
37. Walker, *Alternative Pharmacy*, ibid, p. 225.
38. James Marti, *Alternative Health ibid*, p. 143.
39. Walker, *Alternative Pharmacy*, ibid, p. 225.
40. Walker, *Alternative Pharmacy*, ibid, pp. 225, 227.
41. Walker, *Alternative Pharmacy*, ibid, p. 225.
42. Walker, *Alternative Pharmacy*, ibid, p. 225.

Osteoporosis: Section 1: A raging Epidemic

1. John Robbins, *Diet For A New America*, p. 200.
2. National Osteoporosis Foundation, 2008, www.nof.org/osteoporosis/diseasefacts.htm.
3. John McDougall, *A Challenging Second Opinion*, p. 61.

4. McDougall, *A Challenging Second Opinion, ibid,* p. 62.

5. Lynne Paige Walker, *The Alternative Pharmacy,* p. 91.

6. Neil Nedley, *Proof Positive,* p. 152.

7. Walker, *Alternative Pharmacy* ibid, p. 91.

8. Julian Whitaker, *Whitaker's Guide ibid,* p. 318.

9 Robbins, *Diet, ibid,* p. 189.

10. McDougall, *A Challenging Second Opinion,* p.61.

11. McDougall, *A Challenging Second Opinion,* p. 61.

12. Julian Whitaker, *Whitaker's Guide, ibid,* pp. 314, 315.

13. Whitaker, *Whitaker's Guide, ibid,* p. 314, 315.

14. Whitaker, *Whitaker's Guide, ibid,* p. 314.

15. Robbins, *Diet, ibid,* p. 189.

16. McDougall, *A Challenging Second Opinion,* p. 61.

17. McDougall, *A Challenging Second Opinion,* p. 61.

18. Robbins, Diet, ibid, p. 189.

19. Nedley, *Proof Positive,* ibid, p. 151.

20. Walker, *Alternative Pharmacy* ibid, p. 91.

21. McDougall, *A Challenging Second Opinion,* p. 69.

22. McDougall, *A Challenging Second Opinion,* p. 69.

23. McDougall, *A Challenging Second Opinion,* p. 64.

24. McDougall, *A Challenging Second Opinion, ibid,* p. 64.

25. McDougall, *A Challenging Second Opinion, ibid,* p. 69.

26. McDougall, *A Challenging Second Opinion, ibid,* p. 69.

27. Whitaker, *Whitaker's Guide, ibid,* p. 317.

28. Nedley, *Proof Positive, ibid,* p. 155.

29. McDougall, *A Challenging Second Opinion, ibid,* p. 73.

30. McDougall, *A Challenging Second Opinion, ibid,* p. 74, 75.

31. Whitaker, *Whitaker's Guide, ibid,* p. .317.

32. Whitaker, *Reversing Diabetes,* p. 55.

33. Whitaker, *Reversing Diabetes, ibid,* p. 55.

34. Robbins, *Diet ibid,* p. 191.

35. McDougall, *A Challenging Second Opinion, ibid,* p. 72.

36. McDougall, *A Challenging Second Opinion, ibid,* p. 73.

37. McDougall, *A Challenging Second Opinion, ibid,* p. 73.

38. McDougall, *A Challenging Second Opinion, ibid,* p. 76.

39. McDougall, *A Challenging Second Opinion, ibid,* p. 76.

40. McDougall, *A Challenging Second Opinion, ibid,* p. 76.

41. Nedley, *Proof Positive, ibid,* p. 155.

42. McDougall, *A Challenging Second Opinion, ibid,* p. 76.

43. McDougall, *A Challenging Second Opinion, ibid,* p. 77.

44. Nancy Appleton, *Lick the Sugar Habit,* pp. 57, 58.

45. Appleton, *ibid,* p. 59.

46. McDougall, *A Challenging Second Opinion, ibid,* p. 77.

47. McDougall, *A Challenging Second Opinion, ibid,* p. 77.

48. McDougall, *A Challenging Second Opinion, ibid,* p. 77.

49. Whitaker, *Whitaker's Guide, ibid,* p. 317.
50. Whitaker, *Whitaker's Guide, ibid,* p. 317.
51. Appleton, *Sugar Habit, ibid,* p. 58.
52. Appleton, *Sugar Habit, ibid,* p. 12.
53. Appleton, *Sugar Habit, ibid,* p. 12.
54. Appleton, *Sugar Habit, ibid,* p. 12.
55. Appleton, *Sugar Habit, ibid,* p. 13.
56. Appleton, *Sugar Habit, ibid,* p. 12.
57. Appleton, *Sugar Habit, ibid,* p. 14.
58. Appleton, *Sugar Habit, ibid,* p. 58.
59. Appleton, *Sugar Habit, ibid,* p. 14.
60. Appleton, *Sugar Habit, ibid,* p. 15.
61. Robbins, Diet, *ibid,* p. 196.
62. Appleton, *Sugar Habit, ibid,* p. 15.
63. Appleton, *Sugar Habit, ibid,* p. 16.
64. Appleton, *Sugar Habit, ibid,* p. 16.
65. Appleton, *Sugar Habit, ibid,* p. 57.
66. Appleton, *Sugar Habit, ibid,* p. 58.
67. Robbins, *Diet, ibid,* p. 196.
68. Robbins, *Diet, ibid,* p. 196.
69. Robbins, *Diet, ibid,* p. 196.
70. Robbins, *Diet, ibid,* p. 196.
71. Robbins, *Diet, ibid,* p. 196.
72. Robbins, *Diet, ibid,* p. 197.
73. Whitaker, *Whitaker's Guide, ibid,* p. 317.
74. Whitaker, *Whitaker's Guide, ibid,* p. 317.
75. Appleton, *Sugar Habit, ibid,* p. 57.
76. Appleton, *Sugar Habit, ibid,* p. 58.
77. Appleton, *Sugar Habit, ibid,* p. 58.
78. Appleton, *Sugar Habit, ibid,* p. 58.
79. Appleton, *Sugar Habit, ibid,* p. 58.

Osteoporosis: Section 2: Got Milk?

1. John Robbins, *Diet For a New America,* p.191.
2. Neil Nedley, *Proof Positive,* p. 153.
3. Nedley, *Proof Positive, ibid,* p. 153.
4. Nedley, *Proof Positive, ibid,* p. 153.
5. Nedley, *Proof Positive, ibid,* p. 153.
6. Julian Whitaker, *Whitaker's Guide to Natural Healing,* p. 317.
7. Whitaker, Whitaker's Guide, *ibid,* p. 317.
8. Robbins, Diet, *ibid,* p. 199.
9. Robbins, Diet, *ibid,* p. 193.
10. Robbins, Diet, *ibid,* p. 193.
11. McDougall, A Challenging Second Opinion, *ibid,* p. 68.

12. Robbins, Diet, *ibid*, p. 198.

13. Robbins, Diet, *ibid*, p. 198.

14. McDougall, A Challenging Second Opinion, *ibid*, p. 66.

15. McDougall, A Challenging Second Opinion, *ibid*, p. 66.

16. McDougall, A Challenging Second Opinion, *ibid*, p. 66.

17. McDougall, A Challenging Second Opinion, *ibid*, p. 66.

18. Lynne Paige Walker, *The Alternative Pharmacy*, p. 91.

19. Whitaker, Reversing Diabetes, *ibid*, p. 60.

20. Walker, *Alternative Pharmacy*, *ibid*, p. 91.

21. Walker, *Alternative Pharmacy*, *ibid*, p. . 92.

22. Walker, *Alternative Pharmacy*, *ibid*, p. . 92.

23. Walker, *Alternative Pharmacy*, *ibid*, p. . 92.

24. Walker, *Alternative Pharmacy*, *ibid*, p. . 92.

25. Walker, *Alternative Pharmacy*, *ibid*, p. . 92.

26. McDougall, A Challenging Second Opinion, *ibid*, p. 65.

27. McDougall, A Challenging Second Opinion, *ibid*, p. 66.

28. McDougall, A Challenging Second Opinion, *ibid*, p. 66.

29. McDougall, A Challenging Second Opinion, *ibid*, p. 72.

Osteoporosis Section 3: Sorry, ain't got no Milk (or Soda): Repairing Porous Bones

1. Julian Whitaker, *Reversing Diabetes*, p. 58.

2. Nancy Appleton, *Lick The Sugar Habit*, p. 59.

3. John McDougall, *A Challenging Second Opinion*, *ibid*, p. 77.

4. Neil Nedley, *Proof Positive*, p. 154.

5. Nedley, *Proof Positive*, *ibid*, pp. 153, 154.

6. John Robbins, *Diet For a New America*, p. 196.

7. Robbins, *Diet*, *ibid*, p 195.

8. Whitaker, *Reversing Diabetes*, *ibid*, p. 61.

9. Robbins, *Diet*, *ibid*, p 195.

10. Appleton, *Sugar Habit*, *ibid*, p. 60.

11. Appleton, *Sugar Habit*, *ibid*, p. 60.

12. Appleton, *Sugar Habit*, *ibid*, p. 60.

13. Appleton, *Sugar Habit*, *ibid*, p. 60.

14. Nedley, *Proof Positive*, *ibid*, p. 155.

15. Nedley, *Proof Positive*, *ibid*, p. 155.

16. Nedley, *Proof Positive*, *ibid*, p. 155.

17. Nedley, *Proof Positive*, *ibid*, p. 156.

18. Lynne Paige Walker, *The Alternative Pharmacy*, pp. 92, 93.

19. Walker, *Alternative Pharmacy*, *ibid*, p. 93.

20. Walker, *Alternative Pharmacy*, *ibid*, p. 93.

21. Appleton, *Sugar Habit*, *ibid*, p. 60.

22. Andrew Weil, *Natural Health Natural Medicine*, p. 27.

23. Whitaker, Whitaker's *Guide*, *ibid*, p. 316.

24. Whitaker, Whitaker's *Guide, ibid,* p. 316.

25. Whitaker, Whitaker's *Guide, ibid,* p. 318.

26. Whitaker, Whitaker's *Guide, ibid,* p. 319.

27. Walker, *Alternative Pharmacy, ibid,* p. 93.

28. Whitaker, Whitaker's *Guide, ibid,* p 319.

29. Whitaker, Whitaker's *Guide, ibid,* p 319.

30. F. Batmanghelidj, *Your Body Many Cries For Water,* p.19.

31. Whitaker, Whitaker's *Guide, ibid,* p, 303, 319.

32. Whitaker, Whitaker's *Guide, ibid,* p 305.

ADMISSIONS:

Section 2: Drug Medicine is based on Faulty Science

1. Julian Whitaker, Dr. *Julian Whitaker's Guide to natural Healing,* p. xiii.

2. Bross, *Crimes of Official Science,* 1987, p. 6.

3. Bross, *Crimes, ibid,* p. 7.

4. Bross, *Crimes, ibid,* p. 27.

5. Bross, *Crimes of Official Science,* 1987, p.4.

6. Francis Bacon, *Novum Organum,* Great Books of the Western World, Bk. One, 1952, p. 107

7. Francis Bacon, *Novum Organum,* Bk. One, ibid, p

8. Francis Bacon, *Novum Organum,* Bk. One, ibid, p. 108.

9. Bross Scientific Fraud vs. Scientific Truth, 1991, p. 18.

10. Francis Bacon, *The Advancement of Learning,* Great Books of the Western World, 1952, bk. 2, p. 51.

11. Francis Bacon *The Advancement of Learning,* ibid, pp. 52, 53.

12. Harris Coulter *Divided Legacy, A History of the Schism in Medical Thought, Vol* 1. *The Patterns emerge Hippocrates to Paracelsus,* p. 347.

13. Coulter, *Divided Legacy,* vol.1, *Ibid,* p. 371.

14. Coulter, *Divided Legacy, vol.* 1, *ibid, p.* 371.

15. Coulter, *Divided Legacy, vol.* 1, *ibid, p.* 410.

16. Coulter, *Divided Legacy, vol.* 1, *ibid,* p. 410

17. Coulter, *Divided Legacy, vol.* 1, ibid, p. 410.

18. Bertrand Russell, *History of Western Philosophy,* ibid, p. 546.

19. Stanley Jaki, *The Origin of Science and the Science of its Origin,* 1978, p. 5.

20. Jaki, ibid, p. 16.

21. Coulter, *Divided Legacy, A History of the Schism in Medical Thought, vol. II,* ibid, p. 111.

22. Russell, *History of Western Philosophy,* ibid, p. 560.

23. Coulter, *Divided Legacy, vol. II,* ibid, p. 120.

24. Coulter, *Divided Legacy,* vol. II, ibid, p. 119.

35. Russell, *History of Western Philosophy,* ibid, p. 565.

36. Coulter, *Divided Legacy, vol. II,* ibid, p. 134.

37. Coulter, *Divided Legacy, vol. II,* ibid, p 113.

38. Coulter, *Divided Legacy, vol. II,* ibid, p 113.

39. Coulter, *Divided Legacy, vol. II,* ibid, p. 111.

30. Coulter, *Divided Legacy, vol. II,* ibid, p 113.

31. Coulter, *Divided Legacy,* ibid, p. 113, Sprengel, Histoire de la Medicine, V, 58.

32. Coulter, *Divided Legacy, vol. II,* ibid, p. 118.

33. Coulter, *Divided Legacy, vol. II, ibid,* p. 118

34. Robert Mendelsohn, Confessions of a Medical Heretic, 1979, p. 152

35. Coulter, *Divided Legacy, vol. II, ibid,* p. 150.

36. Coulter, *Divided Legacy, vol. II, ibid,* p. 150.

37. Coulter, *Divided Legacy, vol. II, ibid,* p. 113

38. Coulter, *Divided Legacy, vol. II, ibid,* pp. 58, 162.

39. Coulter, *Divided Legacy, vol. II,* ibid, pp. 181 182.

40. Coulter, *Divided Legacy, vol. II,* ibid, p. 182.

41. Coulter, *Divided Legacy, vol. II* ibid, p. 182.

42 Coulter, *Divided Legacy, vol. II,* ibid, p. 228.

43. Coulter, *Divided Legacy, vol. II,* ibid, p. 229.

44. Coulter, *Divided Legacy, vol. II,* ibid, p. 229.

45. Coulter, *Divided Legacy, vol. II,* ibid, p. 233.

46. Coulter, *Divided Legacy, vol. II,* ibid, p. 322.

47. Coulter, *Divided Legacy, vol. II,* ibid, pp. 331, 332.

48. Coulter, *Divided Legacy, vol. II,* ibid, p. 349.

49. Coulter, *Divided Legacy, vol. II,* ibid, p. 349.

50. Coulter, *Divided Legacy, vol. II,* ibid, p. 367.

51. Hans Ruesch, *The Slaughter of the Innocent,* p. 221.

52. Phillip Frank Philosophy of Science: The Link Between Science and Philosophy, 1957, p. 298

53. Charles Singer, *The History of Science,* 1900, ibid, p. 514.

54. Singer, *The History of Science,* ibid, p. 500.

55. Ruesch, *Naked Empress,* ibid, p. 34.

56. Bross, *Fifty Years of Fraud and Folly,* ibid, p. 1.

57. Ruesch, *Naked Empress,* ibid, p. 66.

58. William Campbell Douglass II, 1997, *Bad Medicine,* p.1

59. Bross, From Crossroads, ibid, p. 87.

60. Coulter, *The Divided Legacy,* vol.3, Ibid, p. 172.

61. Coulter, *The Divided Legacy, vol.* 3, Ibid, p. 179.

62. Coulter, *The Divided Legacy, vol.* 3, Ibid, p. 314.

63. Bross, *Fifty Years of Fraud,* ibid, pp. 9, 56.

Section 3: Instances of Fraud and Bias in Science and Medicine

1. Mendelsohn, *Confessions,* ibid, p. 125.

2. Mendelsohn, *Confessions,* ibid, p. 125

3. Bross, *Fifty Years of Fraud,* ibid, p. 27.

4. Mendelsohn, *Confessions,* ibid, p. 126
5. Mendelsohn, *Confessions,* ibid, p. 126.
6. Douglass, *Bad Medicine,* 1998, p. 11.
7. Douglass, ibid, p. 11.
8. Douglass, ibid, p. 11.
9. Douglass, ibid, p. 11.
10. T. Colin Campbell, *The China Study,* 2006, p. 367.
11. Campbell, ibid, p. 267.
13. Bross, *Fifty Years of Folly and Fr*aud, ibid, p. 102.
14. Bross, *Fifty Years of Folly and Fr*aud, ibid, p. 40.
15. Bross, *Fifty Years of Folly and Fr*aud, ibid, p. 97.
16. Bross, *Fifty Years of Folly and Fr*aud, ibid, p. 53.
17. Bross, *Fifty Years of Folly and Fr*aud, ibid, p. 66.

Section 4: The Symptomatic Treatment of Disease is a Failure

1. George Vithoulkas, *Homeopathy, Medicine of the New Age,* 1992, 31.
2. Coulter, *The Divided Legacy, vol.* 3, Ibid, p. 312.
3. Coulter, *The Divided Legacy, vol.* 3, Ibid, p. 312.
4. James Tyler Kent *Lectures on Homoeopathic Philosophy,* 1900, p. 96.
5. Kent, *Lectures,* ibid, p. 97
6. Vithoulkas, *Homeopathy,* ibid, p. 39.
7. Max Gerson, *A Cancer Therapy,* ibid, cover quotation
8. Gerson, *A Cancer Therapy,* Ibid, p. 20
9. Gerson, *A Cancer Therapy,* ibid, p. 11.
10. Gerson, *A Cancer Therapy,* ibid, p. 11.
11. Gerson, *A Cancer Therapy,* ibid, p. 19.
12. Gerson, *A Cancer Therapy,* ibid, pp. 13, 14
13. Brown, *Aids, Cancer,* ibid, p. 66.
14. Brown, *Aids, Cancer,* ibid, p. 67.
15. Coulter, *The Divided Legacy, vol.* 3, Ibid, p. 50.
16. Coulter, *The Divided Legacy, vol.* 3, Ibid, p. 49 ...
17. Ellen While, *The Ministry of Healing,* 1905, p. 127.
18. Coulter, *The Divided Legacy, vol.* 3, Ibid, p. 48.
19. Ellen White, Testimonies, vol. 3, 1872, p. 138.
20. Gerson, *A Cancer Therapy,* ibid, pp. 89, 90.
21. Gerson, *A Cancer Therapy,* ibid, p. 50.
22 Coulter, *The Divided Legacy, vol.* 3, Ibid, p. 171.
23. Coulter, *The Divided Legacy, vol.* 3, Ibid, p. 59.
24. Coulter, *The Divided Legacy, vol.* 3, Ibid, p. 72.
25. Coulter, *The Divided Legacy, vol.* 3, Ibid, p. 59.
26. Coulter, *The Divided Legacy, vol.* 3, Ibid, p. 67.
27. Coulter, *The Divided Legacy, vol.* 3, Ibid, pp. 66, 67.
28. P. Joseph Lisa, *The Assault, ibid,* p. 29.

29. Mendelsohn, *Confessions,* ibid, p. 179.
30. Douglass, *Bad Medicine*, ibid, p. 6
31. Douglass, *Bad Medicine*, ibid, p. 6
32. Mendelsohn, *Confessions,* ibid, p. 26.
33. Andrew Weil, *Health and Healing*, pp. 96, 97.
34. Mendelsohn, *Confessions,* ibid, p. 39.
35. Physician Desk Reference 1999, p. 922.
36. Mendelsohn, *Confessions,* ibid, p. 42.
37. Douglass, *Bad Medicine*, ibid, p. 4
38. Douglass, *Bad Medicine*, p. 4.
39. Douglass, *Bad Medicine,* ibid, p. 4
40. Douglass, *Bad Medicine*, ibid, p. 6
41. Mendelsohn, *Confessions,* ibid, p. x.
42. Mendelsohn, *Confessions,* ibid, p. xi.
43. Mendelsohn, *Confessions,* ibid, p. 114.
44. Mendelsohn, *Confessions,* ibid, p. 114.
45. Mendelsohn, *Confessions,* ibid, p. 114.
46. Mendelsohn, *Confessions,* ibid, p. 147.
47. Andrew Weil, *Natural Health*, ibid, p. x.
48. Mendelsohn, *Confessions,* ibid, p. 24.
49. Mendelsohn, *Confessions,* ibid, p. 26.
50. Mendelsohn, *Confessions,* ibid, p. 42.

Section 5: The War on Cancer is a Failure

1. Bross, *Fifty Years of Folly and Fraud*, ibid, p. 8
2. Bross, *Fifty Years of Folly and Fraud*, ibid, p. 16.
3. Bross, *Fifty Years of Folly and Fraud*, ibid, p. 6.
4. Bross, *Fifty Years of Folly and Fraud*, ibid, p. 99,
5. Bross, *Fifty Years of Folly and Fraud*, ibid, p. 111.
6. Bross, *Fifty Years of Folly and Fraud*, ibid, p. 111.
7. Bross, *Fifty Years of Folly and Fraud*, ibid, pp. 114, 116.
8. Bross, *Fifty Years of Folly and Fraud*, ibid, p. 112.
9. Bross, *Fifty Years of Folly and Fraud*, ibid, pp. 120, 122.
10. Mendelsohn, *Confessions,* ibid, p. 5
11. Mendelsohn, *Confessions,* ibid, p. 5
12. Mendelsohn, *Confessions,* p. 6.
13. Bross, *Fifty Years of Folly and Fraud*, ibid, p. 93
14. Bross, *Fifty Years of Folly and Fraud*, ibid, p. 92
15. Bross, *Fifty Years of Folly and Fraud*, ibid, p. 85.
16. Bross, *Fifty Years of Folly and Fraud*, ibid, pp.84, 85.
17. Bross, *Fifty Years of Folly and Fraud*, ibid, p. 85.
18. Bross, *Fifty Years of Folly and Fraud*, ibid, p. 85.
19. Bross, *Fifty Years of Folly and Fraud*, ibid, p. 85.
20. Bross, *Fifty Years of Folly and Fraud*, ibid, p. 86, 87.

21. Bross, *Fifty Years of Folly and Fr*aud, ibid, p. 91

22. Bross, *Fifty Years of Folly and Fr*aud, ibid, p. 120.

23. Bross, *Fifty Years of Folly and Fr*aud, ibid, p. 120.

24. Brown, *Aids, Cancer,* ibid, p. 66.

25. Bross, *Fifty Years of Folly and Fr*aud, ibid, p. 83

26. Bross, *Fifty Years of Folly and Fr*aud, ibid, p. 83

27. Bross, *Fifty Years of Folly and Fr*aud, ibid, p. 88.

28. Brown, *Aids, Cancer,* ibid, p.66.

29. Brown, Aids, Cancer, ibid, p. 66.

30. Ruesch, *The Naked Empress,* ibid, p. 68.

31. Ruesch, *The Naked Empress,* ibid, p. 74

32. Ruesch, *The Naked Empress,* ibid, p. 74

33. Bross, *Fifty Years of Folly and Fr*aud, ibid, p. 102.

34. Bross, *Fifty Years of Folly and Fr*aud, ibid, p. 101.

35. Bross, *Fifty Years of Folly and Fr*aud, ibid, p. 102.

36. Bross, *Fifty Years of Folly and Fr*aud, ibid, p. 100

37. Bross, *Crimes of Offici*al Science, ibid, p. 14.

38. Ruesch, *The Naked Empress,* ibid, pp. 65, 66.

39. Ruesch, *The Naked Empress,* ibid, p. 67.

40. Ruesch, *The Naked Empress,* ibid, 66

41. Ruesch, *The Naked Empress,* ibid, 66

42. Ruesch, *The Naked Empress,* ibid, p. 69

43. Ruesch, *The Naked Empress,* ibid, p. 71.

44. Bross, *Fifty Years of Folly and Fr*aud, ibid, p. 104.

45. Bross, *Fifty Years of Folly and Fr*aud, ibid, pp. 117, 118.

46. Bross, *Scientific Fraud,* ibid, pp. 186, 187.

47. Brown, *Aids, Cancer,* ibid, p. 67.

48. Ruesch, *The Naked Empress,* ibid, p. 77.

49. Ruesch, *The Naked Empress,* ibid, p. 77

50. Ruesch, *The Naked Empress,* ibid, p. 72

51. Bross, *Fifty Years of Folly and Fr*aud, ibid, p. 118

52. Bross, *Fifty Years of Folly and Fr*aud, ibid, pp. 90, 91.

53. Bross, *Fifty Years of Folly and Fr*aud, ibid, p. 119.

54. Bross, *Fifty Years of Folly and Fr*aud, ibid, p. 120

55. Bross, *Fifty Years of Folly and Fr*aud, ibid, p. 120.

56. Bross, *Fifty Years of Folly and Fr*aud, ibid, p. 91

57. Bross, *Fifty Years of Folly and Fr*aud, ibid, p. 125.

58. Mendelsohn, *Confessions,* ibid, p. 149.

59. Ruesch, *The Naked Empress,* ibid, p. 17.

60. Ruesch, *The Naked Empress,* ibid, p. 18.

61. Ruesch, *The Naked Empress,* ibid, 18.

62. Bross, *Fifty Years of Folly and Fr*aud, ibid, p. 103.

63. Bross, *Fifty Years of Folly and Fr*aud, ibid, p. 129

64. Brown, *Aids, Cancer,* ibid, p. 66.

65. Brown, *Aids, Cancer,* ibid, p. 74.

66. Ruesch, *The Naked Empress*, ibid, p. 74

67. Ruesch, *The Naked Empress*, ibid, p. 74

Section 6: Nutritional Medicine is Advocated by the best Minds and Medical Geniuses

1. Coulter, *The Divided Legacy, vol.* 3, Ibid, p. 153.

2. Coulter, The *Divided Legacy, vol.* 3, Ibid, p. 154.

3. Coulter, *The Divided Legacy, vol.* 3, Ibid, p. 435.

4. Coulter, *The Divided Legacy, vol.* 3, Ibid, p. 154.

5. Coulter, *The Divided Legacy, vol.* 3, Ibid, p. 154.

6. Coulter, *The Divided Legacy, vol.* 3, Ibid, p. 154.

7. Ruesch, *The Naked Empress*, ibid, p. 66, 67.

8. Coulter, *Divided Legacy, vol. II*, ibid, p. 118.

9. Coulter, *Divided Legacy, vol. II*, ibid, pp. 181, 182.

10. Coulter, *Divided Legacy, vol. II*, ibid, p. 233.

Section 7: Modern Medicine is Controlled by the Petro-Chemical Industry

1. Martin Walker, *Dirty Medicine*, p. xxiii.

2. Eustace Mullins, Murder by Injection, ibid, p. 343.

3. Mullins, *Murder*, bid, p 342.

4. Campbell, *China Study*, ibid, p. 332.

5. Campbell, *China Study*, ibid, p. 332.

6. Campbell, *China Study*, ibid, p. 333.

7. Campbell, *China Study*, ibid, p. 333.

8. Campbell, *China Study*, ibid, p. 333.

9. Campbell, *China Study*, ibid, p. 333.

10. Campbell, *China Study*, ibid, pp. 333, 334.

11. Campbell, *China Study*, ibid, p. 334.

12. Campbell, *China Study*, ibid, p. 334.

13. Ruesch, *Naked Empress*, ibid, p. 37

14. Brown, *Aids, Cancer*, ibid, p. 138.

15. Brown, *Aids, Cancer*, ibid, p. 139.

16. Brown, *Aids, Cancer*, ibid, p. 141.

17. Campbell, *China Study*, ibid, p. 314.

18. Campbell, *China Study*, ibid, pp. 315, 315.

19. Campbell, *China Study*, ibid, p. 315.

20. Campbell, *China Study*, ibid, p. 316.

21. Bross, *Fifty Years of Folly and Fr*aud, ibid, p. 67.

22. Brown, Aids, Cancer, ibid, p. 142.

Section 8: FDA Protects the Medical Monopoly of Pharmaceutical Medicine

1. G. Edward Griffin, *World Without Cancer*, ibid, p 277.
2. Griffin, *World Without Cancer* ibid, p 311.
3. Griffin, *World Without Cancer*, ibid, p. 304.
4. Griffin, ibid, p. 312.
5. Walker, *Dirty Medicine,* ibid, p. 15.
6. Brown, *Aids, Cancer,* ibid, p. 154.
7. Brown, *Aids, Cancer,* ibid, p. 147.
8. Brown, *Aids, Cancer,* p. 147.
9. Brown, *Aids, Cancer,* ibid, p. 145.
10. Brown, *Aids, Cancer,* ibid, p. 148.
11. Douglass, *Bad Medicine,* ibid, p. 5
12. Douglass, *Aids, Cancer,* ibid, p. 5
13. Walker, *Dirty Medicine, ibid,* pp. 203,204.
14. Griffin, *World Without Cancer,* ibid, p. 282.
15. Campbell, *China Study,* ibid, p. 321.
16. Ruesch, *Naked Empress,* ibid, p. 64.
17. P. Joseph Lisa, *The Assault on Medical Freedom,* 1994, p. 32.
18. P. Joseph Lisa, *The Assault, ibid,* p. 32.
19. Ruesch, *The Naked Empress,* ibid, p. 74?
20. Ruesch, The Naked Empress, ibid, p. 11.

CLOSING STATEMENT: A Call for Accountability

Redefining Medical Practice

1. John Eisberg, Esq. *Medical Malpractice Litigation, Art and Science,* page 10.
2. Harris Coulter, *Divided Legacy, vol. 4, ibid,* pp. 564, 565.
3. Restatement Third of Torts, The American Law Institute, 1998, pp. 144, 145.
4. Restatement Third of Torts, ibid, p. 14.
5. Andrew Weil, *Health and Healing,* 1983, p. 97.
6. Weil, *Health and Healing,* ibid, p. 99.
7. Weil, *Health and Healing,* ibid, pp. 98, 99.
8. Francis Bacon, *Novum Organum, Great Books of the Western World,* 1952, p. 108.
9. Francis Bacon, *Novum Organum, ibid,* p. 108.
10. Weil, *Spontaneous Healing,* 1995, pp. 47, 48.
11. Weil, *Spontaneous Healing, ibid,* pp. 48, 49.
12. Weil, *Health and Healing, ibid,* p. 99.
13. Coulter, *Divided Legacy, ibid,* p. 690.
14. Weil, *Spontaneous Healing,* ibid, p. 6
16. Ellen White, *The place of Herbs in Rational Therapy,* 1931.
17. Weil, *Health and Healing, ibid,* p. 108.
18. Weil, *Health and Healing, ibid,* p. 108.
19. Weil, *Health and Healing, ibid,* p. 108.
20. Weil, *Health and Healing, ibid,* p. 109.
21. Weil, *Health and Healing, ibid,* p. 110.
22. Phillip Frank, *Philosophy of Science,* p. 298.

THE VERDICT: Request for an Indictment:

1. Patrick Quillin, *Beating Cancer by Nutrition*, p. 29, 30.
2. Julian Whitaker, *Reversing Heart Disease*, p. 105.
3. Whitaker, *Reversing Diabetes*, p. 108, 109.
4. John McDougall, *A Challenging Second Opinion*, p. 74, 75.
5. Jason Theodosakis & Brenda Adderly, *The Arthritis Cure*, p. 4.
6. Paavo Airola, *There is a Cure for Arthritis*, p. 37.
7. Dean Ornish, *Reversing Heart Disease*, p.57.
8. F. Batmanghelidj, *Your Body's Many cries for Water*, p.1.
9. Batmanghelidj, *Water, ibid, p.* 2.
10. Batmanghelidj, *Water, ibid, p.* 38,39.
11. Batmanghelidj, *Water, ibid, p.* 71.
12. Batmanghelidj, *Water, ibid, p.* 75.
13. Batmanghelidj, *I Water, bid, p.* 115,116.
14. Nancy Appleton, *Lick The Sugar Habit*, p. 51.
15. Maureen Salaman, *Foods That Heal*, p. 65.

AMERICA AT A CROSSROADS.

1. Harris Coulter, Divided Legacy, vol. 4, ibid, p. 570.
2. Coulter, Divided Legacy, *Vol. 4, ibid, p.* 571.
3. Ellen White, *The Use of Drugs in the Care of the Sick*, p.1.
4. White, *The Use of Drugs, ibid,* p. 93.
5. White, *The Use of Drugs,* p. ibid, pp. 93, 94.
6. Weil, *Health and Healing,* 1983, p. 110.
7. Weil, *Health and Healing,* ibid, p. 110.
8. Weil, *Spontaneous Healing,* 1995, p. 13.
9. Weil, *Spontaneous Healing,* ibid, pp. 13, 14.
10. Weil, *Spontaneous Healing,* ibid, p. 14.
11. Weil, *Spontaneous Healing,* ibid, p. 14.
12. Weil, *Spontaneous Healing,* ibid, p. 243.
13. Coulter, Divided Legacy, *Vol. 4, ibid, p.* 603.
14. Campaign against Fraudulent Medical Research, *The Pharmaceutical Drug Racket,* ibid, p. 4.
15. Coulter, Divided Legacy, *Vol. 4, ibid, p.* 619.
16. Stanley Jaki, *The Origin of Science and the Science of its Origin*, pp. 9, 93.
17. Jaki, *Origin of Science* ibid, p. 105.
18. Jaki, *Origin of Science* ibid, p. 21.
19. G. Edward Griffin, *World Without Cancer*, p. 357.
20. Hans Ruesch, *Naked Empress, or the Great Medical Fraud,* 1982, p. 108.

BIBLIOGRAPHY

American Journal of Clinical Nutrition, March 11, 2008. Andrew Weil, Health and Healing, 1983.
Andrew Weil, *Spontaneous Healing,* 1995.
Andrew Weil, *Natural Health, Natural Medicine,* 1995.
Anne E. Frahm with David J. Frahm, *A Cancer Battle Plan,* 1992.
Bertrand Russell, *A History of Western Philosophy,* 1945.
Campaign Against Fraudulent Medical Research, *The Pharmaceutical Drug Racket,* 1993.
Charles Colson and Nancy Pearcey, *How Now Shall We Live.* 1990.
Charles Singer, *A History of Scientific Ideas,* 1900.
Dharma Singh Khalsa, *Brain Longevity,* 1997.
Dan Graves, *Scientists of Faith,* 1996.
Dean Ornish, *Reversing Heart Disease,* 1996.
Dean Ornish, *Stress, Diet. & Your Heart,* 1984.
Donald McAlvany, *The McAlvany Intelligence Advisor,* Nov. 1997.
Ellen G. White Selected Messages, vol. 2, 1958
Ellen G. White, Medical Ministry, 1932.
Ellen While, The Ministry of Healing, 1905.
Ellen White, My Life Today, 1952
Ellen White, *The place of Herbs in Rational Therapy,* 1931
Ellen White, *The Use of Drugs in the Care of the Sick.,* 1897.
Ellen White, Testimonies, vol. 3, 1872.
Ellen White, *The Use of Drugs in the Care of the Sick,* 1954.
Ellen White, *Testimonies to the Church,* vol. 9, 1984
Ellen G. White, *Counsels on Diet and Foods,* 1938.
Ellen White, *Health, or How to Live,* 1952.
Elinor Levy, Ph.D. and Tom Monte, *The Ten Best Tools to Boost Your Immune System,* 1997.
Eustace Mullins, Murder by Injection, 1988.
F. Batmanghelidj, *Your Body's Many cries for Water,* 1992.
Francis Bacon, *The Advancement of Learning,* Book One, p. 1, Great Books of the W estern World, 1952.
G. Edward Griffin, *World Without Cancer,* 1998.
Gary Null, the Vegetarian Handbook, 1987.
George Vithoulkas, *Homeopathy, Medicine of the New Age,* 1992.
Genesis 3:4.
Genesis 3: 15 Gary Null and Carolyn Dean, *Death by Medicine,* 2003.

Francis Bacon, *Novum Organum*, Book One, p. 107, Great Books of the Western World, 1952.

Francis Schaefer, *Escape From Reason* 1968.

Harris Coulter, *Divided Legacy, A History of the Schism in Medical Thought, Vol* 1. *The Patterns emerge Hippocrates to Paracelsus*, 1994.

Harris Coulter, *Divided Legacy: A History of the Schism in Medical Thought*, Vol. 2, 1988.

Harris Coulter, *Divided Legacy:* The Conflict Between Homoeopathy and the American Medical Association, vol. 3, 1973.

Harris Coulter, Divided Legacy, A History of the Schism in Medical Thought, Vol. 4: Twentieth Century Medicine: The Biological Era, 1994.

Hans Ruesch, *Naked Empress, or the Great Medical Fraud*, 1982.

Hans Ruesch, *The Slaughter of the Innocent*, 1983.

Harvey Bigelsen, Robert E. Smith, Ph.D., Phronda Keala Smith, *Your Cure for Cancer*, 1998.

Henry Morris, *Men of Science, Men of God*, 1982.

I. William Lane, *Sharks Don't Get Cancer*, 1993.

Irwin Bross, *Crimes of Official Science*, 1987.

Irwin Bross Scientific Fraud vs. Scientific Truth, 1991.

Irwin Bross, *Fifty Years of Fraud and Folly A In the Name of Science"* 1994.

Isaac Newton's A*Observations upon the Prophecies of Daniel, and the Apocalypse of St. John*; 1991 ed. by Arthur Robinson from the personal copy of Thomas Jefferson's copy of the book now in the library of Congress.

J. A. Wylie, *The History of Protestantism*, 1878.

James Henderson, *The Whisper of the Serpent.*, *MSS*, 2007.

James Marti, *The Alternative Health Medicine Encyclopedia*, 1995.

James Tyler Kent, *Lectures on Homoeopathic Philosophy*, 1900.

James Balch, *Prescription for Nutritional Healing*, 2002.

James A. Duke, Ph.D., *The Green Pharmacy*, 1997.

James W. Anderson, Maury M. Breecher, Dr. *Anderson's Antioxidant, Antiaging Health Program*, 1996.

Jason Theodosakis & Brenda Adderly, *The Arthritis Cure*, 1997.

John Eisberg, Esq. *Medical Malpractice Litigation, Art and Science*, 1982.

John Richardson, Letter to G. Edward Griffin, dated Dec. 2, 1972.

John Robbins, *Diet For a New America*, 1987

John Robbins, *Reclaiming our Health*, 1996.

John McDougall, *A Challenging Second Opinion*, 1985.

John McDougall, *The McDougall Program for a Health Heart*, 1998.

John McDougall, *McDougall Program for Maximum Weight Loss*, 1994.

John McDougall, *A Challenging Second Opinion*, 1985.

Journal of American College of Nutrition, Vol. 19, No. 2, 312S-319S (200).

Julian Whitaker, Reversing Health Risks, 1988.

Julian Whitaker, *Reversing Heart Disease*, 1985.

Julian Whitaker, *Reversing Diabetes*, 1987.

Julian Whitaker, *Whitaker's Guide to Natural Healing*, 1994.

Julian Whitaker, Are you and your doctor making these COMMON MISTAKES with your health? Special Medical Alert, July 1999.

K. Alan Snyder, *If the Foundations are Destroyed,* 1994.

Kenny Ausubel, *When Healing Becomes a Crime: The Amazing Story of the Hoxsey Clinics and the Return of Alternative Therapies,* 2000.

Kevin Trudeau, *Natural Cures "They" Don't Want You to Know About,* 2004

Let's Live Nutrition Insights, May 1998, issue 5 vol. 3.

Let's Live, Nutrition Insights, page 1, Issue 4 vol. 3, April 1988.

Linus Pauling, *Vegetarian Times,* Dec. 1981

Lorraine Day, A*Diseases Just Don't Happen,* video tape series, 1998.

Lorraine Day, A*You Can't Improve on God,* video tape series, 1998.

Louise Tenney, *The Immune System, A Nutritional Approach,* 1988.

Lynn Paige Walker, Ellen Hodgson Brown, J.D. *The Alternative Pharmacy,* 1998.

Martin Walker, *Dirty Medicine.* 1993.

Maureen Salaman, *Foods That Heal,* 1989.

Max Gerson, *A Cancer Therapy, The Powerful Nutritional Therapy that has Healed Thousands,* 1958.

Medicine in the Public Interest, Learning to live with Diabetes, 1984.

Michael Colgan, *Prevent Cancer Now,* 1990

Mike Colgan, *Optimum Sports Nutrition,* 1993.

Nancy Appleton, Lick the Sugar Habit, 1988.

Neal Barnard, *The Power of your Plate,* 1990.

Neal Barnard, *Eat Right Live Longer,* 1995.

Neil Nedley, Proof Positive, How to Reliably Combat Disease and Achieve Optional Health through Nutrition and Lifestyle, 1998.

Norman Cantor and Peter Klein, Seventh-Century Rationalism: Bacon & Descartes, 1969.

Nutrition Nonsense—and Sense, FDA Fact Sheet, July, 1971.

P. Joseph Lisa, *The Assault on Medical Freedom,* 1994.

Paavo Airola, *There is a Cure for Arthritis,* 1988.

Patrick Quillin, *Beating Cancer by Nutrition,* 1994.

Philipp Frank, *Philosophy of Science,* 1957.

Physician's Desk Reference, 1999.

Prevention A*Joints Feel the Weight."* 41:10, February 1989.

Ray Moynihan and Alan Cassels, *Selling Sickness: How the World's Biggest Pharmaceutical Companies Are Turning us All into Patients,* 2005.

Raymond Keith Brown, MD, *Aids, Cancer & the Medical Establishment,* 1986.

Robert Mendelsohn, Confessions of a Medical Heretic, 1979.

Richard Passwater, *Cancer Prevention and Nutritional Therapies,* 1978.

Richard Tarnas, *The Passion of the Western Mind,* 1991.

Richard Schulze, A*Am Evening with Dr. Schulze"* DVD Series, 2007.

S. M. Jones, A*Nutritional Rudiments in Cancer"* 1972.

Stanley Jaki, *The Origin of Science and the Science of its Origin,* 1978.

The Bob Livingston Letter, citing information from Nutrition Action Health Letter, Washington, D.C., February 1999.

Tortora & Anagnostakos, *Principles of Anatomy & Physiology,* 2nd. ed., 1975.

Vernon Foster, *Newstart*, 1990.
Will Durant, *The Story of Philosophy*, 1938.
William Campbell Douglass II, *Bad Medicine*, 1997.
T. Colin Campbell, and Thomas M. Campbell, *The China Study*, 2006.

Index

A

B

E

Eat Right Live Longer, 117
Eclectic Medical Journal, 379
Edison, Thomas 287
Edwards, Charles C., 408
eggs, 55, 61, 85, 95, 165, 218, 329
eicosapentaenoic acid (EPA), 91
Einstein, Albert, 65, 71, 287, 357, 378, 403
Eli Lilly, 382
empirical medicine, 344, 346
empirical science, restoring, 13; nutritional medicine and, 13; of Hippocrates and Bacon, 20, 437; abandoned today, 27, 29, 352, 426, 440; objective standard, 35; rationalism destroyed, 34, 350; fruits of 34; liberates 75; only true science, 342; Dark Ages, 344, 426; cardinal sin agaisnt, 346; considers all facts, 346; Descartes perverted, 351; painful birth of, 350; rationalistic science eclipsed, 350; brilliant minds embraced, 357; conformity to data, 359, 426; modern drug medicine rejects, 360, 420; and false science, 425; creation model produced, 437; benefits to medicine, 437, 438
Enderlein, Gunther, 130, 133, 202, 204
enzymes, 55, 111, 137, 161, 169, 174, 204, 249, 328
epidemic of osteoporosis, 323-325
epidemics of chronic degenerative diseases, 42, 297
epinephrine, 221, 223, 230, 306
Erastus, Thomas (1523-1583), 350
Escape From Reason, 27
Eskimos, 290, 332, 326, 327
Esselstyn, Caldwell, 26, 38
estrogen, trophoblast cell activity, 109; and metabolic dysfunction, 109, 110, 114; breast cancer, 115; excessive and cancer risks, 114, 115; birth control pills, 115; excessive fat, 115; refined sugar increases, 114; obsity increases, 114; high blood sugar, 116; androgen, 116; meat eating, 116; receptors in cancer cells, 152; Tamoxifen, 152; osteoporosis, 324, 334; replacement therapy, 335; menopause 335; bone loss 337; natural replacement 339; phytoestrogen plant foods, 339; FDA errors 338
evolutionary concept, 32, 163, 205, 347, 350, 362, 401
exercise, Hippocrates, 9; nutritional therapy, 38, 39, 192, 212, 245, 259, 298, 430; immune system, 45; lack of and diseases, 55, 213, 218; excessive, 83, 256; osteoporosis, 83, 338, 339; arthritis, 97; cancer prevention, 201, 204; glucose absorption, 210; diabetes, 218, 232, 238; high blood pressure, 230, 318; reduces insulin needs, 237; cotrols blood sugar 239; timing, 239; heart disease, 256, 263, 307; reversing heart disease, 279, 281, 318; longevity 293; good health, 300, 434; beta blockers, 314;

F

facts of Scripture, 31
Fall of Man, 10, 351

G

H

Lee, Anne, 179, 180
Lee, John R., 338
Leonardo da Vinci, 286
Ley, Herbert, 409
Lick the Sugar Habit, 65, 69, 80, 175
Lisa, P. Joseph, 380, 415
Livestock and Meat Board, 60, 331
Livingston, Bob, 44
Locke, John, 65, 162, 356, 359, 364
lopressor, 229
lovastatin, 272, 277, 283, 429
low animal fat and protein diet, 37
low protein diet, 94, 120, 217, 285, 338
low-fat vegetarian diet, 286
L-threonic acid, 194
Luer, Carl, 179, 180
lumpectomy, 143, 144, 145, 149
lung cancer rates, 102

M

MacGregor, Graham A.,306
magan, 89
magnesium,and carbohydrate metabolism, 51, 200, 243; arthritic treatment 89; salicylate, 89; white flour depletes, 200; thiazides and loss of, 230; deficient in diabetics, 241; 242; sugar leaches, 243; essential in all functions, 243, 294; asparte, 243; heart attacks, 243; high blood pressure, 243; kidney function, 243; prevents kidney stones, 243; adequate daily intake, 243; calcium magnesium ration, 294; bufferin, 273, 368; diazide depletes, 274; benefits of, assigned to aspirin, 368; aids potassium absorption, 368; blood thiner, 368
magic bullet, 111, 151, 165, 181, 438
Mannatech, 189
Marti, James, 65, 311
mastectomy, 26, 143, 145, 149, 391
materia medica, 375, 434
Max Gerson, nutritional therapy, 37, 374, 391; excess salt, 50, 172; cancer, a metabolic disease, 105; disease clusters, 111, 373; excess sodium and potassium loss, 112, 244; cancer cells irrepairable, 114; animal protein and cancer, 119; liver restoration and cancer treatment, 125; liver dysfunction and cancer, 124, 126, 272; terminal patients, 140; cancer not a local disease, 166; mineral balance, 171; detoxification, 170, 174; vegitarian diet, 174; disease precedes symptoms, 378
Mayo Clinic, 154, 160, 194
McAlvany, Donald, 103, 137
McCarron, David A., 306
McCormack, J. N., 401

N

O

U

V

W

Appendix A

Healthcare Cost-Reduction Act

DRAFT OF PROPOSED BILL

Preamble:
Our nation faces a healthcare-cost crisis that parallels the epidemics of chronic degenerative diseases sweeping across our land and undermining the health and productivity of its citizens. Experts tell us that by the year 2010, the cost of healthcare will consume 28 percent of our GNP and a significant portion of the budget of each state. This fiscal tumor must be lanced, or it will continue to contribute to the bankruptcy of our federal and state treasuries.

Today, California, indeed the United States of America, does not have a healthcare system. In the area of the treatment of chronic degenerative diseases, where most of our healthcare dollars are spent, we have a disease-management system. Managing the signs of chronic degenerative diseases like cancer, heart disease, diabetes, high blood pressure, osteoporosis, and arthritis has become big business. The focus of drug medicine is not to cure or reverse the causes of diseases but to manage the signs and symptoms—at a high cost—with essentially poisonous drugs, whose side effects are often deleterious and require even costlier management to the detriment of the patient and the treasury. It is a national scandal. The interventionist model of healthcare, dominated by drug-medicine, presents a clear and present danger to the health of our nation and its national security. While America has the best trauma and infectious disease medicine in the world, epidemics of chronic degenerative diseases are sweeping the nation, from cancer and diabetes to obesity. These epidemics are sapping the strength of our citizens, our work force, and are significantly adding to our mounting state and federal deficits.

Because the greater portion of our healthcare dollars are spent on managing the signs and symptoms of medical conditions that are primarily lifestyle diseases, our state and national treasuries can realize great savings in healthcare costs if medicine was redirected to placing a greater emphasis on preventing and reversing the underlying causes of these chronic degenerative diseases. The proposed legislation goes to the heart of the problem: retraining doctors to shift their emphasis from disease management to preventing and curing diseases, both in patient care and patient education. This problem must be addressed at its origins.

Firstly, medical schools must offer more classes in preventive medicine and nutritional therapy. Today few of our medical schools offer substantial courses in nutritional medicine. The use of drugs to manage the signs and symptoms of disease overrides all other concerns.

Secondly, the public must be re-educated: Doctors must educate their patients and the general public to take responsibility for their health by adopting healthy lifestyles and more nutritious eating habits. Today the average patient is conditioned by media propaganda and drug advertisements to expect a quick fix of their largely self-perpetuating spiral—the patient is conditioned to disregard the laws of life and health by promises of better health by miracle drugs, and the doctor is expected to meet these demands or lose the confidence of the patient. The winner in this bottomless spiral is the drug companies—not the patient, not the doctor, and not the state and national treasuries.

Thirdly, the standard for determining what constitutes proper medical practice must be redefined to open the door to nutritional medicine that seeks to prevent and reverse the causes of lifestyle disease. Today nutritional physicians are excluded from fully participating in patient care. They are often ostracized, ridiculed, or penalized for removing the patient from a dependency on a lifetime use of palliative drugs. Yet they are the very ones saving the state and national treasuries countless millions in healthcare costs. Physicians practicing nutritional therapy, judiciously utilizing drugs in emergency cases, must be given a seat at the table. The playing field must be leveled so they can compete in the marketplace of healthcare.

Fourthly, the definition of a medically safe product or procedure must be altered. It must be brought into conformity with the definition of other safe/unsafe products. The general definition of what constitutes an unsafe product utilizes the reasonably safe alternative design model. For some mysterious reason, this definition is excluded from medical practice and medical product manufacture—the result is to create a monopoly for drug medicine and the exclusion of nutritional modalities in the treatment of chronic degenerative diseases.

Finally, the public consumption of harmful foods must be addressed. While it may not be proper to command behavior, incentives may be devised to influence behavior into the right channels. Today health science has identified the cause of 80 percent-plus of diseases people now have—the ones that cost 80 percent-plus of our medical dollars. This is not a mystery that needs to be researched or pondered. The medical and scientific literature identifies a major cause of our chronic degenerative diseases to be a lack of whole foods in the diet combined with the excessive consumption of red meat, poultry, dairy and junk foods, whose main ingredients are overly refined foods, including white sugar, white flour, and pasta. The jury is not still out on these issues. The facts are clear and the evidence is legion. What we have is a failure of government to stand up to the manufacturers of harmful foods and regulate the industry so that the health of its citizens is protected.

Proposed Bill:

To amend the relevant sections of the Education Code to make it mandatory that our medical schools teach substantial classes in nutritional medicine/therapy. Note: Hippocrates, the Father of Medicine, stated that if a doctor does not know the relation between food and disease, how can he ever hope to help his patients? For a physician to "first do no harm," he must be properly educated so that he can both medically help and educate his patients.

To amend the relevant sections of the Education Code to provide that a doctor shall take a specified number of units of continuing education in diet or nutritional therapy to get his/her license renewed. Note: Similar requirements are in existence for elder care, AIDS, cancer/hospice, pain management, etc.

To amend the relevant sections of the Medical Code to redefine proper medical care: It should be medical negligence for a physician to only manage the signs/symptoms of chronic degenerative diseases, without also attempting to cure or arrest the underlying causes of the diseases by means which include nutritional medicine/therapy, lifestyle changes, and change of poor nutritional eating habits. Note: The state and federal treasury will greatly benefit if, while judiciously utilizing conventional medicine to stabilize and preserve the life of the patient, the physician explores nutritional means and lifestyle changes to reverse or arrest the underlying cause of the chronic degenerative disease he/she is treating. The evidence is clear that physicians are contributing to the epidemic of chronic degenerative diseases by their disdain for nutritional therapy while relying excessively on drug medications that leave the underlying disease intact, often aggravate it, and often result in the onset of new diseases to be treated by yet more poisonous drugs.

To amend the relevant sections of the Civil Code to redefine a safe/unsafe medical product or procedure as follows: A) A medical product is defective in design when the foreseeable risks of harm posed by the product could have been reduced or avoided by the adoption of a reasonable alternative design by the seller or other distributor, or a predecessor in the chain of distribution, and the omission of the alternative design or procedure renders the product or procedure not reasonably safe. B) A medical procedure is defective in implementation when the foreseeable risks of harm posed by the procedure could have been reduced or avoided by the adoption of a reasonable alternative procedure or practice by the physician, and the omission of the alternative procedure or practice renders the procedure not reasonably safe. Note: The standard for medical conduct must be based on commonsense. If a practice or procedure results in death or more suffering than the disease, it must be condemned outright. Most importantly, the opinions of the nutritional and herbal physicians who base their practice on sound empirical principles that successfully prevent or reverse chronic degenerative diseases must be admitted as competent evidence as to what constitutes proper medical care.

To amend the relevant sections of the Consumer Code as follows: It shall be unlawful for a manufacturer or producer of foods designed for sale or distribution for profit to the public, to put into the marketplace products whose main ingredients are either of the following or combinations of them: refined sugar, refined flour, white rice, high-fats and trans-fats. Note: Today the fast food and junk food industries have severed all connection between food production and nutrition. America is being malnourished by the failure of the FDA and the several states to see that wholesome foods are put into the marketplace. When combined with poor lifestyle choices, the result is an exponential rise in metabolic diseases such as obesity, diabetes, heart disease, and cancer.

To amend the relevant sections of the Education Code to provide that A) nutrition education from grade school to higher education shall utilize a food pyramid that places greater emphasis on the consumption of whole foods, fruits and vegetables, and less on red meats, poultry, dairy and junk foods; B) fast foods and junk foods consisting primarily of refined foods, high-fats and trans-fat foods, and refined sugar shall not be sold in public schools or by facilities one-half mile from such schools. Note: The evidence is clear that refined foods are slow poisons that result in poor academic performance of schoolchildren, while contributing to obesity and other diseases.

Plan of Action

In order to change the healthcare model in every state of the Union from one of intervention by means of potentially dangerous drugs to one of prevention and cure of chronic degenerative diseases, the author urges the reader to take the following urgent actions:

1. E-mail a copy of this Healthcare Cost-Reduction Act to your local state and federal government representative and urge them to sponsor legislation to change our healthcare model. Send this e-mail to your local newspaper editor, radio, and TV talk show hosts to promote publicity for the legislation. A copy of the proposed bill can be found at www. Healthcarecostreductionact.org.

2. Purchase copies of *Indicted!* and send copies to your local state and federal government representatives, urging them to take action, and also to your local newspaper editor, radio, and TV talk show hosts to generate publicity and backing for this legislation. Purchase copies at www. indicted.us.

3. Send a copy of *Indicted!* to your friends and relatives who are battling with or have survived chronic degenerative diseases by including herbal and nutritional medicine in their treatment, asking them to support potential legislation in their states to change our healthcare model from intervention to prevention and cure. Ask them to purchase and send a copy of *Indicted!* to their treating physicians, urging them to support the inclusion of nutritional therapy in the care of their patients.

4. Contact www.healthcarereform.biz or e-mail us at healthcarereformact@gmail.com and tell us your stories of victory over chronic degenerative diseases by the inclusion of nutritional and herbal therapy in your treatment. Your consent for us to use this information in publications and testimonials is hereby given.

5. Pre-order a copy of the author's follow-up book: *The Whisper of the Serpent: How a False Theory of Knowledge Destroyed Ancient Science and Medicine and Threatens to Destroy Modern Science and Medicine. The Whisper* is a panoramic analysis of over 2,500 years of civil war between nutritional medicine and drug therapy. www.whisperoftheserpent.com

6. Send a donation to CRCL, Inc., a California nonprofit organization promoting humanitarian and educational work worldwide, including

Healthcare Reform, a medical and dental clinic in Haiti, and elementary schools in Haiti, India, and among the Maya Indians of Belize. Contact www.crclinc.org to donate by check, credit card, or to make gifts of property by wills or trust. Note: Fifty percent of the sales from *Indicted!* go to support our worldwide humanitarian and educational work.

7. Organize a local Healthcare Reform Chapter to promote legislation changing our healthcare model from intervention to prevention and cure.

James Henderson, Esq.